An Introduction to Veterinary Medical Ethics

SECOND EDITION

An Introduction to Veterinary Medical Ethics
Theory and Cases

Bernard E. Rollin, PhD

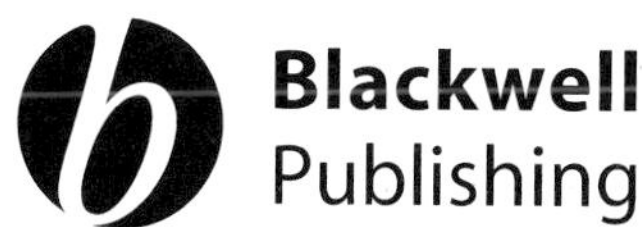

Bernard Rollin, a university distinguished professor of philosophy, biomedical sciences, animal sciences, and university bioethicist at Colorado State University, Fort Collins, where he developed the world's first course in veterinary ethics and animal rights. He is the recipient of the prestigious Henry Spira Award from the Johns Hopkins Center for Alternatives to Animal Testing. In worldwide demand as a speaker, Rollin is widely published; his books include *The Unheeded Cry: Animal Consciousness, Animal Pain, and Science, Farm Animal Welfare* and *Science and Ethics.*

Blackwell Publishing Professional
2121 State Avenue, Ames, Iowa 50014, USA

Orders: 1-800-862-6657
Office: 1-515-292-0140
Fax: 1-515-292-3348
Web site: www.blackwellprofessional.com

Blackwell Publishing Ltd
9600 Garsington Road, Oxford OX4 2DQ, UK
Tel.: +44 (0)1865 776868

Blackwell Publishing Asia
550 Swanston Street, Carlton, Victoria 3053, Australia
Tel.: +61 (0)3 8359 1011

Printed and bound in Malaysia by Vivar Printing Sdn Bhd

First edition, ©1996 Iowa State University Press
Second edition, 2006

Library of Congress Cataloging-in-Publication Data

Rollin, Bernard E.
An introduction to veterinary medical ethics : theory and cases / Bernard E. Rollin.— 2nd ed.
p. cm.
ISBN 978-0-8138-0399-9 (alk. paper)
1. Veterinary medicine—Moral and ethical aspects. 2. Veterinarians—Professional ethics. 3. Animal welfare—Moral and ethical aspects. I. Title.
SF756.39.R65 2006
174'.9636—dc22 2005029131

11 2015

To my wife Linda for all the years
of constructive
criticism and
unqualified support

CONTENTS

PREFACE TO THE SECOND EDITION

Since the first edition of this book appeared in 1999, much has occurred that is relevant to veterinary ethics. In particular, public concern regarding farm animal welfare in confinement has increased dramatically, and with it, public expectation of veterinarian involvement in resolving the issues. Additionally, a social movement for increasing the economic value of companion animals has steadily gained momentum, as have the demands for augmented legal status of these animals. Further, veterinary specialization has continued to grow and is thriving, as has veterinarian experimentation with complementary and alternative medicine. Concern with animal pain and distress and their control has proliferated beyond what I ever dared hope for. All of these, of course, pose major ethical challenges for veterinary medicine.

The new edition reflects these concerns, and contains new material on farm animals, legal status and value of animals, alternative medicine, Aesculapian authority, ethics of critical care, and animal pain, distress, and happiness among other new discussions, which I hope will help the veterinary community engage these issues and, as Plato said, "Make a virtue of necessity."

As always, since I first became involved with veterinary medicine almost thirty years ago, I appreciate and value how the veterinary community has embraced me and treated me as a colleague and as a friend. I am grateful to the thousands of veterinarians who have taken the trouble to write, call, or meet me in person to discuss ethical issues, and who have sent me large amounts of invaluable material I would otherwise have missed. I am also grateful to the veterinary students around the world who have demonstrated an unslakable thirst for discussions of ethics.

The veterinary community and all people concerned with veterinary ethics and animal welfare join me in mourning the passing of Dr. Frank Loew, a titanic figure in veterinary medicine and a beloved friend to many.

Finally, I wish to warmly acknowledge and thank Dr. Doug Hare of the *Canadian Veterinary Journal* for allowing me to write and reprint my columns, and Dr. Tim Blackwell for assembling the cases, and for unfailing counsel and friendship.

PREFACE TO THE FIRST EDITION

This book is the result of more than twenty years of reading, writing, teaching, thinking, lecturing, learning, and talking about veterinary medicine. Entering an area that, for a philosopher, was indeed uncharted territory, I encountered overwhelming kindness, interest, and support from veterinarians to whom philosophy was equally terra incognita. Illustrating a visionary truth enunciated by Dr. Edmund Pellegrino in reference to human medical ethics, my veterinary friends became developing philosophers while I (more slowly) emerged as a closet clinician.

I have been privileged to lecture at most of the veterinary schools in North America and indeed in the English-speaking world, and at many local, regional, national, and specialty associations. And everywhere I went I found the same encouragement, kindness, and enthusiasm for veterinary ethics that I did at Colorado State University. A full acknowledgment would thus constitute a small volume, as I would need to thank every veterinary school faculty member and student who ever asked me a question; every practitioner of companion animal medicine, food animal medicine, equine medicine, or laboratory animal medicine who has engaged me in dialogue; every association that gave me a forum; every editor of a veterinary journal who was willing to let me address the journal's readers. No stranger in a strange land has ever been treated better.

I would like, however, to single out those veterinarians at CSU who have most directly shaped my work: the late and remarkable Dr. Harry Gorman, with whom I taught at CSU the first course ever designed in the world in veterinary ethics; Dr. Dennis McCurnin, who carried on with me after Dr. Gorman's retirement; and Dr. Tony Knight, who has put up with me as a team teacher for longer than anyone else, and who is far more of a philosopher than I will ever be a veterinarian; Dr. Bill Tietz, the dean who gave me a chance; Dr. Robert Phemister, his successor, who nurtured my work; and Dr. Jim Voss, our current dean, who more than anyone else in the world gave me the opportunity to practice what I preach, and who was always there.

Virtually all of the enduring faculty at CSU have patiently taught me for twenty years—Dr. Frank Garry, Dr. Wayne McIlwraith, Dr. Ted Stashak, Dr. Gayle Trotter, Dr. Larue Johnson, Dr. John Cheney, the late Dr. Harold Breen, the late Dr. Bill Banks, Dr. Dick Bowen, Dr. Steve Roberts, Dr. Glenn Severin, Dr. Bob Mortimer, Dr. Ray Whalen,

Dr. Rod Rosychuk, Dr. Bruce Heath, Dr. Wayne Wingfield, Dr. Steve Withrow, Dr. Jim Ingram—have all been true mentors.

Outside of CSU, people have been equally kind, though bothered less by me—Drs. Dave Neil, David Robertshaw, Jackie Grandy, Jerry and Patty Olson, Lloyd Davis, formerly of CSU; Drs. Walt Weirich, Wally Morrison, and Alan Beck of Purdue; Dr. Dale Brooks of the University of California at Davis; Dr. Jim Wilson of the University of Pennsylvania; Dr. Frank Loew, formerly of Tufts and Cornell; Dr. Tom Wolfle of ILAR; Dr. Don Draper of Iowa State.

Dr. Tim Blackwell, the founder and editor of the ethics column in the *Canadian Veterinary Journal*, has been a partner in hundreds of hours of dialogue and deserves at least half of the credit for the column's success. We are both grateful to the veterinarians who sent in the challenging cases we deal with in the column, and to the editors of the *Canadian Veterinary Journal*, who graciously allowed me to reprint these cases.

In a class by itself is the debt I owe to Dr. Lynne Kesel of CSU, briefly my student and for longer my teacher and sounding board, my collaborator on two books, and the person who taught me the most about veterinary medicine.

Among non-veterinarians I am indebted to my philosophy department colleagues, who allowed me to strike off in a direction most philosophers considered odd, and who were always interested, helpful, and supportive.

Most important, I would like to thank my wife, Linda, and son, Michael, who not only discussed with me every ethics case I ever dealt with, but who themselves have become, like me, closet veterinarians, with an abiding interest in, and love for, the field.

Part

I

Theory

Theory

There is an ancient curse that is most appropriate to the society in which we live: "May you live in interesting times." From the point of view of our social ethics, we do indeed live in bewildering and rapidly changing times. In less than thirty years veterinary medicine, reflecting this rapid change, has seen itself transformed from an essentially male profession to a profession soon to be dominated by women. Similarly, the rigid, almost military, rules governing the demeanor, conduct, and deportment of veterinary students have vanished, to be replaced by a laxity literally unimaginable thirty years ago. Whereas sporting a beard, mustache, or long hair was sufficient reason for a faculty member to order a student out of class at my institution as recently as the late 1970s, woe to the instructor who now questions a student's bare feet, halter top, or nose ring. Indeed, the instructor may be so attired.

These changes are of course reflective of changes in society in general, or more accurately, in social ethics. The traditional, widely shared, social ethical truisms that gave us stability, order, and predictability in society for many generations are being widely challenged by women, ethnic minorities, homosexuals, the handicapped, animal rights advocates, internationalists, environmentalists, and more. And all of these changes will inevitably be reflected in veterinary medicine. Most veterinarians now realize, to take a very obvious example, that society is in the process of changing its view of animals, and of our obligations to animals. Laboratory animal veterinarians have probably seen the most clearly articulated evidence of such a changing ethic, but it is also patent to any companion animal practitioners, food animal practitioners, or zoo veterinarians who take the trouble to reflect upon the new social expectations shaping and constraining the way they do their jobs.

It is very likely that there has been more and deeper social-ethical change since the middle of the twentieth century than occurred during centuries of an ethically monolithic period such as the Middle Ages. Anyone over forty has lived through a variety of major moral earthquakes: the sexual revolution, the end of socially sanctioned racism, the banishing of IQ differentiation, the rise of homosexual militancy, the end of "*loco parentis*" in universities, the advent of consumer advocacy, the end of mandatory retirement age, the mass acceptance of environmentalism, the growth of a "sue the bastards" mind-set, the implementation of affirmative action programs, the rise of massive drug use, the designation of alcoholism and child abuse as diseases rather than moral vices, the rise of militant feminism, the emergence of sexual harassment as a major social concern, the demands by the handicapped for equal access, the rise of public suspicion of science and technology, the mass questioning of animal use in science and industry, the end of colonialism, the rise of political correctness—all provide patent examples of the magnitude of ethical change during this brief period.

With such rapid change come instability and bewilderment. Do I hold doors for women? (I was brought up to do so out of politeness, but is such an act patronizing and demeaning?) Do I support black student demands for black dormitories (after I marched in the 1960s to end segregation)? Am I a bad person if I do not wish to hire a transsexual? Can I criticize the people of Rwanda and Bosnia for the bloodbaths they conducted without being accused of insensitivity to cultural diversity? Do I obey the old rules or the new rules? Paradoxically, the appeal to ethics, and the demand for ethical accountability, have probably never been stronger and more prominent—witness the forceful assertion of rights by and for people, animals, and nature—yet an understanding of ethics has never been more tentative, and violations of ethics and their attendant scandals in business, science, government, and the professions have never been more prominent. There is probably more talk of ethics than ever—more endowed chairs, seminars, conferences, college courses, books, media coverage, journals devoted to ethical matters than ever before—and yet, ironically, most people probably believe that they understand ethics far less than their progenitors did. Commonality of values has given way to plurality and diversity; traditions are being eroded; even the church is no longer the staunch defender of traditional ethical norms.

In such a world it is exigent to understand the logical geography of ethics, and to possess the tools with which to negotiate reasonably what is often tortuous and slippery terrain. This is especially true for professionals, because in order to maintain their autonomy, professions must anticipate and accord with changing ethical thought, as we shall shortly see in detail. Our ensuing discussion will provide a conceptual map of the nature and role of ethics in general, and of veterinary ethics in particular. Attempting to analyze difficult ethical cases with many threads or to debate complex ethical issues without such a map is relevantly analogous to attempting to do surgery without an understanding of the basic concepts of anatomy, anesthesia, and asepsis: One can do it, but one literally doesn't know what one is doing and cannot, therefore, adapt to the unexpected. Conversely, once a person has mastered the relevant basic concepts, that person can go well beyond what he or she has hitherto done by rote.

As we shall see, I am not saying that one cannot behave ethically without mastering the conceptual map we shall present. After all, few people make a study of ethics. Most of us just behave properly in an automatic way. And many of our ethical decisions are obvious and straightforward and routine: We don't overcharge a gullible client; we don't attempt to steal another veterinarian's patients; we don't prescribe useless medication; and so on. What we often cannot do, without a conceptual map and a reflective stance on ethics, is see the subtleties and variegated dimensions posed by complex cases; we tend to react to one obvious component and ignore others. Just as it takes training and practice and a conceptual map of medical possibilities to learn differential diagnosis of disease, so too it takes training and practice to dissect all of the ethical nuances of many complex situations.

Detecting ethical questions is, in some ways, like detecting lameness. Prima facie, ordinary people not particularly knowledgeable about veterinary medicine would think that anyone can tell when a horse is lame and which leg is affected. After all, we can do so easily with humans. In fact, when actually confronted with a lame horse, inexperienced laypeople, and even veterinary students, can at best detect that something is wrong (and sometimes not even that), but they can rarely pinpoint the problem. This is exactly analogous to the activity of identifying ethical problems. People (sometimes) know something is problematic, but they have trouble saying exactly what the problem is.

A true case embracing a multitude of ethical issues illustrates the difficulty of recognizing, sorting out, and dealing with ethical questions:

A man brought a small comatose dog with a head injury into our veterinary school clinic. He freely admitted, and even boasted, that he had struck the dog in the head with a frying pan because it barked too much. When the dog did not regain consciousness and the man's wife became upset, he took the dog to his regular practitioner. The veterinarian advised him to take the dog to the veterinary school hospital. The dog died there, and the animal's body was brought to necropsy and presented as a case to a group of students by a pathology instructor.

Coincidentally, one of the veterinary students in that class was an animal control officer, among whose duties was investigating cruelty complaints. With the instructor's permission, the student took the client's name from the file and began to investigate the case, phoning the client's home and speaking with his wife. The client became irate and complained to both the referring veterinarian and to the veterinary school clinician who had taken his case that his right to privacy had been violated. The private practitioner and the veterinary school referral clinician in turn were furious with the student. The student was frightened, was worried about the effect of the incident on his academic and subsequent career, and sought help.

What moral conflicts and problems does this case raise? Initially, the referring practitioner, the veterinary school clinician, and some administrators saw only one issue—the betrayal of client confidentiality by the student. As the case evolved, administrators were also troubled by the involvement of the pathologist who had "betrayed" the identity of the client. Only after much dialogue with an ethicist, the pathologist, and the student did the parties begin to realize that there were many other concurrent issues.

First, there was an animal welfare issue: The client should not be allowed to fatally beat an animal with impunity. In addition, there was a social or moral obligation to report the occurrence of a crime, the same sort of moral obligation (now also a legal one in human medicine) that exists for health care professionals to report suspected child abuse. Furthermore, there was the moral (and legal) question of whether one could invoke confidentiality in a public teaching hospital, where it is implicit that cases will be discussed with students as part of their learning process. Lastly, the pathologist argued that, as a veterinary teaching institution, the school had a high moral obligation not to condone that which society as a whole has recognized as immoral and illegal.

Some veterinarians argued that the pathologist was within his rights to reveal the name, but that the student ought not to have acted upon the information. To this point the student replied that, as a law officer, he had a sworn duty (a moral obligation) to enforce the law. Some veterinarians hypothesized that if confidentiality isn't strictly observed, abusers of animals will not bring animals in for treatment. A controversy also arose over the fact that the school clinician had at least obliquely threatened the student with recriminations when he came to the clinic. Others worried that the information about the case and these issues had not been sent back to the referring veterinarian for that party to handle. The issue of a conflict of interest between being a veterinary student and serving with animal control was also raised.

Ultimately, the situation was resolved, at least for future cases, by the university's drafting a formal policy that suspected abuse cases of this sort would automatically be reported to the school and government authorities. One of the noteworthy features of the case was its dramatic teaching value in demonstrating just how complex a single ethical problem or case can be.

This case beautifully illustrates why a conceptual map of ethics can be valuable. People perceive not only with their eyes and ears, but with their expectations, mental sets, preconceptions, habits, acculturations, and theories as well. The clinicians had been trained with a fairly limited ethical conceptual map—they thus perceived only an issue of confidentiality and initially missed the others we noted.

It is worth pausing to illustrate this salient point: We see with more than our eyes. When I teach this idea to my students, I begin with the following child's trick: I ask them to give me a single word for each thing I describe.

I say: What is a cola beverage that comes in a red can?
They say: Coke.
I say: If I tell a funny story, we call that a . . .?
They say: Joke.
I say: If I puff on a cigarette, I . . .
They say: Smoke.
I say: I put some dirty clothes in a tub so they can . . .
They say: Soak.
I then say: What is the white of an egg called?
Most will automatically say: Yolk.

I go on to provide more serious examples of the ways that background, theory, and expectation can determine perception. The famous Rosenthal effect in psychology (Rosenthal, 1966) provides a nice scientific example. Researchers studying rat behavior were told that one of the groups of white rats they would be working with was a special strain of highly intelligent rats. In subsequent studies, the researchers found that the bright rats did better than the ordinary rats in learning trials. In fact, they were all "ordinary" rats—the "brightness" came from the researchers' expectations. Often we experience the same "halo" effect with students in our classes, when we are told by other instructors of a particular student's brightness.

We can all recall the first time we looked at a radiograph. The radiologist pointed to what he said was a fracture, but we saw only dark and light, even though the same stimuli impinged upon our retinas as upon his. As one's knowledge of radiography broadens, however, one *sees* differently, though once again the retinal stimulation is unchanged.

Another amusing example is provided by a "paradox" that used to perplex people in the 1960s and 1970s called "The Boy with Two Fathers," which was presented as follows:

> A father and son are involved in an automobile accident. Both are seriously injured and are rushed to separate hospitals. The son is immediately readied for emergency surgery; at the first sight of him, however, the surgeon says, "I can't operate on this patient—he's my son!" How is this possible?

Twenty and thirty years ago one could perplex almost everyone in a class with this case. Today it falls flat—everyone sees the answer immediately: The surgeon is the boy's mother. Nothing in young people's expectations today precludes the possibility of a female surgeon.

Finally, let me cite a very poignant example from veterinary medicine. In the mid-1980s I was team-teaching a veterinary ethics course with a prominent surgeon. I was discussing the tendency in veterinary medicine (and in science in general) through most of the twentieth century to ignore animal pain. In the midst of my lecture the surgeon stopped me. "My God," he said, "I was trained in the mid-sixties and was taught to castrate horses using succinycholine chloride [a curariform drug]. This is the first time it ever dawned on me that the animals must have been hurting!" I shall return to the relationship between human mind-set and animal pain later in this book.

For now, however, the important point to realize is that the study of ethics provides a way of forcing people, on ethical matters, to go beyond their mind-set and expectations—indeed, that is why many people find it discomfiting. Of course, one can to some extent free oneself from the shackles of univocal perspective by seeking out people with strongly divergent opinions as discussion partners; I often recommend to veterinarians that they orchestrate discussion of ethical matters at meetings wherein they can hear a wide variety of viewpoints. But this alone will not fully assure a deepened perception in the absence of an understanding of what we have called the "logical geography" of ethical or moral questions. Hearing differing opinions is not enough; one must also understand the criteria by which one judges and critically assesses divergent opinions, else one runs the risk of creating a Babel of incommensurable ethical voices—a chorus of individual opinions with no way to generate the consensus that viable ethics requires in a community, and no method for changing others' opinions in a rational way. So it is to an examination of the nature of ethics to which we must now turn.

Social, Personal, and Professional Ethics

There are two very different senses of "ethics" that are often confused and conflated and that must be distinguished at the outset to allow for viable discussion of these matters.

The first sense of ethics I shall call $ethics_1$. In this sense ethics is the set of principles or beliefs that governs views of right and wrong, good and bad, fair and unfair, just and unjust. Whenever we assert that "killing is wrong," or that "discrimination is unfair," or that "one oughtn't belittle a colleague," or that "it is laudable to give to charity," or that "I think abortion is murder," one is explicitly or implicitly appealing to $ethics_1$—moral rules that one believes ought to bind society, oneself, and/or some subgroup of society, such as veterinarians.

Under $ethics_1$ must fall a distinction between social ethics, personal ethics, and professional ethics. Of these, social ethics is the most basic and most objective, in a sense to be explained shortly.

People, especially scientists, are tempted sometimes to assert that unlike scientific judgments, which are "objective," ethical judgments are "subjective" opinion and not "fact," and thus not subject to rational discussion and adjudication. Although it is true that one cannot conduct experiments or gather data to decide what is right and wrong, ethics, nevertheless, cannot be based upon personal whim and caprice. If anyone doubts this, let that person go out and rob a bank in front of witnesses, then argue before a court that, in his or her ethical opinion, bank robbery is morally acceptable if one needs the money.

In other words, the fact that ethical judgments are not validated by gathering data or doing experiments does not mean that they are simply a matter of individual subjective opinion. If one stops to think about it, one will quickly realize that very little ethics is left to one's opinion. Consensus rules about rightness and wrongness of actions that have an impact on others are in fact articulated in clear social principles, which are in turn encoded in laws and policies. All public regulations, from the zoning of pornographic bookstores out of school zones to laws against insider trading and murder, are examples of consensus ethical principles "writ large," in Plato's felicitous phrase, in public policy. This is not to say that, in every case, law and ethics are congruent. We can all think of examples of things that are legal yet generally considered immoral (tax dodges for the superwealthy, for instance) and of things we consider perfectly moral that are illegal (parking one's car for longer than two hours in a two-hour zone).

But, by and large, if we stop to think about it, there must be a pretty close fit between our morality and our social policy. When people attempt to legislate policy that most people do not consider morally acceptable, the law simply does not work. A classic example is, of course, Prohibition, which did not stop people from drinking, but rather funneled the drinking money away from legitimate business to bootleggers.

So there must be a goodly number of ethical judgments in society that are held to be universally binding and socially objective. Even though such judgments are not objective in the way that "water boils at 212°F" is objective (that is, they are not validated by the way the world works), they are nonetheless objective as rules governing social behavior. We are all familiar with other instances of this kind of objectivity. For example, it is an objective rule of English that one cannot say, "You ain't gonna be there." Though people, of course, do say it, it is *objectively* wrong to do so. Similarly, the bishop in chess can objectively move only on diagonals of its own color. Someone may, of course, move the bishop a different way, but that move is objectively wrong, and one is not then "playing chess."

Those portions of ethical rules that we believe to be universally binding on all members of society, and socially objective, I will call the *social consensus* ethic. A moment's reflection reveals that without some such consensus ethic, we could not live together, we would have chaos and anarchy, and society would be impossible. This is true for any society at all that intends to persist: There must be rules governing everyone's behavior. Do the rules need to be the same for all societies? Obviously not—we all know that there are endless ethical variations across societies. Does there need to be at least a common core in all of these ethics? That is a rather profound question I shall address later. For the moment, however, we all need to agree that there exists an identifiable social consensus ethic in our society by which we are all bound.

Now, the social consensus ethic does not regulate all areas of life that have ethical relevance; certain areas of behavior are left to the discretion of the individual or, more accurately, to his or her *personal ethic*. Such matters as what one reads, what religion one practices or doesn't practice, how much charity one gives and to whom, are all matters left in our society to one's personal beliefs about right and wrong and good and bad. This has not always been the case, of course—all of these examples were, during the Middle Ages, appropriated by a theologically based social consensus ethic. And this fact illustrates a very important point about the relationship between *social consensus ethics* and *personal ethics*. As a society evolves and changes over time, certain areas of conduct may move from the concern of the social consensus ethic to the concern of the personal ethic, and vice versa. An excellent example of a matter that has recently moved from the concern of the social ethic, and from the laws that mirror that ethic, to the purview of individual ethical choice is the area of sexual behavior. Whereas once laws constrained activities like homosexual behavior, adultery, and cohabitation, these things are now left to one's personal ethic in western democracies. With the advent during the

1960s of the view that sexual behavior that does not hurt others is not a matter for social regulation but, rather, for personal choice, social regulation of such activity withered away. About ten years ago the mass media reported, with much hilarity, that there was still a law on the books in Greeley, Colorado, a university town, making cohabitation a crime. Radio and TV reporters chortled as they remarked that, if the law were to be enforced, a goodly portion of the Greeley citizenry would have to be jailed!

On the other hand, we must note that many areas of behavior once left to one's personal ethic have been since appropriated by the social ethic. When I was growing up, paradigm cases of what society left to one's personal choice were represented by the renting or selling of one's real property, and by whom one hired for jobs. The prevailing attitude was that these decisions were your own damn business. This, of course, is no longer the case. Federal law now governs renting and selling of property, and hiring and firing.

Generally, as such examples illustrate, conduct becomes appropriated by the social consensus ethic when how it is dealt with by personal ethics is widely perceived to be unfair or unjust. The widespread failure to rent to, sell to, or hire minorities, which resulted from leaving these matters to individual ethics, evolved into a situation viewed by society as unjust, and led to the passage of strong social ethical rules against such unfairness. As we shall see, the treatment of animals in society is also moving into the purview of the social consensus ethic, as society begins to question the injustice that results from leaving such matters to individual discretion.

The third component of ethics_1, in addition to social consensus ethics and personal ethics, is *professional ethics*. Members of a profession are first and foremost members of society—citizens—and are thus bound by all aspects of the consensus social ethic not to steal, murder, break contracts, and so on. However, professionals—be they physicians, attorneys, or veterinarians—also perform specialized and vital functions in society. This kind of role requires special expertise, special training, and involves special situations that ordinary people do not face. The professional functions that veterinarians perform also warrant special privileges, for example, dispensing medications and performing surgery. Democratic societies have been prepared to give professionals some leeway and assume that, given the technical nature of professions and the specialized knowledge their practitioners possess, professionals will understand the ethical issues they confront better than society does as a whole. Thus society generally leaves it to such professionals to set up their own rules of conduct. In other words, the social ethic offers general rules, creating the stage on which professional life is played out, and the subclasses of society comprising professionals are asked to develop their own ethic to cover the special situations they deal with daily. In essence society says to professionals, "Regulate yourselves the way we would regulate you if we understood enough about what you do to regulate you!" Because of this situation, professional ethics occupies a position midway between social consensus ethics and personal ethics, because it neither applies to all members of society nor are its main components left strictly to individuals. It is, for example, a general rule of human medical ethics for psychiatrists not to have sex with their patients.

The failure of a profession to operate in accordance with professional ethics that reflect and are in harmony with the social consensus ethic can result in a significant loss of autonomy by the profession in question. One can argue, for example, that recent attempts to govern health care by legislation is a result of the human medical community's failure to operate in full accord with the social consensus ethic. When hospitals turn away poor people or aged stroke victims, when pediatric surgeons fail to use anesthesia on infants, or when doctors give less analgesia to adolescents than to adults with the same lesion (Rollin, 1997), they are not in accord with social ethics, and it is only a matter of time before society will appropriate regulation of such behavior. In veterinary medicine, social fear of the irresponsible use and dispensing of pharmaceuticals recently threatened the privilege of veterinarians to prescribe drugs in an extralabel fashion—a privilege whose suspension would have in a real sense hamstrung veterinarians. Because so few drugs are approved for animals, veterinary medicine relies heavily on extralabel drug use.

Ethics$_1$ and Ethics$_2$

Thus far we have looked at ethics$_1$—the set of principles that governs people's views of right and wrong, good and bad, fair and unfair, just and unjust—and found that ethics$_1$ can be further divided into social consensus ethics, personal ethics, and professional ethics. Now we must consider a less familiar secondary notion ethics$_2$. Ethics$_2$ is the logical, rational study and examination of ethics$_1$, which may include the attempt to justify the principles of ethics$_1$, the seeking out of inconsistencies in the principles of ethics$_1$, the drawing out of ethics$_1$ principles that have been hitherto ignored or unnoticed, engaging the question of whether all societies ought ultimately to have the same ethics$_1$, and so on. This secondary sense of ethics—ethics$_2$—is thus a branch of philosophy. Most of what we are doing in this book is ethics$_2$, examining the logic of ethics$_1$. Socrates' activities in ancient Athens were a form of ethics$_2$. Whereas we in society learn ethics$_1$ from parents, teachers, churches, movies, books, peers, magazines, newspapers, and mass media, we rarely learn to engage in ethics$_2$ in a disciplined, systematic way unless we take an ethics class in a philosophy curriculum. In one sense this is fine—vast numbers of people are diligent practitioners of ethics$_1$ without ever engaging in ethics$_2$. On the other hand, failure to engage in ethics$_2$—rational criticism of ethics$_1$—can lead to incoherence and inconsistencies in ethics$_1$ going unnoticed, unrecognized, and uncorrected. Although not everyone needs to engage in ethics$_2$ on a regular basis, there is value in at least some people monitoring the logic of ethics$_1$, be it social consensus ethics, personal ethics, or professional ethics. Such monitoring helps us detect problems that have been ignored or have gone undetected and helps us make ethical progress. I shall shortly analyze some of the reasons why ethics$_1$ is likely to stand in need of constant critical examination.

What is "philosophy" of which we have said ethics$_2$ is a part? To tell someone that one is a "professional philosopher" or even a "philosophy teacher" is to risk a wide variety of undesirable responses, ranging from "Isn't everyone a philosopher?" to "Where is your couch?" to glassy-eyed stares, to serious conversational lulls, to questions about crystals and the prophecies of Nostradamus. To many of my nonphilosophy colleagues I am a sort of secular preacher, in whose company one refrains from telling off-color jokes, even though *I* do not refrain from telling them.

In fact, one can provide a fairly straightforward and clear account of philosophical activity that goes a long way toward breaking the stereotype and also helps people in *any* discipline understand why philosophy is relevant to them. As Aristotle long ago pointed out, all human activities and disciplines rest on certain assumptions and concepts that are taken for granted. As in the paradigmatic case of geometry, we must assume certain notions without proof, for it is upon these notions that all subsequent proof is based. If we could prove our foundational assumptions, it would need to be on the basis of other assumptions that are either taken for granted or proved on the basis of other assumptions. Because the latter tack would lead to a never-ending hierarchy of assumptions and proofs—what philosophers call an infinite regress—certain things are simply assumed.

All disciplines and activities make such assumptions: Science assumes that we can identify causes and effects. Art assumes that certain objects are works of art and others are not. History assumes that we can reconstruct the past. Mathematics assumes that certain things count as proof and others do not. The law assumes that people are to be held responsible for certain actions wherein they acted freely. Some schools of ethology assume that animals are conscious beings; others assume they are physiological machines.

In all of these examples it is obvious, on reflection, that certain basic challenges can be directed toward all of these implicit or explicit assumptions. What makes certain things works of art and others not? (Marcel Duchamp humorously asked this question when he submitted a urinal to a Paris sculpture exhibition in the early twentieth century.) Why do we accept someone's brain tumor as exonerating criminal behavior, but not someone's childhood experiences? What about that person's genes? How do we decide which of two incompatible but well-researched historical reconstructions to accept? How do we decide which approach to animal behavior is the correct approach? Is it the one that gives primacy to behavior, the one that gives primacy to evolutionary explanations, the one that invokes consciousness, or the one that invokes neurophysiology? Ought we or ought we not accept a computer proof by exhaustion of Euler's conjecture? This is the terrain in which philosophy operates.

People who raise such basic, conceptual questions about fundamental concepts and assumptions are functioning as philosophers, whether or not they are professionally involved in philosophy. Because most people at some time or another ask such questions, most people have their philosophical moments. Much progress in human thought and behavior has been accomplished by such thoughtful questioning of what is taken for granted by others. For example, one of Einstein's major contributions in developing special relativity was a philosophical critique of notions that physicists since Newton had taken for granted—namely, that one can talk intelligibly of absolute space, absolute time, absolute simultaneity, independent of who is recording or measuring these things. Indeed, it is for this reason that a major book on Einstein's work is entitled *Albert Einstein: Philosopher/Scientist*.

As Plato noted, what we assume about right and wrong, good and bad, justice and injustice, fairness and unfairness, constitutes the most important assumptions we make as individuals, societies, or subgroups of societies, such as the professions. Our vision of the good, of what is right and wrong to do, underlies everything we do at all levels—be it the social level of policies about taxation and redistribution of wealth, what science we do and don't fund (research into environmental preservation versus research into the relationship between race and intelligence), our views of punishment and rehabilitation, et cetera, or be it at the level of individual action.

One sometimes encounters skepticism about philosophical ethics from people who assert that ethics is "just opinion" or "isn't based on facts" and therefore can't be rationally criticized or rationally taught. A moment's reflection, and some judicious examples, should allow us to bury this skeptical nuisance for the remainder of our discussion.

Let us look at clear examples of how social, personal, and professional ethics can be rationally criticized. Consider the social ethic: Those of us who are over forty have lived through a period of social-ethical self-examination regarding our treatment of blacks. We were taught from the time that we were children that all humans should be treated equally regardless of race, creed, or color. Yet we also knew that black people were treated quite differently, most clearly in the segregated states. The society, at the instigation of rational critics, reasoned that separate was inherently unequal, and thus that segregation, however widely practiced, was incompatible with our consensus ethic. Indeed, if the social ethic could not be rationally criticized, we could make no social progress.

By the same token, one can criticize personal ethics. As I said earlier, one's religious beliefs are a matter of personal ethics. Yet one can still rationally criticize the content of another's beliefs. For example, I often ask my audiences how many of them are Christians and, if they are, to hold up their right hands. I also ask the same audiences how many of them are ethical relativists, explaining that an ethical relativist is a person who believes that there are no objective ethical truths, that everyone's opinion is equally valid. I ask the relativists to hold up their left hands. Many people end up holding up both hands. But this is *logically* impossible! One can't be a Christian and a relativist at the same time, because a Christian must believe that certain things are absolutely right and wrong—for example, the Ten Commandments—whereas a relativist asserts that nothing is absolutely right or wrong.

Finally, one can rationally criticize professional ethics in many ways. Two personal examples come to mind. In the mid-1970s I wrote some articles criticizing veterinary ethics, as embodied in the American Veterinary Medical Association (AVMA) Code of Ethics, for failing to deal with many of the issues society expected veterinary ethics to deal with, such as whether one should euthanize a healthy animal for owner convenience, when one should control pain in animals, and whether veterinarians have a social obligation to lead in changing practices that hurt animals. Instead, much attention was devoted to questions of etiquette—how big one's sign can be, what form one's yellow pages ad should take, whether or not one can advertise, and so on (Rollin, 1978). As Dr. Harry Gorman pointed out to me, society got tired of the bickering about advertising, and the decision about its acceptability was made by the courts, not by veterinarians.

A second example concerns the treatment of animals in research. Also beginning in the 1970s, I attempted to persuade researchers that, though how they treated animals had essentially been left by society to the discretion of their professional and personal ethics, their behavior was not in accord with emerging social ethics on animal treatment and was, in fact, at odds with it. I argued that researchers were living on borrowed time. If society knew about some of the practices that were rife in research, such as the systematic failure to use analgesics for postsurgical pain, the multiple use of animals for invasive procedures in teaching, and general poor care, then society would appropriate the treatment of animals in science into the social ethic, no longer leaving it to the professionals. Sure enough, that is what occurred, and what needed to occur.

There is a fundamental lesson here for veterinarians and, indeed, for all professionals. If we wish to continue to run our own professional lives—and ideally we should, because we understand the issues occasioned by our own activities better than anyone else does—then we must be highly sensitive to the issues in our professions, be very anticipatory in dealing with them, and let the public know what we are doing. Veterinary medicine, like human medicine and most other professions, has not done as well as it should or can in any of these three ways.

Veterinary medicine should be teaching ethics throughout veterinary school curricula so that graduates are highly sensitized to the issues they might encounter, both as individual veterinarians and as members of the profession. Too many schools fail to teach ethics, so practitioners and organized veterinary medicine get blindsided by concerns they do not see coming. For example, we know that animal welfare issues are of paramount concern for the social ethic. We also know that society looks to veterinary medicine for answers: Federal law singles out laboratory animal veterinarians as the key to laboratory animal welfare; the AVMA euthanasia recommendations are integral to federal law; the recommendations of the AVMA Panel on Pain and Distress, on which I was privileged to serve, are unofficially part of the law; and Congress requests advice from the AVMA on issues pertaining to the genetic engineering of animals. Thus cognizance of animal welfare issues, and recommendations for their resolution, should be a top priority for organized veterinary medicine and for veterinary practitioners.

Indeed, veterinarians are literally starved for ethical discussion. Almost all veterinarians are "closet moral philosophers" whose philosophical interest is evident whenever they are given the opportunity to "come out of the closet." I know this from my personal experiences of speaking to veterinary audiences—our discussions will almost invariably continue for as long as they are allowed to. For fifteen years I have written a column for the *Canadian Veterinary Journal* on ethical issues facing veterinarians, and surveys by the journal indicate that, except for the scientific articles, the ethics column is by a significant margin the most popular feature of the journal. A survey of veterinary school graduates indicated that the area in which they believe they need a good deal more training in veterinary schools is ethics (James F. Wilson, personal communication, 1994), and this finding was buttressed by a solicitation of reader response in the *Journal of the American Veterinary Medical Association (JAVMA)*. For this reason I have long argued that ethical and social issues should get much more play at the local, national, and international levels of veterinary medicine and in veterinary schools, journals, and conferences. This change is in fact slowly taking place but should proceed more rapidly still.

Once veterinary medicine understands the issues, it should do more to handle major veterinary ethical controversies in an anticipatory, proactive way. The farm animal welfare issue is a good example. It is now clear that a reform of intensive agriculture is being demanded in most western societies to make the industry more animal friendly—even people within the industry now admit that this must be done. Veterinarians should be leading this movement, because they understand the needs of both animals and producers and care for both. I shall return to animal welfare issues later in this discussion.

Another example of a problem area in ethics that it would behoove veterinary medicine to engage in more forcefully is the issue of dealing with practitioners whose behavior violates accepted ethical norms. For example, I heard from a graduate about a case in which a practitioner routinely prescribed fecal examinations for pets, did not bother to examine them, and then charged for deworming. When the young veterinarian who had taken a job in that practice approached the local association and complained, he was told, "Oh, hell, Dr. X has been doing that for years—what can we do?"

The reluctance to implicate a colleague—to "squeal" or "rat," as I was brought up to think of it—is understandable. However, if you do not clean up your own house, society will do it for you by passing laws and regulations. In other words, the control of such conduct will be removed from veterinarians and placed in the hands of the law—law written by non-veterinarians who do not understand veterinary practice, law that can well restrict and erode veterinary autonomy in a detrimental way.

Finally, veterinary medicine could do more to publicize its involvement in ethical and social issues. For that matter, all professions could. The public should understand how the profession polices itself; they should understand that veterinary medicine is actively attempting to solve the pet overpopulation problem; and they should understand the role of veterinarians in changing questionable agricultural practices and in engaging the welter of animal use issues in society. I will discuss many of these problems later in this book.

We can similarly dispatch the claim sometimes made by skeptics to people like myself that "you cannot teach ethics," an ultimately ambiguous statement. If the argument is that "one cannot teach $ethics_1$," this is simply false. Parents, friends, churches, peers, movies, books, veterinary faculty, all teach $ethics_1$, often without knowing it. For example, when surgery was taught by use of multiple survival procedures in veterinary schools in the 1970s, an $ethics_1$ message was transmitted to students about the value of animal life and suffering—though most surgery faculty didn't realize they were communicating such an implicit moral message, and most probably would not have explicitly done so. Not only is it possible, then, to teach $ethics_1$, it is inevitable, though we may not do so consciously, coherently, or defensibly. I shall discuss later the sense in which one can rationally approach teaching $ethics_1$.

On the other hand, if by asserting "one cannot teach ethics" one means one cannot teach $ethics_2$ (that is, how to reason about $ethics_1$), this is also patently false. In fact, teaching $ethics_2$ is the task of this book!

Ethical Vectors in Veterinary Medicine

How and where do ethical issues manifest themselves in veterinary medicine? Before we begin to discuss the variety of ethical pulls on veterinarians, it is important to make a fundamental clarification too often overlooked. Understandably, television, movies, magazines, newspapers, novels, plays, and so on are drawn to ethical issues as a source of controversial and interesting subject matter. And this is not altogether bad. Many citizens have learned a good deal about human medical ethics from the relentless attention it has attracted from mass media. Indeed, the medical community has historically been forced to pay greater attention to ethical issues by virtue of the media attention they attract. By the same token, the media have inevitably tended to portray ethical decisions as *dilemmas*—very dramatic situations wherein one is faced with two extreme, mutually exclusive choices that exhaust all possibilities, yet neither of which seems wholly correct or incorrect. (Etymologically, "di-lemma" means "two horns"—whichever direction you turn, you are "impaled" on a horn.) A classic example of a genuine dilemma occurred when a human hospital was faced with one more patient who needed a kidney machine than the hospital had such machines: How do you choose which patient will live and which will die? The high drama in true dilemmas has led many people to equate "ethical decisions" with "ethical dilemmas." Fortunately for veterinarians' peace of mind, most ethical choices in veterinary medicine, or for that matter in any field, are not dilemmas. In fact, most of our choices are straightforward: I, as a veterinarian, choose not to overcharge the very rich client even though I could use the money for a new set of saddlebags for my Harley-Davidson; I choose to treat an animal belonging to an indigent client for cost and allow the client to pay me over time; I don't seduce a beautiful, neurotic client even though she is sending signals. (This is not of course to say that there are *never* dilemmas in veterinary medicine. Clients who want a veterinarian to euthanize a healthy animal often create dilemmas for clinicians.)

This excessive emphasis on dilemmas has some pernicious consequences. Most mischievous, perhaps, is that people are led to expect that ethical issues will present themselves as overly dramatic Scylla versus Charybdis impasses! Such a tendency may, in turn, lead to people ignoring the ethical dimensions of obvious, less dramatic situations. Equally significant, and of inestimable social importance, is that people begin seeing ethical issues as unbridgeable gulfs, with "us" on one side and "them" on the other. The paradigm for ethical issues and their resolution becomes an image of two heavily armed camps fighting to the death. We are left to think of all ethical conflicts as analogous to the abortion debate—one side says the issue is killing babies, the other says the issue is a woman's control over her body; there is no room for debate.

In fact, this tendency is a socially mischievous and inaccurate gestalt on ethical issues. In the first place, it obscures the important fact that we are far more ethically alike than different. Although a Japanese sumo wrestler may appear vastly different from a Russian ballerina, we know that if we X-ray them both, the differences will appear as nothing next to the striking anatomical similarities. Similarly, if we take two apparently culturally dissimilar people from our society—say, a Montana cowboy and a Brooklyn Chasidic Jew—and we "X-ray" them morally, we find far more in common (besides the hat!) than not. And this should not surprise us. We are all reared in the same social consensus ethic, under the same rules and laws, educated within similar core curricula. We are shaped by the same books, movies, and television shows, immersed in the same ideals. We take pride in our love for the same social/political/ethical system. For every major ethical dispute in society—like abortion or capital punishment—there are literally thousands of ethical agreements.

Thus, ethical dilemmas and polarizations are the exception rather than the rule. Certainly abortion represents such a dichotomy, as does capital punishment. But after mentioning these and a few others, we quickly exhaust the list. We may disagree about many things, but there is usually room for a middle way between extremes. Indeed, given the diversity of interest groups pressing for solutions to ethical disagreements in society, and given our commitment to democracy, *inevitably* social solutions will be a result of conflicting forces and thus represent a compromise. As animal activist Henry Spira often and aptly noted, despite our rhetorical tendency to articulate forcefully what seem to be irreconcilable differences, all social revolutions in the history of the United States have in fact been incremental, not catastrophic. Were this not the case, we could not live comfortably together. Despite the apparent major differences between us on ethical matters, then, we should recall Pogo's dictum: "We have met the enemy, and *they* is us."

In fact, the art of ethical resolution, on both a social and a personal ethical level, is the art of finding a middle way—a *via media*—between apparently irreconcilable differences. As many of the ethical cases cited in this book show (for example, see Case 7, the fetotomy case), successful ethical resolution involves "passing between the horns" of an apparent dilemma. Later in this book I will discuss the issue of laboratory animals as a highly emotionally charged example of polarized positions—that is, the medical community's demand that research be allowed to go on in a totally unrestricted way, as opposed to the animal advocates' demand that it be abolished as unjust—and how the issue was ameliorated (but not totally resolved) in the middle.

Before veterinarians can resolve ethical issues, however, they must, as I mentioned earlier, be able to identify and dissect out all of the relevant ethical components. And as we saw in the case of the dog hit with the frying pan, this is not always easy, given the human predilection to perceive with one's expectations. Nor do most people have the time to engage in extensive dialogue in order to garner a multiplicity of perspectives on a given case. For these reasons it is valuable to have some procedure for zeroing in on the relevant ethical components in a given case. Fortunately, this is not hard to do.

Like all professionals, veterinarians find themselves enmeshed in a web of moral duties and obligations that can and often do conflict. In the first place, veterinarians obviously have an obligation to their clients. Second, veterinarians have an obligation to their peers in the profession. Third, veterinarians have, in virtue of their special social role, an obligation to society in general. Fourth, as is often forgotten, veterinarians, like all human beings, have an obligation to themselves. Fifth, and most obscurely, veterinarians have an obligation to animals.

Let us examine each of these issues in more detail. Clearly, veterinarians have moral duties to their clients. For example, they have prima facie obligations to keep contracts, to tell the truth, to explain options, not to cheat, to maintain confidentiality, and so forth. When stated in the abstract, these are self-evident truisms; placed in real-life contexts, however, these maxims are not so clear. For example, some veterinarians believe they are not morally obliged to keep a contract to euthanize a healthy animal if the client has refused to consider other options. Others believe that it is not necessary to tell the truth if the truth is very painful, as for example, when an elderly couple asks if their terminal animal could have been saved if they had brought it in when they first observed symptoms instead of "hoping it would go away." Some veterinarians would argue that one should not explain all therapeutic options to a client if one believes the client will automatically choose the cheapest—not the best—option (see Case 3). And, as the case of a client using illegal food additives demonstrates, the issue of keeping confidences is not always open-and-shut (see Case 4).

Similar problems arise when one begins to consider one's obligations to peers. Veterinarians are obliged to protect the profession and treat other veterinarians in a collegial way. But how does this relate to the veterinarian who is incompetent (see Case 59)? To the veterinarian who is practicing scientifically questionable alternative medicine? To the veterinarian who is misleading the public (see Cases 19 and 36)? To the veterinarian who has missed an obvious diagnosis (see Case 45)? What does one do when one knows that a colleague is abusing drugs or alcohol? When one merely suspects? What does one do in cases wherein rules established by the profession conflict with common sense (see Case 34)?

And what of a veterinarian's obligations to society? Public health obligations clearly exist, but as we can see in the case of the growth promotant (Case 4), these can conflict with confidentiality. Similarly, as I discuss later in detail, society seems to expect veterinarians to lead in animal welfare. Yet it seems to many veterinarians that fulfilling these social obligations can well mean betrayal of their clients. For example, until federal law was passed, many laboratory animal veterinarians were frustrated by the fact that researchers consistently ignored their advice on animal care; yet they also believed they could not advocate for relevant legislation as long as the medical research community was opposed to it. By the same token, organized veterinary medicine will rarely criticize aspects of confinement agriculture that society finds increasingly objectionable—indeed, they often feel compelled to defend it! Again, in some states, veterinarians, as health care professionals, are obliged to report suspected child abuse but are not required to report suspected animal abuse. Yet strong arguments can be marshaled in favor of a moral obligation on the part of veterinarians to report the latter (see Case 41). Although society expects all professionals, including veterinarians, to self-regulate in a way that accords with the social ethic, the profession, like all professions, feels strongly inclined to band together and protect its own—which, of course, creates ethical conflict.

The veterinarian's obligation to himself or herself may seem straightforward, but, alas, here too there are problems. Every veterinarian confronts the problem of people who cannot afford treatment, or who bring in an injured unowned animal. How much can you, as a professional, do for free or at cost? (I once heard a practice management consultant affirm that veterinarians make as much money as they think they deserve!) Similarly, if you are good at what you do, you can end up working twenty-four hours a day. How much time do you owe clients? Animals? Peers? How much leisure do you owe yourself? Your family? Are you obliged to risk your position with the veterinary community by exposing a colleague engaged in blatantly unethical behavior that everyone else chooses to ignore?

Finally, of course, we must turn to the veterinarian's obligations to animals. These obligations are far from clear, because society is only now beginning to articulate a social ethic for animals that goes beyond the very restricted issue of cruelty. Indeed, it is this very matter of "flying by the seat of one's pants" when it comes to obligations to animals that makes veterinary ethics, in my view, the most interesting of all professional ethics. The problems are legion. Do I euthanize a healthy animal? Do I respect a client's wish not to euthanize a suffering animal? How important is controlling animal pain? What are my obligations to individual animals when my basic job is herd health? What of the claim, made by a veterinary student of mine whose whole life was spent as a rancher, that there is something morally odd about keeping animals healthy only to slaughter them? And, of course, there is what I have elsewhere called the fundamental question of veterinary ethics (Rollin, 1978, 1981): To whom does the veterinarian owe primary obligation: animal or owner? Ought the model for the veterinarian be the pediatrician or the car mechanic?

As we can see even from our brief sketch of these issues, the potential for tension across the categories is endless. Can I lie to a client to save an animal? Do I expose a colleague's drinking to protect clients and animals? Do I violate confidentiality to preserve public health? Should I support such sports as horse racing and rodeo, which may cause animal suffering? Should I go to my son's softball game or perform surgery on an unowned, injured animal? Should I risk the ire of ranchers I serve by criticizing hot-iron branding and castration without anesthesia? What is the role, if any, of organized veterinary medicine in raising the moral status of animals?

The key point here, let us recall, is that before one can resolve ethical problems, one must recognize all the ethically relevant components of a situation (the same relation one finds between medical diagnosis and treatment). And a good way to begin doing this is to measure the given situation against all the categories we have discussed. When evaluating any situation, one should routinely ask, "Does it contain elements of obligation to client, peers, animals, society, or self?" In this way one is certain to have at least thought about all possible domains of ethical concern. (As mentioned earlier, another way to make sure that one has unearthed all morally relevant nuances of a situation is to seek dialogue with others who bring to the discussion different paradigms and perspectives. For this reason it is wise to cultivate dialogue partners from varying interest groups, though the natural human tendency is to seek conversation only with like-minded people.)

In any event, let us suppose that one has dissected a given situation into its morally relevant components. What happens next? Can we give a rational account of how one comes to a reasonable resolution? Second, and equally important, what happens when two parties, both well intentioned, disagree about how ethical matters are to be resolved? What happens when the two parties are two individuals disagreeing about personal ethics? What happens when the two parties disagree about the form social ethics should take (for example, on whether or not there should be restrictions on animal use in science)?

The Anatomy of Ethical Decision Making

There are, of course, many situations that may have diverse ethical components, yet whose resolution is clearly dictated by the social ethic. To take a simple example, if a client owes me money, I cannot jump him on the street and search his wallet for my just recompense. Similarly, if I believe that a person is not raising his or her child properly, I cannot kidnap the child. On the other hand, many of the situations people face in a field like veterinary medicine are not so clearly defined, which is why they are vexatious and challenge individuals to apply rationally the components of one's personal ethic, or an admixture of personal and social ethics; it is why they challenge the profession as a whole to reach a consensus on professional ethics, or even to change the existing social ethic. Most of the cases we deal with in the *Canadian Veterinary Journal* are issues involving areas left to one's personal ethic; however, the column on whether veterinarians should be mandated to report cruelty involves changing the social consensus ethic (see Case 41). Similarly, the cases of widespread illegal food-additive use involve an issue that must be addressed by the whole profession or by a significant subgroup thereof (see Case 4). Other such cases might involve the profession speaking out against cosmetic surgery in dogs, or against the steel-jawed trap, or against horse-tripping, all of which have in fact recently occurred. As we shall see, there is going to be increasing social pressure for the veterinary profession to address animal use and welfare issues.

So let us now look at how individuals can rationally make ethical decisions, and how they can rationally convince (or attempt to convince) others with whom they have putative disagreement. In the first place, as I stated earlier, one must attempt to define all ethically relevant components of the situation. Assuming that the situation is thus analyzed, and the answer not dictated by the social ethic, what does one do next? Let us here take a hint from the philosopher Wittgenstein and ask ourselves how we learned about right and wrong, good and bad. As children, we might, for example, reach over to steal our brother's chocolate pudding and be told by our mother, "No! That is wrong!" In other words, this is how we learn that certain actions are wrong, or right, as when we are praised for sharing our chocolate pudding with our brother. As we get older, we gradually move from learning that forcibly taking the chocolate pudding away from brother is wrong on this particular occasion, to the generalization that taking it on any occasion is wrong, to the more abstract generalization that taking something from someone else without permission is wrong, to the even more abstract notion that stealing is wrong. In other words, we ascend from particulars to generalizations in our moral beliefs, just as we do in our knowledge of the world, moving from "Don't touch this radiator," to "Don't touch any hot objects," to "Hot objects cause burns if touched."

Let us call the ethical generalizations that we learn as we grow *moral principles* (or $ethics_1$ principles). Although we originally learn such moral principles primarily from parents, as we grow older, we acquire them from many and varied sources—friends and other peers, teachers, churches, movies, books, radio and television, newspapers, magazines, and so on. We learn such diverse principles as "It is wrong to lie," "It is wrong to steal," "It is wrong to hurt people's feelings," "It is wrong to use drugs," "Stand up for yourself," and, of course, many others. Eventually, we have the mental equivalent of a hall closet chock-full of moral principles, which we (ideally) pull out in the appropriate circumstances. So far this sounds simple enough. The trouble is that sometimes two or more principles fit a situation yet patently contradict one another. It is easy to envision a multitude of situations wherein this dilemma might occur.

For example, we have all learned the principles not to lie and not to hurt others' feelings. Yet these may stand in conflict, as when a co-worker or wife asks me, "What do you think of my new three-hundred-dollar hairdo?" and I think it is an aesthetic travesty. Similarly, many of my male students growing up on ranches also face such tension. On the one hand, they have been brought up as Christians and taught the principle

"Turn the other cheek." On the other hand, they have also been taught "not to take any crap and to stand up for yourself." As a third example, a female colleague tells of suffering a great deal of anguish when dating, as she had been taught both to be chaste and not to make others feel bad. Veterinarians also obviously face conflicting principles—indeed, one need go no further than the Veterinarian's Oath to see a clear conflict. For example, there is certainly a tension between the injunction to "advance scientific knowledge" and the injunction to "ameliorate animal suffering," as scientific knowledge often advances by creating animal suffering.

When faced with such conflicts, many of us simply don't notice them. As one of my cowboy students said to me once about the internal conflict between turning the other cheek and not being bullied: "What's the problem, doc! 'Turn the other cheek' comes out in church, the other one comes out in bars." Obviously, this response is less than satisfactory!

The key to resolving such contradictions lies in how one prioritizes the principles in conflict. Obviously, if they are given equal priority, one is at an impasse. So one needs a higher-order theory to decide which principles are given greater weight in which sorts of situations, and to keep us consistent in our evaluations, so that we do the same sorts of prioritizing in situations that are analogous in a morally relevant way. In this regard one can perhaps draw a reasonable analogy between levels of understanding in science (that is, knowledge of the world) and ethics. In science one begins with individual experiences (for example, of a moving body); one then learns a variety of laws of motion (celestial motion, Kepler's laws, terrestrial motion), and one finally unifies the variegated laws under one more general theory from which they can all be derived (Newton's theory of universal gravitation). Similarly, in ethics one begins with awareness that particular things are wrong (or right), moves to principles, and then ascends to a theory that prioritizes, explains, or provides a rationale for both having and applying the principles. Theories can also help us identify ethical components of situations wherein we intuitively surmise there are problems but can't sort them out.

The Nature of Ethical Theory

Construction of such ethical theories has occupied philosophers from Plato to the present. It is beyond the scope of this discussion to survey the many diverse theories that have been promulgated. On the other hand, it is valuable to look at two significantly different systems that nicely represent extremes in ethical theory, and that, more important, have been synthesized in the theory underlying our own consensus social ethic.

Ethical theories tend to fall into two major groups: those stressing goodness and badness, that is, the results of actions; and those stressing rightness and wrongness, or duty, that is, the intrinsic properties of actions. The former are called *consequentialist*, or *teleological*, theories (from the Greek word *telos*, meaning "result," "end," or "purpose"). The latter are termed *deontological* theories (from the Greek word *deontos*, meaning "necessity" or "obligation")—in other words, what one is obliged to do. The most common deontological theories are theologically based, wherein action is obligatory because commanded by God.

The most well-known consequentialist theory is *utilitarianism*. It has appeared in a variety of forms throughout history but is most famously associated with nineteeth-century philosophers Jeremy Bentham and John Stuart Mill (Bentham, 1961; Mill, 1961). In its simplest version utilitarianism holds that one acts in given situations according to what produces the greatest happiness for the greatest number, wherein *happiness* is defined in terms of pleasure and absence of pain. Principles of utilitarianism would be generalizations about courses of action that tend to produce more happiness than unhappiness. In situations wherein principles conflict, one decides by calculating which course of action is most likely to produce the greatest happiness. Thus, in the trivial case of the ugly hairstyle mentioned previously, telling a "little white lie" will likely produce no harm, whereas telling the truth will result in hostility and bad feeling, so one ought to choose the former course of action.

There are many problems with this sort of theory, but they lie beyond the scope of this discussion. The only point here is that adherence to such a theory resolves conflict among principles by providing a higher-order rule for decision making.

Those of us who grew up with very liberal parents will quickly recognize the utilitarian approach. Suppose you approach such parents in a quandary. You are thinking of entering into an adulterous relationship with a married woman. You explain that she is terminally ill—despised and abandoned by her vile, abusive husband who does not care what she does, but who nonetheless sadistically blocks a divorce—and she is attempting to snatch a brief period of happiness before her demise. These parents might well say, "Adultery is generally wrong, as it usually results in great unhappiness. But in this case perhaps you both deserve the joy you can have together. . . . No one will be hurt."

On the other hand, those of us who grew up with German Lutheran grandparents can imagine a very different scenario if one approached them with the same story. They would be very likely to say, "I don't care what the results will be—adultery is always wrong! Period!" This is, of course, a strongly deontological position. The most famous rational reconstruction of such a position is to be found historically in the writings of the German philosopher Immanuel Kant (Kant, 1959). According to Kant, ethics is unique to rational beings. Rational beings, unlike other beings, are capable of formulating universal truths of mathematics, science, and so on. Animals, lacking language, simply do not have the mechanism to think in terms such as "all X is Y." As rational beings, humans are bound to strive for rationality in all areas of life. Rationality in the area of conduct is to be found in subjecting the principle of action you are considering to the test of universality, by thinking through what the world would be like if everyone behaved the way you are considering behaving. Kant called this requirement "the Categorical Imperative," that is, the requirement of all rational beings to judge their intended actions by the test of universality. In other words, suppose you are trying to decide on whether you should tell a little white lie in an apparently innocuous case, like the ugly hairdo dilemma. Before doing so, you must test that action by the Categorical Imperative, which enjoins you to "act in such a way that your action could be conceived to be a universal law." So before you lie, you conceive of what would occur if everyone were allowed to lie whenever it was convenient to do so. In such a world the notion of telling the truth would cease to have meaning, and thus so, too, would the notion of telling a lie. In other words, no one would trust anyone.

Thus, universalizing a lie leads to a situation that destroys the possibility of the very act you are contemplating, and therefore becomes rationally indefensible, *regardless of the good or bad consequences in the given case.* By the same token, subjecting your act of adultery to the same test shows that if one universalizes adultery, one destroys the institution of marriage, and would thereby in turn render adultery impossible! Thus, in a situation of conflicting principles, one rejects the choice that could not possibly be universalized.

Kant goes on to draw some other implications from his account, including the conclusion that one should always treat other rational beings as "ends in themselves, not merely as means," but these are irrelevant to our example. While Kant's theory also is open to some strong criticisms, these too need not be discussed here. The point is that both personal and social ethics must be based in some theory that prioritizes principles to assure consistency in behavior and action. Having such a theory helps prevent arbitrary and capricious actions.

Whatever theory we adhere to as individuals, we must be careful to assure that it fits the requirements demanded of morality in general: It must treat people who are relevantly equal equally; it must treat relevantly similar cases the same way; it must avoid favoring some individuals for morally irrelevant reasons (such as hair color); it must be fair, and not subject to whimsical change.

Obviously, a society needs some higher-order theory underlying its social consensus ethic. Indeed, such a need is immediately obvious as soon as one realizes that every society faces a fundamental conflict of moral concerns—the good of the group or state or society versus the good of the individual. This conflict is obvious in almost all social decision making, be it the military demanding life-threatening service from citizens, or the legislature redistributing wealth through taxation. It is in society's interest to send you to war—it may not be in yours, as you risk being killed or maimed. It is in society's interest to take money from the wealthy to support social programs or, more simply, to improve quality of life for the impoverished, but it arguably doesn't do the wealthy individual much good.

Different societies have of course constructed different theories to resolve this conflict. Totalitarian societies have taken the position that the group, or state, or Reich, or however they formulate the corporate entity, must unequivocally and always take precedence over the individual. The behavior of the Soviet Union under Stalin, Germany under Hitler, China under Mao, and Japan under the emperors all bespeak the primacy of the social body over individuals. On the other end of the spectrum are anarchistic communes, such as those of the 1960s, that give total primacy to individual wills and see the social body as nothing more than an amalgam of individuals. Obviously, societies along the spectrum are driven by different higher-order theories.

Before discussing the theoretical structure by which our society and other western democratic societies respond to this problem, we are obliged to consider a problem that has been a thorn in the side of ethics since antiquity. This is the position known as *ethical relativism*, which asserts that all ethical positions are equally valid, and that no society (or individual) can be said to have a better ethic than another. The Sophists in ancient Greece, for example, would point out that although incest was a heinous moral offense in Greece, it was the rule among the Egyptian royal family. One still finds this relativistic position among college freshmen and among scientists who see ethics as "opinion," rather than fact.

There are many refutations of relativism; here we will consider two.

1. *Relativism is self-defeating.*
   Relativism asserts that all ethical positions are equally valid or true. In saying this, the relativist admits that his own position has no special validity, and that the ethical position that *denies* the legitimacy of relativism is as true as relativism. Thus, if relativism is correct, its absolute correctness cannot be asserted by its defenders.

2. *There exist criteria for judging competing ethics.*
   It is certainly true that there are differences in people's (and societies') ethical approaches. That in itself, however, does not mean that all approaches are equally valid. Perhaps we can judge different ethical views by comparing them to the basic purposes of ethics, and to the reasons that there is a need for ethics in the first place.

As mentioned early in this discussion, rules for conduct are necessary if people are to live together—which of course they must. Without such rules, with people doing whatever they wish, chaos, anarchy, and what Hobbes called "the war of each against all" would ensue. Some idea of what such a world would be like may be gleaned from what happens during wars, floods, blackouts, and other natural or human-made disasters. A perennial source of friction and drama, such situations lead to looting, pillaging, rape, robbery, outrageous black-market prices for such necessities as food, water, and medicine, and so on.

What sorts of rules best meet the needs dictated by social life? We know through ordinary experience and common sense what sorts of things matter to people. Security regarding life and property is one such need. The ability to trust what others tell us is another. Leaving certain things in one's life to one's own choices is a third. Clearly, certain moral constraints, principles, and even theories will flow from these needs. Rational self-interest dictates that if I do not respect your property, you will not feel any need to respect mine. Because I value my property and you value yours, and we cannot stand watch over it all the time, we "agree" not to steal and adopt this agreement as a moral principle. A similar argument could be mounted for prohibitions against killing, assault, and so on. By the same token, the prohibition against lying could be based naturally in the fact that communication is essential to human life, and that a presupposition of communication is that, in general, the people with whom one is conversing are telling the truth.

By the same token, as we have seen Kant emphasize, certain conclusions can be drawn about morality from the fact that it is based on reason. We would all agree that the strongest way someone can err rationally is to be self-contradictory. To be sensible, or rational, we must be consistent. According to some thinkers, something very like the Golden Rule is a natural consequence of a requirement for consistency. In other words, I can be harmed in certain ways, helped in others, and wish to avoid harm and fulfill my needs and goals—and I see precisely the same features in you and the same concerns. Thus if I believe something should not be done to me, I am led by the similarities between us to conclude that neither should it be done to you, by me or by any other human being. In fact, it is precisely to circumvent this plausible sort of reasoning that we focus on differences between ourselves and others: color, place of origin, social station, heritage, genealogy, anything that might serve to differentiate you from me, us from them, so I don't have to apply the same concerns to others as to me and mine. The history of civilization, in a way, is a history of discarding differences that are not relevant to how one should be treated, like sex or skin color. In sum, some notion of justice—treat equals equally—has been said to be a simple deduction from logic.

In support of this argument, one can say that at least a core of common principles survives even cross-cultural comparison. For example, some version of the Golden Rule can be found in Judaism, Christianity, Islam, Brahmanism, Hinduism, Jainism, Sikhism, Buddhism, Confucianism, Taoism, Shintoism, and Zoroastrianism. And it stands to reason that certain moral principles would evolve in all societies as a minimal requirement for living together. Any society with property would need prohibitions against stealing; communication necessitates prohibitions against lying; murder could certainly not be freely condoned; and so on.

In any case, even if one is philosophically drawn to relativism, one must, like it or not, obey the consensus social ethic. So we now return to the main thread of our discussion, namely, the nature of the ethical theory operative in our and other democratic societies and how it resolves the tension between the individual and society.

In my view, our society has developed the best mechanism in human history for maximizing both the interests of the social body and the interests of the individual. Although we make most of our social decisions by considering what will produce the greatest benefit for the greatest number, a utilitarian/teleological/consequentialist ethical approach, we skillfully avoid the "tyranny of the majority" or the submersion of the individual under the weight of the general good. We do this by considering the individual as, in some sense, inviolable. Specifically, we consider those traits of an individual that we believe are constitutive of his or her *human nature* to be worth protecting at almost all costs. We believe that individual humans are by nature thinking, speaking, social beings who do not wish to be tortured, want to believe as they see fit, desire to speak their mind freely, have a need to congregate with others of their choice, seek to retain their property, and so forth. We take the human interests flowing from this view of human nature as embodied in individuals and build protective, legal/moral fences around them that insulate those interests even from the powerful, coercive effect of the general welfare. These protective fences guarding individual fundamental human interests even against the social interest are called *rights*. Not only do we as a society respect individual rights, we do our best to sanction other societies that ride roughshod over individual rights.

In essence, then, the theory behind our social ethic represents a middle ground or synthesis between utilitarian and deontological theories. On the one hand, social decisions are made and conflicts resolved by appeal to the greatest good for the greatest number. But in cases wherein maximizing the general welfare could oppress the basic interests constituting the humanness of individuals, general welfare is checked by a deontological theoretical component, namely, respect for the individual human's nature and the interests flowing therefrom, which are in turn guaranteed by rights.

The practical implications of this theory are manifest. Consider some examples. Suppose a terrorist has planted a time bomb in an elementary school, placing the lives of innocent children in jeopardy. Suppose further that there is no way to defuse the bomb without setting it off unless the terrorist, whom we have in custody, tells us how to do so. But he refuses to speak. Most of us would advocate torturing the terrorist to find out how to neutralize the bomb; after all, many innocent lives are at stake. Yet despite the enormous utilitarian costs, our social ethic would not allow it, because the right not to be tortured is so fundamental to human nature that we protect that right at whatever cost.

Similarly, suppose I wish to give a speech advocating homosexual, atheistic, satanic bestiality in a small ranching community in Wyoming. The citizens do not wish me to speak—they fear heart attacks, enormous expenses for police protection, harm to children exposed to these ideas, and other evils. No one in the community wishes to hear me. Despite all this, I could call the ACLU or some such organization, and eventually federal marshals would be dispatched at enormous taxpayer expense to assure my being permitted to speak, even if no one in fact attended my speech.

This, then, is a sketch of our underlying social ethical theory. One may choose any personal ethical theory, but it must not conflict with the precedence of the social ethical theory. Thus I may choose to limit what I read by virtue of my adherence to some theological ethical theory, but if I am a librarian, I cannot restrict what *you* read. We shall shortly return to the consensus social ethical theory just discussed, as it is highly relevant to the new ethic emerging in society about animal treatment, an ethic that is in turn highly relevant to veterinary ethics. First, however, it is important to discuss the general question of how ethics can rationally change, at both the personal and social levels.

Effecting Ethical Change

We now have a clearer idea of how ethical reasoning occurs. When one is confronted with an ethically charged situation, one first of all isolates all of the ethically relevant questions and components. Then one considers whether the issues fall under social ethics, personal ethics, or professional ethics. One then adduces all of the relevant ethical principles that could be applied to the situation or its elements and, if necessary, appeals to one's (or the society's) ethical theory for ordering and prioritizing the principles. It is important to recall that principles do not change with differing situations—principles are like wrenches in one's ethical toolbox. What does change in different situations, of course, is *which* principles apply to the case. The analogy of wrenches is apt. Although one's wrenches do not change from car to car, one needs to look at each car to see if one needs metric or SAE wrenches and, having determined this, which wrenches fit what one needs to adjust.

The very interesting question that now arises is this: How does ethical change in individuals, subgroups of society, and society as a whole occur? As is well known, moral judgments are not verified and falsified by reference to experiment or to gathering new data about the world—indeed, recognition of this fact has led twentieth-century science to conclude erroneously that science is "value-free" in general and "ethics-free" in particular. In any event, the knowledge that ethics is not validated by gathering empirical information has led some people to conclude that the only way to change anyone's (or any society's) ethical beliefs is by emotion and propaganda—and that reason has no role.

The best account of the subtle way in which ethical change occurs in a rational manner is given by Plato (Plato, 1965). Plato explicitly stated that people who are attempting to deal with ethical matters rationally cannot *teach* rational adults, they can only *remind*. Whereas one can teach one's veterinary students the various parasites of the dog and demand that they spit back the relevant answers on a quiz, one cannot do that with matters of ethics_1, except insofar as one is testing their knowledge of the social ethic as objectified in law—what they may not do with drugs, for example. (Children, of course, *are* taught ethics.)

Some years ago I experienced an amusing incident that underscores this point. That year I had a class of particularly obstreperous veterinary students. Throughout the course they complained incessantly that I was only raising ethical questions, not giving them "answers." One morning I came to class an hour early and filled the blackboard with a variety of maxims, such as, "Never euthanize a healthy animal"; "Always tell the whole truth to clients"; "Don't castrate without anesthesia"; "Don't dock tails or crop ears"; and so on. When the students filed into class, I told them to copy down these maxims and memorize them. "What are they?" they asked. "These are the answers," I replied. "You've been badgering me all semester to give you answers; there they are." "Who the hell are you to give us answers?" they immediately chorused.

This illustrates the first part of Plato's point, that one cannot teach ethics to rational adults the same way one teaches state capitals. But what of his claim that though one cannot teach, one can remind?

In answering this question, I always appeal to a metaphor from the martial arts. One can, when talking about physical combat, distinguish between sumo and judo. Sumo, of course, involves two large men trying to push each other out of a circle. If a one-hundred-pound man is engaging a four-hundred-pound man in a sumo contest, the result is a foregone conclusion. In other words, if one is simply pitting force against force, the greater force must prevail. On the other hand, a one-hundred-pound man can fare quite well against a four-hundred-pound man if the former uses judo, that is, turns the opponent's force against him. For example, you can throw much larger opponents simply by "helping them along" in the direction of the attack on you.

When you are trying to change people's ethical views, you accomplish nothing by clashing your views against theirs—all you get is a counterthrust. Far better to show that the conclusion you wish them to draw is implicit in what *they* already believe, albeit unnoticed. This is the sense in which Plato talked about "reminding."

As one who spends a good deal of my time attempting to explicate the new ethic for animals to people whose initial impulse is to reject it, I can attest to the futility of ethical sumo and the efficacy of moral judo. One excellent example leaps to mind. Some years ago I was asked to speak at the Colorado State University Rodeo Club about the new ethic in relation to rodeo. When I entered the room, I found some two dozen cowboys seated as far back as possible, cowboy hats over their eyes, booted feet up, arms folded defiantly, arrogantly smirking at me. With the quick-wittedness for which I am known, I immediately sized up the situation as a hostile one.

"Why am I here?" I began by asking. No response. I repeated the question. "Seriously, why am I here? You ought to know, you invited me."

One brave soul ventured, "You're here to tell us what is wrong with rodeo."

"Would you listen?" said I.

"Hell no!" they chorused.

"Well, in that case I would be stupid to try, and I'm not stupid."

A long silence followed. Finally someone suggested, "Are you here to help us think about rodeo?"

"Is that what you want?" I asked.

"Yes," they said.

"Okay," I replied, "I can do that."

For the next hour, without mentioning rodeo, I discussed many aspects of ethics: the nature of social morality and individual morality, the relationship between law and ethics, the need for an ethic for how we treat animals. I queried them as to their position on the latter question. After some dialogue they all agreed that, as a minimal ethical principle, one should not hurt animals for trivial reasons. "Okay," I said. "In the face of our discussion, take a fifteen-minute break, go out in the hall, talk among yourselves, and come back and tell me what *you guys* think is wrong with rodeo—if anything—from the point of view of your own animal ethics."

Fifteen minutes later they came back. All took seats in the front, not the back. One man, the president of the club, stood nervously in front of the room, hat in hand. "Well," I said, not knowing what to expect, nor what the change in attitude betokened. "What did you guys agree is wrong with rodeo?"

The president looked at me and quietly spoke: "Everything, Doc."

"Beg your pardon?" I said.

"Everything," he repeated. "When we started to think about it, we realized that what we do violates our own ethic about animals, namely that you don't hurt an animal unless you must."

"Okay," I said, "I've done my job. I can go."

"Please don't go," he said. "We want to think this through. Rodeo means a lot to us. Will you help us think through how we can hold on to rodeo and yet not violate our ethic?"

To me that incident represents an archetypal example of successful ethical dialogue, using recollection, and judo rather than sumo!

This example has been drawn from an instance that involved people's personal ethics; the social ethic (and the law that mirrors it) has essentially hitherto ignored rodeo. But it is crucial to understand that the logic governing this particular case is precisely the same logic that governs changes in the social ethic as well. Here also, as Plato was aware, lasting change occurs by drawing out unnoticed implications of universally accepted ethical assumptions.

An excellent example of this point is provided by the Civil Rights movement in general, and more particularly by Lyndon Johnson's shepherding of the monumental Civil Rights Act of the 1960s. As an astute politician, and particularly as an astute southern politician, Johnson had his finger on the pulse of how American segregationists were thinking. He realized that the social zeitgeist had progressed to the point that most Americans, even most Southerners, accepted two fundamental premises, one ethical and one factual. The ethical assumption was that all humans should be treated equally in society, and the factual assumption was that blacks were humans. The problem was that many people had never bothered to put the two premises together and draw the inevitable conclusion, namely, that blacks should be treated equally. Johnson believed that if this simple deduction were put into law at that particular time, most people would "remember" and be prepared to bow to the inevitable conclusion. Had he been wrong, the Civil Rights Act would have been as meaningless as Prohibition, where a small subgroup of society attempted to force (sumo) its ethic on everyone else.

We have, in fact, over the last forty years, lived through a good deal of Platonic ethical recollection regarding the ignored consequences of our accepted social ethic. We have seen that ethic rightfully extended not only to blacks, but to women and other disenfranchised minorities, when there was no morally relevant basis for withholding that ethic. To deny an otherwise qualified woman admission into veterinary school, for example, on the grounds that she is a woman (a practice that was rife in these schools until the late 1970s) is as much a violation of the implications of our social ethic as is segregation. Nonetheless, getting people to recollect is a long, hard process, despite the simplicity of the argument on paper. But, still and all, social recollection has occurred, and we have become very much sensitized to remembering those groups of people hitherto disenfranchised and ignored.

The importance of judo—or recollection—cannot be overestimated. Too often we clash like linemen over ethical matters. We forget that, as remarked earlier, our ethical similarities, like our anatomical ones, are far greater than our differences. We are all brought up under the same laws, and the same Judeo-Christian ethic; we watch the same movies and television programs, read the same newspapers and magazines, and share major portions of a culture. It is thus reasonable to assume that, if I detect something morally problematic, you will as well—*if* the problem is presented to you in such a way that you willingly, reflectively examine your own moral response rather than erect defenses.

Thus social ethical change as well as personal ethical change proceeds optimally by recollection. In the next section I will illustrate how recollection is currently generating a consensus social ethical answer to the most vexatious question in veterinary ethics—the moral status of animals.

The Fundamental Question of Veterinary Ethics

As indicated earlier, perhaps the most difficult moral problem that confronts veterinarians today concerns the veterinarian's obligation to the animal. Whereas all other moral tugs—obligations to clients, peers, society, and self—are pretty clearly outlined in the social ethic, the question of one's duties toward animals has been virtually ignored by society and by the consensus social ethic until very recently. What I have elsewhere called the fundamental question of veterinary ethics amounts to this (Rollin, 1978): Does the veterinarian have primary allegiance to client or animal? Are animals moral objects in themselves, or are they of moral concern only as *someone's* animals? Is the ideal model for the veterinarian the garage mechanic or the pediatrician? If a person brings a car to a mechanic and the mechanic determines that the vehicle will cost five thousand dollars to repair, it is perfectly permissible for the owner to declare "Five thousand dollars? The hell with it! Junk it!" On the other hand, if a parent brings a child to a pediatrician and the physician determines that the child needs five thousand dollars' worth of surgery, the pediatrician certainly doesn't allow the parent to say, "The hell with the kid! Junk 'em! I can make another one."

In my experience of working with veterinarians all over the world for over two decades, I have found that well over 90 percent of veterinarians are inclined toward the pediatrician model. The impediments to articulating this ideal, however, have been manifold. In the first place, the social ethic has traditionally dictated something closer to the mechanic model, as I shall soon discuss in detail. In short, society has not been, at least historically, much interested in the treatment of animals. Second, veterinary medicine in the twentieth century fell victim to an ideology that has dominated twentieth-century science and medicine. This ideology asserts that science is "value-free," and thus severely limits the scientist's and the physician's addressing of moral issues that science and medicine occasion and encounter.

In our traditional social ethic (and in the legal system reflecting that ethic even today), animals are property, and their treatment is fundamentally left to the individual, or more accurately, to the individual's personal ethic. This state of affairs naturally leads to a mechanic model. Thus if a pet owner wishes to euthanize a healthy animal for some trivial reason, the veterinarian is powerless to intercede. If a farmer does not wish to spend the money to treat a disease or injury, the veterinarian can do little to contravene that decision. Until very recently, if researchers did not wish their animals to receive postsurgical analgesia, the veterinarian could not compel them to provide pain relief. If a zoo kept animals under conditions seriously incompatible with their biological and behavioral needs, the zoo veterinarian (if there even was one) could do nothing. Racetrack veterinarians were traditionally expected by owners to administer drugs to the animals that would enhance performance, even if they hurt the animal's long-term health and well-being, and so on.

Thus, the treatment of animals was essentially left up to owners, with the social ethic virtually mute on animal treatment. The one exception to this was the social prohibition against willful, useless, purposeless, sadistic, outrageous, deliberate infliction of pain and suffering on animals, or wanton neglect, such as not providing food and water. This social ethic of opposition to cruelty is virtually as old as civilization. The Bible condemns cruelty when it forbids yoking the ox and the ass together, or when it prohibits muzzling the ox when it is milling grain. Ancient Greek and medieval philosophers condemned cruelty, and every civilized society in the world has laws against it.

The sources of opposition to cruelty are twofold. In the first place, there is the commonsense recognition that animals can feel pain, fear, hunger, thirst, and other negative experiences. Second, there is the realization, clearly articulated in St. Thomas Aquinas (Thomas Aquinas, 1956), that even if animals in themselves are not worthy of moral concern (Thomas believed that animals didn't have souls), cruelty to animals must be prevented, because those who perform cruel acts will very likely "graduate" to being cruel to people, an insight confirmed by recent scientific study (Kellert and Felthous, 1985).

Thus the social ethic regarding animal treatment has traditionally been very minimalistic, focusing only on the bizarre and deviant, never on ordinary, accepted, "necessary" uses that might occasion pain and suffering. "Accepted" or "normal" practices in agriculture, hunting, trapping, research, and testing have been invisible to the anticruelty laws and ethic. Furthermore, anticruelty laws have not typically been taken very seriously by police and judges, especially given an overcrowded court system. Indeed, many veterinarians who have attempted to prosecute cruelty have found that they lose much time from their practice, only to find the case repeatedly postponed, and the perpetrator, even if found guilty, given a very minimal sentence, as the following anecdote illustrates.

Two of my second-year veterinary students had acquired a kitten, the possession of which violated their apartment lease. The landlord somehow found out about it, let himself into the apartment with a passkey, beat the kitten to death with a hammer, and left the body in a Dumpster. He also left a note for the students, explaining that he had killed the kitten and that they were not allowed to have animals. Understandably upset, the students brought charges against the landlord for cruelty to animals. Some months later he was tried and convicted—and fined twenty-five dollars. As he left the courtroom, he leaned over to the students and said with a grin, "For twenty-five dollars I'd do it again."

Such a situation is not exceptional—any humane society officer can recount similar incidents. These laws have traditionally been given low priority; this is a fortiori the case in an already overcrowded legal system, where plea bargaining on major felonies, to keep things moving through the system, is the norm. Any veterinarians attempting to prosecute cases of cruelty have found it a frustrating business, with much time lost from their practices, and defense attorneys creating endless delays.

For that matter, judges have ruled that even such an activity as a tame pigeon shoot, put on by a civic group as a charity fund-raiser, is not covered by the laws. (A tame pigeon shoot is an event in which tame pigeons are released and participants are sold the opportunity to shoot them. Whoever shoots the greatest number wins a prize.) In that particular case the judge ruled that the people who were sponsoring the event were not sadists and psychopaths, were not likely to move on to shooting people, and were putting on the shoot for a good cause, so the cruelty laws were not relevant, despite the manifest pain and suffering experienced by the animals.

Of late, more attention has been directed at getting police, prosecutors, and judges to take cruelty seriously, as scientific research has confirmed the close connection between animal abuse and the abuse of children and women. Veterinarians have been recognized as key individuals when dealing with cruelty, and a move is afoot to mandate legally the reporting by veterinarians of suspected animal cruelty, in the same way that health care professionals (including veterinarians) must report suspected child abuse in many states. Such a law would help veterinarians get around the ethical tension created by feeling obliged to respect confidentiality and also feeling obliged to report cruelty. Legally mandating such reporting removes the onus from the veterinarian's personal ethic and places it on the social ethic (see Case 41).

The major problem with the anticruelty social consensus ethic, however, is that it is conceptually inadequate both to changing animal uses in society and to changing social concerns about that use. We shall first briefly examine the new patterns of animal use that necessitated the development of a new social ethic for animals in the latter half of the twentieth century.

New Patterns of Animal Use

The end of World War II witnessed the emergence of two major patterns that had profound implications for the traditional social ethic for animals. The first pattern occurred in the area of animal use in biomedical research. From 1900 to 1920 the number of animals used in such research was both low and constant. After 1920 the growth rate increased somewhat, then precipitously increased during and especially directly after World War II, when large amounts of money were pumped into research and drug production. Such activity reached a peak in the 1960s.

The second pattern occurred in agriculture and grew out of the industrialization of animal agriculture. Between World War II and the mid-1970s agricultural productivity, including animal products, increased dramatically. In the hundred years between 1820 and 1920, agricultural productivity doubled. After that productivity continued to double in much shorter and ever-decreasing time periods. The next doubling took fifteen years (1950–1965); the next took only ten years (1965–1975). As Taylor points out, the most dramatic change took place after World War II, when productivity increased more than fivefold in thirty years (Taylor, 1992). Fewer workers were producing far more food. Directly prior to World War II, 24 percent of the U.S. population was involved in production agriculture; today the figure is about 1.7 percent. Whereas in 1940 each farm worker supplied food for eleven persons in the general population, by 1990 each farm worker was supplying eighty persons. At the same time, the percentage of disposable income spent on food dropped significantly between 1950 (30 percent) and 1990 (11.8 percent).

There is thus no question that industrialized agriculture, including animal agriculture, has been responsible for greatly increased productivity. At the same time, it is equally clear that the husbandry associated with traditional agriculture has changed significantly as a result of industrialization. Departments of Animal Husbandry in universities in the United States have changed their names to departments of Animal Science, thereby marking an essential feature of the change.

For our purposes several features of technological agriculture should be noted. In the first place, although the number of workers has declined significantly, the number of animals produced has increased. This trend has been possible because of mechanization, technological advancement, and the consequent capability of confining large numbers of animals in highly capitalized facilities. As a result, less attention is paid to individual animals. Second, technological innovations have allowed us to alter the environments in which animals are kept. Whereas in traditional agriculture animals had to be kept in environments for which they had evolved, we can now keep them in environments that are contrary to their natures but congenial to increased productivity. Battery cages for laying hens and gestation crates for sows are two examples. The friction that is thus engendered is controlled by technology. Whereas crowding of poultry would once have been impossible because of flock decimation by disease, now antibiotics and vaccines allow producers to avoid this undesirable consequence.

A moment's reflection on the development of large-scale animal research and high-technology agriculture will elucidate why these innovations have led to the advent of a demand for a new ethic for animals in society. In a nutshell, these innovations represent a radically different playing field for animal use from what has characterized most of human history, and one wherein the traditional ethic grows increasingly irrelevant.

Recall that the major animal use in society before this period was agriculture (as it is now), which depended on accommodating animals' natures. Inflicting suffering of any sort on the animals was literally counterproductive to the interests of those making a living from the animals, and to the interests of society in general. Thus, society restricted its moral concern to intentional deviant infliction of suffering.

But the situation was drastically changed by post–World War II developments. A thought experiment will make this change clear. Imagine a pie chart that represents all of the suffering that animals experience at human hands today. What percentage of that suffering is a result of intentional cruelty of the sort condemned by the anticruelty ethic and laws? When I ask my audiences this question—be they scientists, agriculturalists, animal advocates, or members of the general public—I always get the same response: only a fraction of 1 percent. Few people have ever witnessed overt, intentional cruelty, which, we may be thankful, is rare.

On the other hand, people realize that biomedical and other scientific research, toxicological safety testing, uses of animals in teaching, pharmaceutical product extraction from animals, and so on, all produce far more suffering than does overt cruelty. This suffering comes from the poisoning of animals to study toxicity; performing surgery on animals to develop new operative procedures; creating, for the sake of controlled observation, disease, burns, trauma, fractures, pain, fear, learned helplessness, aggression—the list is endless. In addition, more suffering is engendered by the way in which research animals are housed, often under conditions convenient for us but inimical to their biological natures. For example, rodents, which are nocturnal, burrowing creatures, are often kept in polycarbonate cages under artificial, full-time light. Indeed, a prominent member of the biomedical research community has argued that the discomfort and suffering of animals used in research, in virtue of being housed under such conditions, far exceed the suffering produced by invasive research protocols.

Now, it is clear that researchers are not intentionally cruel; they are motivated by plausible and decent intentions: to cure disease, advance knowledge, assure product safety, augment their résumés. Nonetheless, they may inflict great amounts of suffering on the animals they use. (This is not, of course, to suggest that *all* animal research involves pain and suffering.) Furthermore, the traditional ethic of anticruelty and the laws expressing it had no vocabulary for labeling such suffering, since researchers were not maliciously intending to hurt the animals. Indeed, this fact is eloquently marked by the exemption of animal use in science from the purview of anticruelty laws.

Those who first recognized this suffering as a concern—by and large the humane societies—lacking any vocabulary to describe it, often labeled researchers as cruel, but such a description was clearly inadequate and in fact served only to shut down dialogue between such concerned people and the research community. A new set of concepts beyond cruelty and kindness was needed to discuss the issues associated with the burgeoning use of animals in research.

Precisely the same point is true regarding criticism of confinement in industrialized agriculture. As we shall see, society eventually became aware that new kinds of suffering were engendered by this new sort of agriculture. Once again the producers could not be categorized as cruel, yet were responsible for new kinds of animal suffering on at least three fronts:

1. The rise of production diseases, that is, diseases originating from the new ways the animals were produced. For example, liver abscesses in cattle are a function of certain animals' response to high-concentrate, low-roughage diet, a diet that characterizes feedlot production. (This is, of course, not the only cause of liver abscesses.) Although a certain percentage of the animals get sick and die, the overall economic efficiency of feedlots is maximized by the provision of such a diet.
2. Less care and concern for each animal. The huge scale of industrialized agricultural operations—and the small profit margin per animal—militate against the sort of individual attention per animal that characterized much of traditional agriculture.
3. Physical and psychological deprivation for animals in confinement. In industrialized agriculture this means lack of space, lack of companionship for social animals, inability to move freely, boredom, austerity of environments, and so on, all of which will be discussed in detail elsewhere. Since the animals have evolved for adaptation to extensive environments, but are now placed in much-truncated environments, such deprivation is inevitable. This was not a problem in traditional, extensive agriculture.

What is noteworthy here is that these sources of suffering, like the sources of suffering in research, are again not captured by the vocabulary of cruelty, nor are they proscribed or even acknowledged by the laws of the anticruelty ethic. Furthermore, they typically did not arise under the traditional agriculture and ethic of husbandry. Therefore, the rise of massive uses of animals in science and the (roughly) contemporaneous rise of intensive agriculture have engendered significant amounts of new suffering for animals that could not be conceptually encompassed or even discussed in terms of the traditional social ethic proscribing cruelty. At the same time, as public awareness of this suffering has increased, the concern for its alleviation and mitigation have grown exponentially. Thus the need for a new ethic and a new set of ethical concepts adequate to these technological innovations now exists.

The emergence of the new ethic in response to changes in agricultural and research use of animals was facilitated by a variety of sociocultural factors that are worthy of mention.

The Urbanization of Society

Along with the development of confinement agriculture came a significant movement of population from rural communities to urban and suburban areas. Inevitably, the vast majority of the population lost direct connection with the nature of agriculture. Although agriculture has changed dramatically during the past fifty years, public understanding of these changes was at first minimal, and most of the population still schematized agriculture in terms of the small, extensive unit typified in "Old MacDonald's

Farm." This stereotypical agrarian ideal was perpetuated by a variety of factors, not the least of which was agriculture's own self-promotion, as in the Perdue Company's advertisement boasting of raising "happy chickens" under what was depicted as barnyard conditions. Public consciousness was therefore shocked by its encounter with the realities of confinement agriculture. This was most obvious in Great Britain, where Ruth Harrison's 1964 book, *Animal Machines* (Harrison, 1964), introduced the British public to the realities of industrialized agriculture, and galvanized social concern to such an extent that the British government was forced to appoint a Royal Commission, the Brambell Commission, to examine the issue and make recommendations. At the same time, attempts to articulate new moral categories that went beyond cruelty were sparked in Britain primarily by the growing awareness of confinement agriculture.

The same sort of concern about the discord between the public agrarian ideal and the realities of confinement agriculture surfaced in Sweden in the late 1980s, sparked by a campaign led by children's book writer Astrid Lindgren, who was appalled by the realities of confinement. Her concern struck a responsive chord in Swedish society, which, in 1988, passed legislation that severely restricted confinement agriculture. I shall discuss this development shortly, for it provides a very concrete example of the new ethic applied to agriculture in the political arena.

Augmenting the persistence of the agrarian ideal in urbanized society was a new way of looking at animals. Once again, a thought experiment will clarify this point expeditiously. Imagine traveling back in time one hundred years and stopping people on the street in either an urban or a rural setting. Imagine further subjecting these people to a word-association test, wherein they state the first word that comes to mind when you prompt them with a word of your own. Suppose you say "steam"—they might say "engine." You then say "animal." Most people living at that time would probably respond with "cow," "horse," "food," "farm," or the like. Were one to attempt this experiment today, however, the response would be very different. One would undoubtedly hear such responses as "dog," "cat," "pet," "friend"—the vast majority of the pet-owning population see their animals as "members of the family." In other words, a primarily utilitarian view of animals has been superseded by a more personal and comradely view. Veterinary medicine has witnessed the same change as the preponderance of practitioners have found themselves working with companion animals rather than food animals.

Media Exploitation

The aforementioned view of animals, coupled with a lack of daily dependence upon or interaction with or knowledge of animals of the sort farmers had for most of the population, has made animals a source of endless fascination to the general public. People care about animals but know little about them, even their pets. Books, movies, newspapers, and television are quick to exploit this fascination and to augment it with both accurate and inaccurate anthropomorphic accounts of animals, which an uninformed public cannot critically assess.

That "animals sell papers," as one reporter told me, has been proved repeatedly. Thus media coverage of animals, and of human exploitation and abuse of animals, finds a perennially interested and responsive audience. Concern about the welfare of animals used in science, agriculture, and other areas has been fueled by extensive press coverage. For example, the media coverage of the 1984 University of Pennsylvania atrocities against laboratory animals in baboon head injury studies, as documented on videotape by the researchers themselves, rapidly accelerated public concern about animals used in research and thereby assured passage of the federal legislation I shall shortly discuss.

Social Context

Since the 1950s we have witnessed the rise of an ethics of social concern for traditionally ignored and exploited segments of the population: blacks, native peoples, women, the handicapped, children, non-industrialized populations, the mentally ill, unsuspecting humans used in research, endangered species and ecosystems, and so on. *Exploitation* became a dirty word, and new generations were significantly sensitized to any sort of injustice or unfairness. A growing ecological consciousness stressed our kinship with other inhabitants of "spaceship Earth." It was thus inevitable that this sort of mind-set would eventually encompass the issue of animal suffering at human hands. Indeed, many leaders in the crusade for a new ethic for animals are veterans of other social struggles—civil rights, the labor movement, feminism, and so on. The treatment of animals is thus perceived as contiguous with a wide variety of other socioethical concerns.

Rational Articulation of a Moral Base

Hegel once remarked that the job of philosophers is to articulate in an explicit and rational fashion currents of thought that are inchoately surfacing in society in general. Beginning in the 1970s, philosophers have done just that with regard to the social ethic for animals. Departing from the traditional twentieth-century tendency of philosophers to talk only to other philosophers, a series of philosophers has spoken to society at large and helped to shape, articulate, and draw out the emerging ethic for animals. Significantly, very few philosophers have defended the status quo regarding animal use; one who did, Michael A. Fox—who wrote a moral defense of animal use in research (Fox, 1986)—rapidly repudiated his own argument.

Again deviating from the standard stereotype, many of these philosophers writing on the moral status of animals have addressed their remarks to the general public and have garnered a good deal of attention. Peter Singer's seminal *Animal Liberation* has been steadily in print since 1975 (Singer, 1975) and is in its second edition; Bernard Rollin's *Animal Rights and Human Morality* (Rollin, 1981) has been in print since 1981 and is in its third edition. These and other philosophers, along with scientists, attorneys, and other professionals concerned about the issues, have done much to provide a rational lens focusing in a rational way on what would otherwise be unfocused and uninformed moral indignation and sentiment.

In summary, then, these are the salient issues: Both changes in society and changes in animal use have led to the need—and demand—for a new ethic for animals that goes beyond the issue of cruelty alone. Before the mid–twentieth century, the major use of animals in society was agricultural, specifically extensive, husbandry-based agriculture. People who used animals put those animals in environments for which they were evolved and adapted, then augmented the animals' natural ability to cope with additional food, shelter, protection from predators, and so on. The biblical shepherd who leads the animals to green pastures is the lovely paradigm case of this approach. Producers did well if and only if animals did well. This is what Temple Grandin has aptly called "the ancient contract"—as ranchers say, "We take care of the animals and they take care of us." No producer could, for example, have attempted to raise one hundred thousand egg-laying chickens in one building—he would have had all his animals succumb to disease in weeks.

In contrast, when "Animal Husbandry" departments became "Animal Science" departments in the 1940s and 1950s, industry replaced husbandry, and the values of efficiency and productivity, above all else, entered agricultural thinking and practice. Whereas traditional agriculture was about putting square pegs in square holes, round pegs in round holes, and creating as little friction as possible while doing so, "technological sanders" such as antibiotics and vaccines allowed us to produce animals in environments that didn't suit their natures but that were convenient for us. For example, we can now raise one hundred thousand chickens in one building. Technological sanders led to Colonel Sanders.

Similarly, the rise of significant amounts of research and toxicity testing on animals in the mid–twentieth century also differs from the ancient contract; we inflict disease on animals, wound, burn, and poison them for our benefit, with no benefit to them.

When animal use was agriculture governed by husbandry, the activity was essentially self-policing—if one hurt the animals, one hurt oneself. Thus the only social ethic necessary regarding animal treatment was the prohibition of cruelty, to deal with sadists and psychopaths. With the mid-twentieth-century changes in animal use, and the loss of the ancient contract, a new ethic was required if society wished to deal with animal suffering not captured by the notion of cruelty. There is nothing irrational about seeking such an ethic—it would, indeed, be immoral and irrational not to.

Articulating a New Ethic for Animals

I spoke earlier of Plato's notion of recollection, and of the philosopher's job of helping to effect such recollection. My own work over the past twenty-seven years has been based on Plato's insight. During the mid-1970s it became clear to me (and to many of my veterinary colleagues) that social attitudes regarding animals were changing, though we were unable to articulate the nature of that change. I thus saw my task in this area as twofold:

Task 1: to attempt to understand the sources of and reasons for the new and increasing social concern for animals

Task 2: to attempt to articulate the nature of that ethic in a manner that would be accessible to all members of society, from animal users to animal activists

In the foregoing discussion I summarized the social and conceptual bases of the demand for a new ethic, thus completing task 1. But what of task 2? Here Plato's insight is operative in two ways. First of all, I needed to examine the ethical principles we all already shared, to see which of them could plausibly be extended or adapted to apply to animals. In other words, given that ethics always builds on and grows out of previously held ethical beliefs, I found it necessary to identify the beliefs that society was likely to apply to animals. Second, having done so, I needed to articulate in a detailed and formal way the logic of how these previously held ethical notions could legitimately be applied to animals.

The latter task, as Hegel pointed out, is one appropriately undertaken by philosophers: Hegel believed that social thought evolves in progressive ways through different historical periods. At any given period, then, social thought takes a certain form, though the average member of society probably cannot articulate that form. Thus the job of a philosopher is, as Hegel put it, to make thought "conscious of itself," in other words, to explicitly articulate in a clear way what form social thought is taking at any given historical moment.

One need not subscribe to Hegel's entire theory of history to benefit from his insight, and to use it to amplify Plato's notion of ethical recollection. In my work I attempted to show very explicitly how certain elements of our social ethic could logically be extended to apply to animals. In other words, I reconstructed what I thought followed about the forms of animal treatment from our ethic for treating humans. In my writings and lectures I tried to put this reconstruction in language any ordinary citizen could understand. Once this was done, I tried to determine if my reconstruction captured and articulated the feelings of people who were concerned about animal treatment, whether as advocates or opponents of animal rights, or just as ordinary citizens. Gratifyingly, my work has elicited from a wide variety of people—veterinarians, cattle ranchers, swine producers, animal advocates, researchers, and many others—confirmation that I have created a fair articulation of social thought. Far more gratifying, the overwhelming majority of people believed that the ethic my reconstruction expressed was difficult to argue against and had moral validity, at least as an ideal.

At long last I can now turn to an explicit statement of what I believe to be the emerging ethic for animals in society. Let us recall the two classical types of ethical theory defined earlier in this discussion—the consequentialist approach of utilitarianism, emphasizing results of action, and the deontological theory exemplified by Kant. We saw that our social consensus ethic has its own implicit theory, an interesting amalgam of both these conflicting approaches. Our social ethic functions mostly by making decisions in a utilitarian way, assessing the greatest good for the greatest number, but it also contains a strong deontological component—the concept of rights—designed to protect individuals from being harmed and oppressed for the sake of the general welfare. Specifically, rights protect those elements we believe to be essential to a person's human nature—speech, religious belief, assembly, property, and so on—from being eroded for utilitarian considerations. Thus the concept of rights strikes a happy balance between individualistic anarchy and totalitarian oppression of individuals for the sake of the group, the Volk, the Reich—whatever term one might use. It is basically this notion of rights that society inexorably extended to animals in the face of the societal changes previously described. Recall that the last fifty years or so have in fact been dominated by concerns with rights—the rights of blacks, women, gays, other minorities, students, the handicapped, indigenous peoples, and so on. In fact, even our foreign policy has been colored by concern for the basic human rights of foreign populations. So extensive has been our social concern with rights that it was inevitable that this notion be called upon when people sought a new moral language about animal treatment.

Furthermore, the notion of rights is extremely appropriate to assessing the new uses of animals emerging in the twentieth century. First of all, the core notion of human nature is readily exportable to animals. If anything, it is probably easier to grasp the nature of a dog or a pig than to encapsulate "human nature." Furthermore, the notion of animal nature—what, following Aristotle, I call *telos* (Rollin, 1981)—fits both ordinary common sense and scientific knowledge. In biological terms, the animal's nature is encoded in its genome and expressed in its environment. Few people who work with animals would deny that there is a "pigness" to a pig, a "dogness" to a dog.

Indeed, in my view, public awareness of the systematic violation of animal *telos* and the suffering it entails in confinement agriculture, research, zoos and circuses, and elsewhere has inexorably led to the public demand for a new ethic! People across society, from ranchers to urban dwellers, are shocked by veal calves in crates, laying hens in battery cages, sows in severe confinement. The issue of the violation of *telos,* we must stress, did not surface in the area of agriculture, or in any other large-scale way, until the mid–twentieth century. When the overwhelming use of animals in society was agricultural, and agriculture was based on husbandry, violations of animal nature were inconceivable and would be committed only by a sadistic or cruel human being; certainly not by anyone trying to make a profit. Animal *telos*—and thus animal rights—was automatically respected in traditional animal use. (Zoos are an obvious exception to this generalization.) Today's new uses, and today's social concern for animals, call forth the social demand for guarantees that animals' natures not be violated and the rights flowing from those natures be guaranteed, if necessary, in the law.

This is the sense in which the vast majority of the public believes animals have rights—the core of the new ethic. A survey taken in the United States in 1989 shows that 80 percent of the general public believe that animals have rights, whereas the same percentage believe that it is permissible for humans to use animals for human benefit (Kane and Parsons, 1989). A British survey shows that more than 95 percent of the British public believe that animals have rights (Richard Ryder, personal communication, 1997). And over 90 percent of the ten thousand or so western cattle ranchers to whom I have lectured also believe that animals have rights, because they have never deviated from the husbandry-based contract that respects animal *telos.* This is also the notion captured by a survey that shows that 93 percent of the U.S. public believe we are obliged to concern ourselves with how food animals live their lives, even though they are destined to die for human use. And an Associated Press survey of 1995 shows that two-thirds of the U.S. public agree with the notion that "an animal's right to live free of suffering should be just as important as a person's" (Reynells, 1996).

This, then, is my reconstruction of the new ethic for animals emerging in society. It is based in the notion of rights, because that is our key ethical concept for protecting individuals' interests from being submerged for the sake of the general welfare. It is a notion that can easily be exported to cover animal use. The ethic I describe is not, by and large, abolitionist in the sense of affirming that humans should not use animals; it is, rather, intended to preserve the fairness of our ancient contract. On the other hand, it is abolitionist about many uses that are thought to be frivolous and yet produce significant animal suffering: Activities such as trapping, prairie dog shoots, cosmetics testing, roadside zoos, animal shows, Mexican rodeos, and so on have already felt the strength of the new ethic.

Why do we need to export the concept of rights to animals? Why can't we simply continue to talk of animal welfare and reserve the concept of animal rights for radical abolitionism? The answer is simple. The notion of animal welfare has historically been employed by animal users to mean the fulfillment of those needs and wants of an animal *compatible with and demanded by our use of that animal.* In extensive, husbandry-based agriculture, that meant satisfying all the needs flowing from the animal's nature, as we saw—so concern with animal welfare effectively *meant* concern for animals' rights. But in industrialized agriculture it means fulfilling only those needs necessary for keeping the animals productive. So producers can now ignore animal needs and interests that don't affect production: space, movement, social instincts, for example. In essence, then, *the notion of animal rights is an augmentation of the traditional notion of animal welfare in the face of this century's technological, profit-oriented changes in animal use.*

Veterinarians and the New Social Ethic for Animals

In over twenty years of working with veterinarians, I have found that the vast majority of them (over 90 percent) would readily agree to something like the emerging social ethic just described. Yet organized veterinary medicine in North America on the national, state, and local levels has tended to avoid taking this ethic and running with it; and veterinary associations have not been leaders in pressing the ethic forward. There are a number of reasons for this situation.

First of all, those involved in organized veterinary medicine believe that the profession must follow the lead of those it serves. Because confinement agriculturalists have not embraced the new ethic, veterinarians who serve agriculture do not wish to antagonize those who hire them.

This, of course, is a reasonable concern. The irony occurs when veterinarians are more zealous in defending agricultural practices than are the producers they are trying to protect. Dr. Hugh Lewis, former dean of the Purdue College of Veterinary Medicine, related a striking story to me. On assuming the deanship, he sent letters to all of the major groups using veterinary services in the state of Indiana, inquiring about their satisfaction with the service the school provided. He received a very interesting response from the swine producers. They indicated that they were very happy with the medical help provided by the school. The problem, they said, was animal welfare. "We expect veterinarians to tell us when we are pushing the animals too hard for society to accept. Instead, they tell us that whatever we do is fine, and we get blindsided by public opinion!" Exactly the same thing occurred in the early 1980s with agribusiness and a major state veterinary association.

The point is that veterinarians do not serve their agricultural clients well by *not* leading in welfare—or rights—improvement. A friend, after all—as one rancher told me—is one who tells you what you *need* to hear, not what you *want* to hear. A failure to tell those in agriculture (or other animal users, such as the equine industry) where they are out of harmony with the social ethic can ultimately hurt these industries more than telling them the truth. Veterinarians can help change socially unacceptable agricultural and other animal use practices before society gets fed up with such practices and bans them or severely restricts them (as in Sweden) regardless of economic impact on producers.

Further, failure of veterinarians to advocate for animals is not only potentially harmful to animals and producers, it can also severely damage veterinarians' credibility in society. At the moment, surveys indicate that society holds veterinarians in high esteem—higher, in fact, than physicians. Society also, not surprisingly, expects veterinarians to be animal advocates (the pediatrician model we discussed earlier). Thus, when organized veterinary medicine issues a report asserting that there are no morally questionable systems in contemporary animal agriculture, only a few "bad managers" (as the AVMA Animal Welfare Committee did some years ago), this does a good deal of harm to the credibility of veterinarians with the general public. In the twenty-five years I have worked with agriculturalists, I have never met a farmer or rancher who would make such an assertion! Similarly, when organized veterinary medicine refused until the mid-1990s to condemn the steel-jawed trap, society tended to lose confidence in veterinary seriousness about animal treatment.

The second reason that organized veterinary medicine has been loath to spearhead social concern about animal treatment and its attendant ethic is a widespread belief that this new ethic is inimical to veterinary medicine. Indeed, in some versions of this notion, the idea that animals have rights is a harbinger of the death of veterinary medicine. If animals have rights, the story goes, people will not be able to own them, keep them as pets, raise them for food, or do research on them. And this, in turn, would mean no work for veterinarians. Thus veterinarians must uncompromisingly defend the status quo.

This belief is, of course, total nonsense. Assuming that the emerging consensus social ethic was totally and radically abolitionist, there might be a concern, though even here, there would presumably be more work for veterinarians as society became increasingly attentive to the health and well-being of all animals in nature. But the key point, as already demonstrated in this book, is that the emerging ethic does not proscribe animal use, except in a few limited areas; it is, rather, overwhelmingly concerned with assuring that the animals we do use live decent and happy lives. And far from being a threat to veterinarians, such a social stance is clearly going to increase the demand for veterinary intervention greatly! For example, as we shall shortly see, the new ethic's concern for the welfare of laboratory animals has resulted in a precipitous increase in salary, status, and job satisfaction for laboratory animal veterinarians.

A final reason that veterinary medicine has not aggressively pressed forward the new ethic for animals is a deeply philosophical one that I have explored at length in my book *The Unheeded Cry* (Rollin, 1998). In the early twentieth century, science attempted to separate itself clearly from any speculative activities such as theology and philosophy. Unfortunately, many speculative and unfounded notions had entered science by the late nineteenth century—"life force" in biology, and absolute space and time in physics, are two salient examples. To banish such speculation, science became strongly positivistic, operating on the presupposition that only that which can be empirically observed, experimentally tested, or operationally defined can be legitimately admitted into science. This hard-line criterion, it was believed, would banish pseudoscience and speculative metaphysics from the scientific arena.

Unfortunately, however well intentioned the emphasis on testability was, scientists, researchers, and theorists ended up throwing out numerous healthy babies with the bathwater. One of the casualties was the idea of consciousness—because we cannot experience the consciousness of others, or verify its existence, talk of mental life was banished from science, and psychology became the study of overt behavior. John B. Watson, the founder of this approach (known as behaviorism) in fact came perilously close to asserting that we don't have thoughts, we only think we do. I shall discuss the ethical consequences of behaviorism later in this essay.

For our purposes here, the most profound consequence of extreme positivism was to exclude value judgments in general, and ethical judgments in particular, from the purview of scientific activity. Science, it was proclaimed, was "value-free" and "ethics-free." Science, as even recent biology textbooks have proclaimed, does not make ethical judgments—it can only supply relevant data for society so that *society* can make informed ethical judgments. This sort of position dominated science for about seventy years. Scientific textbooks, journals, conferences, and courses did not talk about the ethical issues scientific activities occasioned, whether in human research, animal research, or biosafety. Thus, when society challenged the medical community on animal use in research, the responses were essentially non sequiturs: "Look at all the benefits we've given you. Now shut up and let me do what I want with my animals." Consequently, science ran afoul of the social ethic, inevitably leading to laws or regulations restricting scientific autonomy. This is especially true today, when people are as sensitized as humans have ever been to "unfairness," "injustice," and ethical issues in general.

This sort of ethical naïveté consistently clashed with ordinary common sense, as when, in 1989, the head of the National Institutes of Health (NIH), arguably the chief spokesperson for biomedical research in the United States, asserted that although issues such as genetic engineering were always controversial, "research should not be hampered by ethical considerations" (*Michigan State News*, 1989). Such a statement betokened the extent of the influence of positivism on the scientific community.

The development of scientific veterinary medicine in the twentieth century coincided with the advent of positivism and its distancing of science from ethics. Thus veterinarians too were taught to see science and medicine as value-free and divorced from moral positions. Medicine, human and veterinary, was largely taught as applied science; science tended toward the reductionism of physics, chemistry, and molecular biology as an ideal, further marginalizing the place of ethics in medicine. And thus, in both human and veterinary medicine, for most of the twentieth century, medical ethics became largely a matter of intraprofessional etiquette, establishing codes of conduct for peers. Thus in the 1970s, when I first examined the AVMA's Code of Ethics, I found scores of entries dealing with advertising and none dealing with the euthanasia of healthy animals. And when, in the early 1980s, the AVMA finally created an Animal Welfare Committee, it did so more as a reaction to increasing international social pressure than out of genuine moral reflection. Further, the influence of the positivistic denial of ethics was clearly present in the remarks chartering the committee, wherein it was asserted that "AVMA positions [on welfare] should be concerned primarily with the scientific aspects of the medical well-being of animals, rather than the philosophical or moral aspects" (American Veterinary Medical Association, 1982).

Thus, in sum, we can see that a variety of factors militated against veterinarians spearheading a new ethic for animals: First of all, society as a whole did not really demand a new ethic until very recently; certainly this demand has evolved only in the last two decades. Second, if society in general didn't press for such an ethic, the subgroups in society using animals—agriculture, research, toxicology—and correlatively paying for veterinary services a fortiori, did not. Interestingly enough, this was true also of companion animal owners who by and large tended to focus on the positive side of human animal interactions. And, third, the pervasive ideology governing science, in which veterinary medicine shared, served to distance veterinary medicine from any reflection at all on societal moral issues.

How Veterinary Medicine Should Respond to the New Ethic: The Case of Animal Research

Must we say, then, that veterinary medicine has lost the opportunity to lead as society develops what we have called the new ethic for animals? I do not believe that this is the case, for reasons I shall now detail. In my view veterinary medicine can still seize leadership in this area and, by doing so, can both do good and do well.

The best example of how veterinary medicine can lead in moving the new ethic forward, respond to public concern about animal use, and benefit significantly from doing so can be found in the area of animal research. Because I was part of the Colorado group that developed the federal laws guaranteeing proper treatment of animals used in research, I can provide a firsthand, participant's account of how these laws came about.

In 1976 I was approached by the laboratory animal veterinarian at Colorado State University, Dr. David Neil, and asked if I would join a small group assembled to bring laboratory animal use into harmony with social concerns about animals. We met for about three years, first attempting to reconstruct the emerging social ethic, generating some form of societal recollection, and then attempting to make that recollection operative in research. At the time, there were, in essence, no constraints on research use of animals. Although the National Institutes of Health had promulgated excellent guidelines for animal research, these were neither enforced nor observed. And though a federal Animal Welfare Act was passed into law in 1966, the act was concerned only with licensing animal dealers and setting standards for cage size; it was virtually silent on pain and suffering and their control, which was ever-increasingly emerging as the public's main concern about experimentation.

In addition to our laboratory animal veterinarian, the group included an attorney, Robert Welborn, who was associated with the humane movement, and a veterinary researcher, Dr. Harry Gorman, who had over forty years of distinguished service in surgical and aerospace-related animal research, and who had helped found the accreditation body for laboratory animal veterinarians.

Our task was to write viable legislation that would assure the minimization of pain, suffering, and distress; eliminate multiple surgical procedures; create housing for laboratory animals more suited to the animals' *telos*; assure meaningful oversight of research animal use; and eliminate the positivistic ideology that distanced researchers from the moral dimensions of their activities. At the same time we wished to avoid "cops in the lab," or creating an onerous, proliferative bureaucracy. In the end we decided on mandating local institutional animal care committees both to review research protocols and to inspect facilities and the delivery of animal care. These committees, we concluded, should consist of both researchers and laypeople, including persons concerned with animal welfare. The committees would have the power to reject, amend, or terminate protocols. Most significant for our purposes, each research institution would be required to have a veterinarian knowledgeable in research and laboratory animal care, and that veterinarian was to be the operational or executive arm of the committee.

Interestingly enough, and indicative of the unwillingness of veterinarians to lead in animal welfare, we were not supported by laboratory animal veterinary associations, despite the fact that these groups believed they had the expertise to improve both research and animal care and regularly complained of being ignored by researchers. Less surprising, we were strongly opposed by the medical research establishment, whose members were accustomed to laissez-faire in animal use, and who asserted that any constraints imposed on research for the benefit of animals would imperil human health. Thus, when I published a book in 1981 describing our approach (Rollin, 1981), I was compared to a Nazi and called an "apologist for the lab trashers" in a review in the *New England Journal of Medicine* (Visscher, 1982). In the same week I was called a "sellout" by radical animal activists for "accepting the reality of science," essentially dissolving my distress at the earlier cut, and buttressing my belief that our approach was mainstream and practicable, as it had been so viciously attacked by both extremes.

In 1982 I was called before Congress to define our legislative proposal, the bill having been introduced by Representatives Pat Schroeder and Doug Walgren. And in 1985 not one, but two versions of our approach were carried by Senator Bob Dole and Representative George Brown and passed. One made the aforementioned NIH Guidelines into law, the other amended the Animal Welfare Act significantly to control pain and suffering. This was a great surprise to me and demonstrated the strength of social concern about animals. In 1980 I had predicted that nothing would pass until 2010!

Twenty years later the laws appear to have been beneficial. The medical community now admits that the new legislation has in fact helped good research by helping to minimize stress and pain variables that have biological consequences and could skew research results. Animal advocates, too, generally admit that progress has been made, and there are fewer scandals about and media exposés of horror stories in research facilities.

Most important for purposes of our discussion, however, has been the effect on laboratory animal veterinarians. Before the law, as one prominent laboratory animal veterinarian bitterly commented, "we were glorified shit cleaners" and were paid accordingly. Since the passage of the laws, the salaries of such veterinarians has soared. Six-figure salaries were common after 1985, and in 1986 I was told by the director of a laboratory animal veterinarian training program that all three veterinary graduates who emerged from a two-year training program got jobs with starting salaries of fifty thousand dollars or more. (To become eligible for board certification, one needs to enter at least a *six-year* training program.) Job security and job satisfaction for laboratory animal veterinarians increased precipitously with the advent of the laws, and no longer is their advice ignored.

The key points are clear: As the moral status of animals rises in society, so too does the social status and remuneration of those whose profession is to care for animals—veterinarians. Further, society was willing, indeed eager, to charge veterinarians with assuring the welfare of animals used by society. And third, whereas society wishes to use animals, it also wants legislated assurance that the sort of fair contract represented in husbandry agriculture is being preserved. And, remarkably, two major government officials involved with implementing the laws, one at NIH and one at USDA/APHIS (the agency that enforces the Animal Welfare Act), both veterinarians, have told me that they see these new laws as embodying some very basic and minimal moral rights for animals! I believe that the model of research animal welfare is a weathervane assuring future changes in animal use in other areas, and that in these areas, too, veterinarians will be expected by society to lead with rational reform—a leadership that can answer social concerns as well as benefit both veterinarians and animals. Veterinarians are in fact the natural midwives for change, as they are professionally committed to the well-being of animals, while at the same time appreciative of the realities and necessities of various forms of animal use.

Veterinarians and Farm Animal Welfare

I suspect—though I can't prove—that traditional veterinary involvement in animal agriculture also played a part in the profession's failure to lead, at least initially, in the movement for a new social ethic. Until relatively recently most veterinarians worked in agricultural practice. Given the nature of husbandry-based agriculture, including its respect for the *telos* of animals, welfare was not a major issue.

Probably the major welfare issue regularly arising in a traditional agricultural practice, and directly relevant to veterinary medicine, had to do with treatable diseases whose treatment was not economically feasible. For example, calves might suffer from scours, for which there was effective therapy. But the cost of the therapeutic regimen often exceeded the value of the animals, so some farmers would invariably elect to euthanize the animals. (I say "some" because other farmers and ranchers would treat, out of a sense of moral obligation to the animals.) The key point is that if such a situation did arise, the veterinarian would certainly see (and feel) the moral tension of being able to heal but not being allowed to do so. Whereas some veterinarians would treat the animals at cost or below, others became inured to economic constraints on assuring welfare. This situation, too, probably made veterinarians feel as if they could not do much to advance welfare in the face of harsh economic realities and constraints.

I have already discussed the change in the nature of agriculture that took place in the mid–twentieth century, wherein traditional, extensive agriculture based in husbandry gave way to highly technological, intensive, industrialized activity. I have pointed out in general the deleterious consequences of this change. But it is worth exploring this point in a bit more detail.

In industrialized agriculture, as in traditional agriculture, producers certainly do not try to cause animal suffering. Nonetheless, as we have seen, there are three major forms of suffering that inexorably emerge from the new agricultural technology.

We have seen that the first source of suffering for animals used in industrialized agriculture is *production diseases*, that is, diseases that are largely a result of the way in which the animal is produced. Under husbandry agriculture these were virtually nonexistent, as any system that would lead to disease in farm animals would impair productivity and thus the economic success of the producer. This is not the case in industrialized agriculture, however, for here one may create conditions that do lead to disease, yet maximize the economic productivity of the operation as a whole, even while some animals do get sick.

An example will make this clear. Beef cattle in feedlots are fed high-concentrate (grain) and low-roughage diets. The result is that some 2 percent or more of the animals develop liver abscesses, thereby causing both sickness and economic loss of the carcasses. However, the gain and growth associated with the other 98 percent of the animals who do not develop abscesses far outweigh this loss, rendering it economically irrelevant. This is the logic of production diseases. Animals are put in contexts not optimal for them. Some animals get sick, while the majority, though stressed, manage to survive, grow, reproduce, produce milk, and so on, sometimes despite being sick. The productivity of those who cope outweighs the loss associated with those who cannot.

Any intensive agricultural system is going to generate production diseases because of the lack of congruence between the animals' biological natures and the conditions under which they are kept. In addition to liver abscesses and rumen acidosis in beef cattle, we can cite the examples of environmental mastitis in dairy cattle, laminitis and lameness in dairy cattle, foot and leg problems and respiratory disease in swine, urinary tract disease in swine, porcine stress syndrome, flip-over syndrome in poultry, foot and leg problems and bone breakage in poultry, LDA (left displaced abomasum) in dairy cattle, hypocalcemia and other metabolic problems in dairy cattle, and many others.

The second source of suffering in intensive agriculture has to do with the austere, deprived, and truncated environments in which confinement-reared animals are kept. These environments are characterized by lack of space, lack of companionship (or the opposite, overcrowding), inability to move, boredom, lack of stimulation, lack of ability to express natural behaviors, and so on. Thus animals' psychological and biological natures are frustrated, and the powers they have evolved in order to cope are nullified.

The extent to which this deprivation generates a serious moral and welfare issue can be gleaned from comparing the behavior of farm animals such as pigs and chickens in the extensive conditions for which they evolved with the behavioral possibilities (or lack thereof) in confinement.

A summary of "natural" swine behavior can serve as a guide to identifying problematic areas in the confinement agricultural rearing of swine. Wood-Gush and Stolba

(1981) studied pig behavior under open conditions in a "park" consisting of a pine copse, gorse bushes, a stream, and a swampy wallow. Small populations of pigs, consisting of a boar, four adult females, a sub-adult male and female, and young up to about thirteen weeks of age, were studied over three years. The researchers observed not only the behavior patterns of the animals but also how the pigs used the environment in carrying out their behavior.

It was found that pigs built a series of communal nests in a cooperative way. These nests displayed certain common features, including walls to protect the animals against prevailing winds and a wide view that allowed the pigs to see what was approaching. These nests were far from the feeding sites. Before retiring to the nest, the animals brought additional nesting material for the walls and rearranged the nest.

On arising in the morning, the animals walked at least 7 meters before urinating and defecating. Defecation occurred on paths so that excreta ran between bushes. Pigs learned to mark trees in allelomimetic fashion (by imitation). The pigs formed complex social bonds between certain animals, and new animals introduced to the area took a long time to be assimilated. Some formed special relationships—for example, a pair of sows would join together for several days after farrowing, and forage and sleep together. Members of a litter of the same sex tended to stay together and to pay attention to one another's exploratory behavior. Young males also attended to the behavior of older males. Juveniles of both sexes exhibited manipulative play. In autumn, 51 percent of the day was devoted to rooting.

Pregnant sows would choose a nest site several hours before giving birth, a significant distance from the communal nest (6 kilometers in one case). Nests were built, sometimes even with log walls. The sow would not allow other pigs to intrude for several days but might eventually allow another sow with a litter, with which she had previously established a bond, to share the nest, though no cross-suckling was ever noted. Piglets began exploring the environment at about five days of age and weaned themselves at somewhere between twelve and fifteen weeks. Sows came into estrus and conceived while lactating (Wood-Gush and Stolba, 1981).

One of Wood-Gush's comments is telling: "Generally the behavior of . . . pigs, born and reared in an intensive system, once they had the appropriate environment, resembled that of the European wild boar" (Wood-Gush, 1983, p. 197). In other words, there is good reason to believe that domestic swine are not far removed from their nondomestic counterparts.

Thus, comparison of behavioral possibilities in confinement with those in the rich, open environment that pigs have evolved to cope with seems a reasonable way at least to begin to assess the welfare adequacy of confinement systems. If confined environments generate behavioral disorders in the animals, which they do, this represents additional reason to believe that there are serious problems with these environments.

Consider the sow. Given the complexity of sow behavior just described, and given that the recommended size for sow gestation stalls or crates is 2 feet wide, 7 feet long, and 3.3 feet high, and given further that the sow spends her entire reproductive life in such stalls (farrowing crates are about the same size), one can see that the degree of restriction of movement and behavior is morally unacceptable, given the ethic outlined above. One could generate a similar argument regarding hens in battery cages. The interested reader who wishes to study these issues in greater detail should consult my *Farm Animal Welfare* (Rollin, 1995).

The third form of suffering in confinement stems from the huge scale of industrialized operations, which makes detecting, let alone treating, individual animal problems impossible—a far cry from the individualized husbandry that characterized traditional agriculture. The value of each animal is furthermore so small that it does not pay to treat individuals. The latter point is well illustrated by one of the cases sent to me for comment in the *Canadian Veterinary Journal*:

> You (as a veterinarian) are called to a five-hundred sow farrow-to-finish swine operation to examine a problem with vaginal discharges in sows. There are three full-time employees and one manager overseeing approximately five thousand animals. As you examine several sows in the crated gestation unit you notice one with a hind leg at an unusual angle and inquire about her status. You are told, "She broke her leg yesterday and she's due to farrow next week. We'll let her farrow in here and then we'll shoot her and foster off her pigs." **Is it ethically correct to leave the sow with a broken leg for one week while you await her farrowing?** (See Case 10.)

Before commenting on the case, I spoke with the veterinarian who had experienced this incident, a swine practitioner. He explained that such operations run on tiny profit margins and on a minimal overextended labor force. Thus, even when he offered at least to splint the leg at cost, he was told that the operation could not afford to expend the manpower needed to separate this sow and care for her! At this point, he said, he realized that confinement agriculture had gone too far. He had been brought up on a family hog farm, where the animals had names and individual husbandry, and the injured animal would have been treated or, if not, euthanized immediately. "If it is not feasible to do this in a confinement operation," he said, "there is something wrong with confinement operations!"

These major sources of suffering in confinement can be augmented by others: Employees in huge confinement operations are often minimum-wage laborers with no animal husbandry knowledge nor animal "savvy." Inevitably, they do not know how to handle or move animals in the most expeditious way and often resort to heavy-handed muscling or hotshotting (use of electric prods). Further, many feel no ethical obligation toward, nor empathy with, the animals.

Another problem arising from confinement agriculture is the tendency to alter animals surgically to fit unnatural environments. Thus battery chickens are debeaked to avoid their cannibalizing one another. Under more natural conditions, they have room to escape. Debeaking in turn creates neuromas, leading to chronic and severe lifelong pain. Docking of tails of confined piglets provides another relevant example.

Some measure of the moral discomfort occasioned by these confinement systems can be gleaned from the following anecdote. I was lecturing to some two hundred independent confinement swine producers in Canada on the new ethic for animals. In closing, I asked them if they agreed with the new ethic, explaining that in my view the ethic was essentially an attempt to restore the fairness of husbandry. I asked for a show of hands, stressing that if they raised their hands they were, in essence, condemning their own systems. After a brief pause every hand in the room was raised! When the extension veterinarian later asked them why, they said that I had "put them in touch with their good part." (Recall the earlier discussion of recollection.) If producers react this way, there is little doubt how the general public would respond.

In addition to the deep-structural animal welfare problems created by confinement agriculture, there are a number of management practices that also generate significant problems. The most obvious arise in the beef industry and include castration and dehorning without anesthesia or analgesia, hot-iron branding, spaying of heifers in the field without anesthesia, and surgical creation of heat-detection bulls known as "gomers" or "sidewinders." (These are bulls that mount cows in heat and thereby identify them but cannot breed them. Their penises are cut off or sewn to the body wall.) An example of such a problem in the dairy industry is tail docking of dairy cattle, allegedly to prevent mastitis (see Case 24). A parallel example from the swine industry is castration of young males without anesthesia, and, in breeding operations, the castration of mature males not chosen to be retained as breeders, also without anesthesia or analgesia.

Clearly, there is much to be done in the area of agricultural animal welfare. Have veterinarians fulfilled social expectations that they provide leadership in effecting change? In my view the answer is equivocal. Certainly organized veterinary medicine on a national level has had little to say about these matters. But locally and internationally, veterinarians have met the challenge with courage and intelligence.

The Federation of European Veterinarians has championed reform of confinement agriculture in Europe. In Sweden the major architect of revolutionary legislation that essentially abolishes high-confinement agriculture and demands that animals be kept under conditions befitting their biological natures was a veterinarian, Dr. Kristina Forslund. (The overwhelming support the law received in Sweden provides further evidence that there is, indeed, an emerging social ethic for animals.)

In the United States and Canada most of the improvements made by veterinarians have been at the state and local levels. In Colorado a cattle veterinarian, Dr. Don Klinkerman, galvanized by discussions of farm animal welfare, drafted and garnered support for a piece of strong legislation addressing the problem of shipping "downer" cattle to sale barns. In southern Michigan Dr. George Bergman has helped swine producers raise pigs under semiextensive, nonconfinement conditions. This has not only helped the animals, but also helped small farmers compete with highly capitalized confinement units. In Ontario Dr. Tim Blackwell has helped develop and market humane pork.

These examples come from my own limited experience. We can be morally certain that many other veterinarians are doing innovative and courageous things to advance farm animal welfare. But there is a great deal more that all farm practitioners and veterinary associations can do. They can work, for example, to develop cost-effective anesthetic and analgesic regimens for castration and dehorning and can educate clients, both ethically and pragmatically, about these techniques. (Sadly, some academic veterinarians have refused to help swine producers develop such regimens, fearing liability for human and animal health, and failing to take pain very seriously.) As herd health managers, they can contribute to the design of confinement buildings when such buildings are recapitalized so as to make these facilities more "animal friendly." They can educate farmers, as Dr. Bergman does, on semiextensive alternatives to intensive systems. They can learn more about animal behavior and handling, so as to help clients better manage animals for the sake of better welfare, which can in turn lead to greater profit. (The work of Dr. Temple Grandin, animal scientist, is a beacon in this area.) They can help galvanize farmer groups to take farm animal welfare issues more seriously. And, if legislation is necessary in order to change problematic practices, they can, like Dr. Klinkerman, lead in its conceptualization and actualization. In short, they should become proactive and outspoken animal advocates. As we saw earlier, no favor is done to farmers if veterinarians fail to speak out on the social ethic and its implications.

If veterinary medicine and animal agriculture fail to address social concerns about fair animal welfare, these concerns will not—and should not—go away. Inevitably well-meaning people who are not knowledgeable about agriculture or about animals will attempt to solve these problems legislatively. The result could be laws that harm farmers and veterinarians while not helping animals. People could, for example, attempt to apply the Swedish law to the United States, failing to note the huge differences in the economic substrata of the two countries. But inevitably society will demand, as it did in animal research, both the control of pain in farm animals and the provision of living environments that suit their natures.

It is worth stressing that backing off from totally intensive agriculture could not hurt either small farmers or veterinarians. Confinement agriculture has tended to lead to large corporate domination of poultry, egg, and swine production, and driven out small farmers without the capital to compete. The same thing seems to be happening in dairy as well. This in turn leads to the dissolution of rural communities, the rural way of life, and rural agrarian values such as independence, community, and hard work. Veterinarians have also suffered from confinement agriculture. Whereas one hundred thousand sows spread out among scattered, small, semiextensive operations requires many veterinary practitioners, one hundred thousand sows in one operation requires one veterinarian, or even one veterinary consultant. Similarly, 1 million cattle spread out over northern Colorado provides work for far more veterinarians than the same number concentrated in Monfort's feedlot. In addition, modern confinement agriculture has virtually eliminated veterinarians' working with individual animals, for the emphasis is ever-increasingly on herd health. For many veterinarians, not focusing on individual sick animals goes against the grain. (There are still, of course, many situations wherein food animal practitioners do doctor individuals, for example, prize bulls, breeding farms, and so on.)

In my view, attending to the welfare of agricultural animals in a manner that takes note of economic realities and yet provides the animals with a pain-free (or close to pain-free) and decent life consonant with their natures is the major challenge facing veterinary medicine in the twenty-first century. This challenge may be less difficult to meet than it appears, for it is not merely animal welfare that militates in favor of change in intensive animal agriculture. Environmental concerns, such as the proper, environmentally sound disposition of hog manure, also militate in favor of change, as do social concerns about small farmers and rural ways of life. The public has already spoken legislatively against large, corporate hog farms for environmental reasons.

Recent Progress

Some movement by veterinary medicine in the direction of standing up for farm animal welfare occurred in 2003–2004. In the first place, general social concern with the issues became manifest. In May 2003, a Gallup poll indicated that fully 75 percent of the American public wished to see proper care and treatment of farm animals assured by legislation (Gallup, 2003). Although what we called "the new ethic for animals" had begun to develop and manifest itself in the United States across many animal uses beginning in the 1970s, and despite the fact that farm animal welfare has been a major European concern since the Brambell commission was chartered in 1964, the U.S. public has remained largely ignorant of animal agriculture. There are a variety of reasons for this. In the first place, the majority of urban Americans are geographically removed from such agriculture. If one lives in New York City or Boston or Los Angeles, one may never have had occasion to see a farm or farm animal. Then too as, interestingly enough, both agricultural interests and animals activists have pointed out, the public does not wish to connect food—steaks, bacon, hamburgers—with living animals that are slaughtered. (One of my close friends is fond of making a distinction, only semi-facetiously, between tuna that lives in the sea, and tunafish that comes in cans.) So there exists a kind of studied disinterest even in educated consumers.

Furthermore, agricultural interests have done their best in their advertising to underscore what most Americans stereotypically think of as farms: the idyllic, pastoral nineteenth-century extensive units where cows and sheep and pigs and goats and chickens romp happily together in barnyards and Elysian fields near a red barn—the stuff of Bugs Bunny cartoons and children's books. Two outrageous example of this misdirection can easily be found. The first is the "California happy cows" advertisement, loosely based in the famed Carnation "contented cow" campaign. The California dairy cows are shown happily lolling in endless green fields. In actual fact, of course, the average cow in California lives in a full-confinement mega-dairy, which can hold six thousand animals that never see a blade of grass growing in a field. One of my friends, a lifelong dairy veterinarian, feels his blood pressure rise whenever he sees this advertisement.

An even more outrageous example were the ads that for about fifteen years on the East Coast showing a red sun rising over a large red barnyard in which chickens happily picked at the ground adjacent to other farm animals while a sonorous voice overintoned "At Megafarms [not the real name], we raise happy chickens." I recall returning to my old Columbia University neighborhood in the 1980s from Colorado, and visiting some of my old former graduate student friends. "Are you still into animal issues?" they asked me. "Yes," I said, "Why do you ask?" "Because we are too," they intoned. "We buy Megafarm's chickens, because they raise happy chickens!" Megafarms, of course, was in fact one of the largest confinement, industrialized producers in the United States!

Furthermore, the news media do not cover farm animal welfare issues. Though I have been interviewed many times by newspapers and newsmagazines about "factory farming," the stories rarely appear. Only once, I recall, a reporter did a detailed story for the *Christian Science Monitor* that actually ran. When *Time* magazine ran a story on the expulsion of hog factories from Colorado by the voters for environmental pollution, animal welfare was never mentioned in the published story, though I was interviewed at length about the issues.

Even if a citizen were seized by a desire to visit a confinement swine or poultry operation, he or she would find it as difficult to get into as Fort Knox! On one occasion, my son and I were on a motorcycle tour in desert Utah when, from the top of a hill, we spotted sunlight reflecting off some distant buildings. Wondering what these were, we carefully rode until we found an unmarked dirt road that led to the facility. We eventually encountered a guardhouse and a gate blocking the road. "Must be a military facility, way out here," I said. We approached the guard to inquire. He was effusive. "Nope, not the military. This is Mega Hog Farms—we produce as much shit per year as the city of LA!" he said proudly.

Despite these formidable barriers to alleviating public ignorance about farm animal welfare, the public is beginning to learn. In California, veterinarians, the majority of whom are in small animal practice, found themselves fielding inquiries from their clients about sow stalls and other confinement agricultural issues; the clients assumed that the veterinarians were knowledgeable about all animal issues. Since many California veterinarians were "tracked" in their education and learned little about agriculture, they looked to organized veterinary medicine for guidance. Unfortunately, what they reported back to the clients was far from satisfying. For example, organized veterinary medicine had proclaimed no substantial animal welfare issues in U.S. agriculture—only some "bad managers"—and also had affirmed that sow stalls were fine since they had been around for a while. (When I talk to veterinary groups, I point out that sow stalls have only been around for about forty years. By that logic, extensive rearing of pigs must be two hundred fifty times better, since it has been around for ten thousand years!) Needless to say, clients were dissatisfied.

It was then that Drs. Donald and Jon Klingborg, father and son and both leaders in California veterinary medicine, took action. Both are dairy veterinarians and thinking men. They were worried about loss of veterinarian credibility among clients if nothing intelligent was forthcoming from veterinary medicine about farm animal welfare. So they proceeded to devote a day at an annual conference of the California House of Delegates in 2003 to the issue of farm animal welfare, where I and veterinary ethicist Jerry Tannenbaum gave presentations on the issues and on veterinary medicine's failure to address them. We then broke into smaller groups and had three hours of discussions, from which emerged a proposal to develop CVMA principles for farm animal welfare. After a year of discussion, the principles were announced, which really moved the issues forward. Here they are as announced in October 2004 (California Veterinary Medical Association, 2004):

THE CALIFORNIA VETERINARY MEDICAL ASSOCIATION'S EIGHT PRINCIPLES OF ANIMAL CARE AND USE

Preamble:

As veterinarians, we endorse the following eight principles founded on our education, experience, commitment to and compassion for animals:

Principles:

1. Animals are sentient beings with wants and needs that may be different from those of humans, and are worthy of respect from individuals and society.
2. Animals' interest should be given thoughtful consideration by individuals and society when determining acceptable care and use. This requires the balancing of scientific knowledge and ethical, philosophical, and moral values.
3. Acceptable care and use of an animal may not always serve the individual animal, but should be balanced by the greater benefits to other animals, humans, or society.
4. Animals should be used purposefully, whether for food and fiber, recreation, companionship, transportation, work, education, or the advancement of scientific knowledge.
5. Animals should be provided with water, nutrition, and an environment appropriate to their care and use, with consideration for their safety, health, and species-specific biological needs and behavioral natures.
6. Animals should be cared for in ways that minimize fear, pain, suffering, and distress.
7. Through an owner's actions, animals should be provided with timely and appropriate preventive medical, dental, and surgical care, and an effort should be made to ensure that animals reproduce responsibly.
8. Animals should be provided a humane death.

This is certainly the beginning of a proper ethic for farm animals. It remains to be seen if organized veterinary medicine will take this ball and run with it, given the natural role of veterinarians as leaders in animal welfare we have discussed. Under the presidency of Dr. Bonnie Beaver, the AVMA has begun to revisit some animal welfare issues, including farm animal issues. Such grassroots action as occurred in California can only help stimulate further action.

Meanwhile, the commercial sphere has grown increasingly conscious of farm animal welfare issues. The restaurant chain Chipotle has made it a matter of principle to buy animal products as much as possible only from nonconfinement producers, and such natural food grocery chains as Sunflower, Whole Foods, and Wild Oats offer the public a readily obtainable option for buying humane products. Grass-fed humane beef cooperatives have sprung up, and filling that niche market may well present a viable survival strategy for Western ranchers. Approximately fifteen of my veterinary students planning to enter ranch practice have continued the veterinary ethics course I teach with Dr. Tony Knight for three more semesters, addressing such issues as local anesthesia for branding, forming cooperatives, and alternatives to castration without anesthesia, as a result of their realization that veterinarians must lead in helping to preserve small agriculture, and that humane systems represent a viable strategy for doing so.

Veterinarians and Companion Animal Welfare

Most veterinarians in practice work with companion animals. What are the implications of the new ethic for such veterinarians, and for such animals? In the face of the movement in social thought described in this book, one would expect that the treatment of companion or pet animals would have been the focus of major criticism and reform, for, in many ways, mistreatment of such animals can be looked upon as the most glaring example of baseless animal abuse. In the case of animals used in research, some have argued that suffering and loss of life are justified by the benefits that accrue to both human beings *and* animals by way of such research. Similarly, in the case of agriculture and other product uses of animals, others argue that humans benefit from the supply of food or clothing, and such benefit in itself justifies harming the animals.

Those who harm animals in research or in pursuit of profit, at root, do not stand in any sort of relationship of bonding with these animals. This is not to deny that many farmers do indeed bond with their animals, though this is unlikely in large-scale confinement operations. Rather, such bonding is not presuppositional to the relationship. It can be argued that those who profit from animals are committed to the welfare of the animals only so far as that welfare affects their profit. Again, I am not suggesting that this is always the case. Those who operate family ranches, small dairy farms, and family farms are notable exceptions, in that they often do bond with their animals. Similar points can be made regarding zookeepers, some hunters, and some of those who train or keep animals for circuses.

In the case of companion animals, however, the situation is quite different. First, few people justify having companion animals by appeal to profit or the advancement of knowledge. Here I am speaking of pets—not working animals such as guard dogs, sheep dogs, racing dogs, or sled dogs, for which the relationship with the human owner can indeed be "strictly business": "You guard my property; I keep you fed and fit." But if most pet owners were asked to schematize their relationship with their pets, they would undoubtedly (and do) compare it with that which develops (or ought to develop) between members of a family. There is no inherent need to inflict pain, suffering, and death on companion animals. Indeed, given the nature of the relationship with companion animals, one would ideally do as much as possible to forestall the animal's pain, suffering, and death, much as in the case of one's children. Furthermore, and perhaps most important, there is a bonding between human beings and animals intrinsic to the companion animal relationship, in the absence of which there is little point to keeping companion animals.

Companion animals are kept to bond with human beings, to give and receive love, loyalty, and companionship, and to enrich and deepen the texture of one's life. The nature of the relationship in its ideal form is not one of exploitation and profit, but one of reciprocity. Despite this idealistic conceptual analysis, however, it is well known that human beings violate their part of the contract. As I have explored in detail elsewhere (Rollin, 1981), the ways in which we fail to uphold our obligations to these animals are legion. We euthanize somewhere between 12.2 and 20.3 million healthy companion animals a year. Many of these animals are killed because owners are ignorant of the most basic aspects of the animal's behavior and cannot deal with treatable behavior problems. Also, they are often ignorant of the animal's basic needs, such as feeding, exercise, preventive medicine, and play, despite the fact that they spend billions of dollars annually on their pets. Additionally, hundreds of genetic diseases of dogs and cats are perpetuated by our own selfish aesthetic predilections embodied in various breed standards.

In short, a major area of animal abuse in society is to be found in our treatment of companion animals, where there isn't even a semblance of justification for the abuse. Pet owners are not trying to extract profit from the animals or to use them as tools for some other human end, such as the advancement of knowledge. The abuse isn't an unfortunate by-product of some selfish goal; in fact, it is directly contrary to the intrinsic goals of pet ownership, that is, bonding with the animal, giving and receiving love, and making the animal an integral part of one's life. Thus, one can argue that the readily documentable pet abuse prevalent in society represents the worst sort of animal abuse, for it is totally wanton, senseless, and useless—and in direct contradiction to the basic raison d'être for having pets.

In the face of these reflections, one would expect that the new ethic described herein would focus intense scrutiny on the morally questionable aspects of companion animals in society, especially since over 50 percent of U.S. households have pets. One would expect massive news media coverage of pet abuse, analogous to media coverage of animal research. One would expect major trends toward legislation designed to curtail unbridled pet ownership and the abuse that follows in its wake. One would expect mass rejection of the senseless killing of millions of animals a year, and of the widespread ignorance of these animals' needs. Yet this has not occurred, even on a small scale. How can this be explained?

Clearly, it is easier to criticize the exotic, the patently exploitative, or the unfamiliar than to criticize oneself. I recall railing at an audience of scientists on one occasion about their failure to provide postoperative analgesia for animals used in experimental studies. "How can you possibly ignore the animal's pain?" I thundered. "How can the medical community operate on neonates without anesthesia?"

"Did you have your child circumcised?" asked one of the audience.

"Yes," I replied. "So what?"

"Did you worry about anesthesia or analgesia?" she asked.

Despite my professional interest in pain and its alleviation, I was shamefacedly forced to confess that the thought had not even crossed my mind!

This lack of sensitivity means that the new ethical searchlight for animals, hitherto used to poke into corners dark and mysterious to the average person, must be used to illuminate areas too familiar and too discomfiting to be noticed. Yet we are unlikely to do this ourselves, given human nature. I easily perceive all blemishes of others, even at night, while mine remain invisible to me, even in the full light of day.

If the new ethic is to effect any change in our treatment of pet animals, its attention must be focused on the moral aspects of our behavior toward them. Animal welfare organizations, veterinarians, and the news media have tended to stress the positive side of having companion animals, whereas radical animal-rights advocates have often dismissed the entire notion of owning companion animals as tantamount to slavery. Neither approach is likely to galvanize public attention. The former adds to our social tendency toward self-congratulation; the latter is rejected as absurd. If the average person were asked to cite the moral problems associated with pet ownership, the standard response probably would be spaying and neutering, and animals running loose. Somehow the public must be made aware that the problem is of far greater scope and complexity.

Fundamentally, as in so many socioethical problems, the root lies in the fact that most people have never thought about it. Herein lies an opportunity for veterinarians, the natural champions of companion animals in society—even as pediatricians have historically been the natural advocates for children—to lay the groundwork for meaningful social change.

Hitherto, veterinarians have been in an ambiguous position vis-à-vis the new social ethic for animals, largely because until recent years veterinary medicine has been primarily a service profession to agriculture. In the first place, veterinarians have been forced by their social roles, whatever their personal ethical predilections, to look at animals first and foremost in terms of the economic interest of the producer. Veterinarians have always pursued the welfare of animals, but always against the background constraints of profit and loss for the agriculturalists who hired them. Insofar as the new ethic has tended to stress the interests of animals irrespective of the economic benefit to producers, it has struck a discordant note with veterinarians whose training was based in an agricultural model. Similarly, with challenges to the scientific use of animals, laboratory animal veterinarians have welcomed legislative backing for their care and husbandry recommendations, but have been chary of anything questioning the basic notion of using animals in science. In large part they identify their role with the advancement of science and tend to believe that science cannot proceed without animal use.

None of this ambiguity and divided loyalty exists in the companion animal area, which now constitutes the vast majority of veterinary practice. Pet owners are not trying to use animals for profit; they simply want the best for their animals. Few, as Plato says, do evil knowingly; most of them are merely ignorant. Let me cite some simple examples. Many pet owners believe that an animal cannot adapt to a new owner and, therefore, demand euthanasia if they cannot keep it (see Case 13). Others truly believe surrendered animals will all be placed in good homes by humane societies, not knowing that most of the animals will be killed. Owners may not know that certain abnormal behavior can be eliminated or prevented by proper training, understanding, and use of the animal's natural behavior. Consequently, euthanasia for behavior problems is a major cause of death in pet animals. Many authorities believe that euthanasia for behavioral problems is the single largest cause of death for pets; but it is difficult to get owners who surrender animals to admit to this on survey forms. Thus many owners may say that they are surrendering the animal because they have too many animals. Presumably, at least in some cases, they surrender the animal that has behavior problems. Many other animal owners have no idea of the personalities and physical and psychological quirks associated with certain breeds of purebred dogs. Vast numbers of pet owners have no notion of training animals and work on folk misinformation ("rub his nose in it if he makes a mess in the house") or patent absurdities (beat or reprimand the dog for not coming when it finally comes); others anthropomorphize the animals to deleterious excess. It is hard to blame people for their ignorance of animals. Pet care and husbandry, after all, are usually not taught in schools. What they learn are often old wives' tales and half-truths. ("Big dogs need more space to exercise than do little dogs.") What must be done, however, is to put in place a mechanism for providing the requisite education relevant to caring for these animals and for looking at their treatment in terms of the emerging new ethic. In my view the task of public education naturally falls to the lot of the veterinarian. In accepting this task, veterinarians would be in a position to do good and to do well.

The problem of pet abuse will not be solved exclusively or even primarily by technological advances. Although one can develop methods to spay and neuter multitudes of animals in simple and ingenious ways, this alone will not stop people from euthanizing animals for trivial reasons, failing to understand and provide for animals' needs, or continuing to proliferate genetic disease as a by-product of aesthetic traits. These problems can be attacked only by changing the way people think, or more accurately, by getting them to think at all. Physicians and veterinarians in all human cultures possess what sociologists have called Aesculapian authority, the authority that comes with the ability to heal, as we shall shortly discuss. Pediatricians have put that authority to good use. Parents who bring children to pediatricians sometimes are subjected to lectures on all aspects of child care and rearing, from nutrition and exercise, to disciplining children, to drug use. Not only can one not escape such lectures, one pays for them. Often one is not getting scientific information that the physician acquired at great effort but, rather, a small sermon on matters of ethics in dealing with children—discussions of right and wrong regarding how they ought to be treated. This is not necessarily bad, for sermons delivered with the backing of Aesculapian authority are often effective in getting us to do the right thing, even if the physician's training and medical expertise are irrelevant to licensing his or her pronouncements regarding the right and wrong of child rearing.

This educational function must be more aggressively engaged by companion animal veterinarians. One of my veterinarian friends has ingeniously set an innovative example for the way this idea can work by reserving one evening a week for clients who do not have animals. They pay him well, and gladly, to advise them on sundry matters related to acquiring a pet—for example, species, breed, training, housing, health, nutrition, and behavior. They then become clients. Everyone wins. The client's fear and trepidation about acquiring an animal is eased, and the client usually ends up with a suitable pet, not one purchased impulsively. The animal is not abused or made to suffer out of ignorance. The veterinarian performs a valuable function consonant with his or her reason for entering the profession and is paid for it. If, in the course of such education, the veterinarian, like the pediatrician, slips in a few ethical pronouncements about owner obligation and responsibilities—backed by Aesculapian authority—who can fault him or her? As I have argued elsewhere, valuational (including ethical) commitments are inescapable in medicine and, indeed, in science as well.

Such a paid educational function should continue in practice as an integral part of pet care. There is no reason that veterinarians should not advise clients regarding proper training or resolution of behavior problems, thereby helping to alleviate animal suffering and animal death; yet many veterinarians have been content to surrender this morally important dimension of animal care to increasing numbers of non-veterinary animal behaviorists. It is absurd that such people, in a field wherein anyone can hang out a shingle and there is little quality control, can siphon income away from veterinary practices. Few veterinarians are content with merely giving shots and prescribing medication. Educating clients is an extremely valuable function, which can enliven and challenge one's professional life.

In addition, communities might choose to pay veterinarians to provide free lectures or short courses on all aspects of pet acquisition, husbandry, behavior, nutrition, ethics, and care. Such lectures could reach a wide audience and could be funded with pet license fees. This money would be well spent and might, indeed, be recouped many times over by a subsequent diminution in animal control and euthanasia costs. Attendance at such a short course could be made a precondition for pet ownership, even as people are required to take hunter safety courses before getting hunting licenses.

Many veterinarians, of course, are already doing these sorts of things. But it would be plausible for organized veterinary medicine to place greater emphasis on this educational function and, in particular, for veterinary schools to lay far more stress on building the groundwork for such activity. For example, detailed emphasis on all aspects of animal behavior, from the animal's nature, to how one trains, to how one treats and changes undesirable behavior, should pervade veterinary curricula. Currently, many veterinary education programs treat companion animal behavior as something one simply picks up, or as something adequately dealt with in an elective course that few students take. Yet most veterinarians will certainly be faced with more client problems concerning animal behavior than with many of the physical problems on which greater curricular emphasis is placed; thus, much animal suffering and death can be averted by a veterinarian's mastery of that corpus of information.

There are, then, obvious potential pecuniary advantages accruing to veterinarians by virtue of getting involved with social-ethical issues relevant to companion animals. If nothing else, there is additional income potential in educational opportunities—instructing clients before they acquire an animal, helping clients deal with behavioral problems, teaching the general public as a necessary condition for pet licensure. But there are two more subtle advantages that, in my view, outweigh the direct financial benefits.

Subtle Advantages of Pursuing Companion Animal Welfare

The first advantage of the veterinarian's involvement in companion animal welfare is best introduced by an anecdote. During the 1970s I worked closely with a group at the Columbia University College of Physicians and Surgeons, The Institute of Thanatology. This institute was dedicated to illuminating aspects of death, dying, and grief that had been neglected in medicine. At one point I was asked to suggest topics wherein thanatology could be relevant to veterinary medicine. From my experiences with veterinarians in the mid to late 1970s, I unhesitatingly suggested the issue of dealing with client grief. (On one notable occasion I had watched a veterinarian inform a woman that her prize bitch and all her puppies had died during a caesarean delivery. As the woman fell forward in a partial faint into the veterinarian's arms, he awkwardly backpedaled away from her until this bizarre dance was abruptly terminated when he crashed into a wall.) On the strength of that suggestion we planned such a conference.

Our attendance was excellent, and we presented a full program. The first morning we had four successive speakers, followed by an hour for questions. A hand shot up, and we recognized an elderly veterinarian. "I know how to deal with client grief," he snapped. "If I didn't, I wouldn't have survived very long in practice! What I need to know is how to deal with *my* grief. I went into veterinary medicine to care for animals, and I am constantly being asked to kill them for trivial reasons!"

He was, of course, talking about the constant demand on veterinarians to provide convenience euthanasia of healthy animals for clients going on vacation and not wanting to pay boarding fees, or clients tired of an adult dog and wanting a puppy, or clients who have redecorated and the dog doesn't match the color scheme, or clients who can't handle the animal's barking, urinating, defecating, or other behavior problems they themselves have almost certainly created, or clients who have gone through psychotherapy and declare that they are "no longer a poodle person, but a Doberman person." (All of the above are real examples!) The entire audience echoed his anger and frustration. Within a year we had orchestrated a conference on convenience euthanasia—one far better attended than the first!

The stress and pain of killing healthy animals (or being asked to kill them even if one refuses to do so) is, in my experience, the most demoralizing part of companion animal practice. In fact, this stress is so qualitatively different from what is normally called occupationally "stressful"—meeting deadlines, flagpole sitting, investing other people's money—that I have called it *moral stress*, because it arises out of a fundamental conflict between one's reasons for going into animal work and what one is in fact doing, or being asked to do (Rollin, 1986). Such stress affects not only veterinarians, but also humane society workers and animal control officers. (Most of the latter would like to see their own jobs rendered obsolete!)

I first learned about this unique sort of stress when I lectured at a conference on euthanasia sponsored by the American Humane Association in the early 1980s. The comprehensive program covered everything from the physiological elements of death to practical "wet labs" in the use of barbiturates for euthanasia. One speaker—a clinical psychologist speaking on stress management—was particularly eagerly awaited. Unfortunately, the psychologist was totally naive about the euthanasia of healthy animals. "What is the most stressful part of it?" he asked rhetorically. "When you push the hypodermic in? No problem! All you have to do is visualize something pleasant—a beach, a tropical island, a mountain scene." He was lucky to leave without being torn limb from limb.

On the basis of many conversations with people involved with the euthanasia of healthy animals, I developed my theory of moral stress, which has in fact served as a basis for counselors and therapists treating highly stressed individuals in humane and veterinary work (Rollin, 1986). Unlike other sorts of stress, moral stress does not peak and diminish. It is cumulative and unrelenting, for one is torn by unbearable tension (and resultant guilt) about what one believes one should be doing as opposed to what one is in fact doing, with the latter violating one's fundamental moral views.

In my view the only way to alleviate moral stress is by way of moral action that is aimed at eliminating the practice giving rise to the stress. In other words, any veterinarian or humane worker troubled by convenience euthanasia must do everything he or she can conceive of to eliminate convenience euthanasia—that is why, as we mentioned earlier, animal control workers would happily see their jobs vanish. Failure to do this leads to one's being vanquished by the moral stress and eventually leaving the field, or else having one's physical and/or mental health eroded by the stress—hence the proliferation of psychogenic disease, substance abuse, and even marital dissolution among people with unalleviated moral stress. (The normal outlet for stress reduction—talking to loved ones and friends—is closed to people involved with convenience euthanasia. One can hardly come home and say to one's family on a regular basis, "I killed the nicest dog today.")

The emerging social ethic for animals provides veterinarians with the opportunity to mitigate moral stress in a variety of ways. One can educate clients and the general public. One can create innovative legislation and social policies to implement the new ethic as it pertains to companion animals—be it noninvasive control of feral cat populations or reduction of abandoned dogs. One can steer public awareness in the direction of looking into our own back yard and realizing that "loving" our animal companions is not equivalent to treating them properly. One can share with society both one's loathing of convenience euthanasia and the public's responsibility for creating the problem, something both animal welfare organizations and veterinarians have been chary of doing. And one can overcome historical feuding and bickering and make common cause with animal control personnel and animal rights advocates to help end practices that all agree are morally unacceptable. Although reasonable people may disagree about the acceptability of animal research or of rearing animals for food, no one can rationally defend the killing of healthy companion animals, or excuse the pain and suffering foisted upon practicing veterinarians or other animal care workers by ignorant owners.

The latter point, of course, includes the hundreds of genetic diseases perpetuated by breeding standards—collie eye, sheltie eye, hip dysplasia, von Willebrand's disease, and so on. Here, too, veterinarians can play a pivotal role. Given the enormous exposure this issue has had in the last few years (including a cover story in *Time* magazine), this is a very plausible place for veterinarians to assume a leadership role immediately—few if any veterinarians approve of creating genetically diseased animals. If veterinary medicine doesn't lead on this issue, society will act on its own. On March 14, 1997, the *San Francisco Chronicle* reported that "more than 100 breeds could be banned (including St. Bernards, some terriers, some toys) if proposals by the Council of Europe's Convention for the Protection of Pet Animals became law. The idea is to evaluate each kind of dog (and cat) to determine whether it is suffering because of being bred for abnormal characteristics." By 1999, eleven nations had signed the document.

The second sense in which raising the moral status and social value of companion animals can benefit veterinarians arises out of a subtle conceptual point often unnoticed in medicine, human or veterinary. Twentieth-century medicine has tended to be highly *reductionistic*, seeing organisms as essentially bodies, and bodies as biochemical machines. This is part of the scientific ideology or common sense of science discussed earlier. Few physicians or veterinarians would find fault with this model. And most would vehemently reject the assertion that the concept of disease or sickness is inextricably bound up with value judgments, since, as we saw, scientific ideology denies that science makes any value judgments.

Yet a moment's reflection reveals that value judgments do shape our notions of sickness. Let us recall that there exist numerous concepts intelligible only in contrast to other concepts—darkness and light, full and empty, illusion and reality. In the same way, the concept of illness makes sense only when paired with the concept of health. That is, something can be called sick only if we have a concept of health with which to compare it, and from which it deviates in some way. Thus far, the point seems obvious and perhaps trivial. What makes it interesting is the realization that "health" is not simply an empirically detectable property; it is a value notion that can vary from society to society and even across different subgroups within a society.

A very simple illustration of the extent to which the concept of health is based in value judgments can be found in the famous World Health Organization definition of health as "a complete state of mental, physical, and social well-being." Clearly this is a value judgment and an ideal—from the insistence on a "complete state" to the obviously valuational notion of "well-being" (Beauchamp and Walters, 1978).

Or we can make the point another way. If we wish to know what a person weighs, we place him or her on some standardly calibrated scale. Similarly, if we wish to know whether a given organism is infected with streptococci, there are standard procedures to follow that will provide a clear-cut answer. But if we wish to know whether an individual is healthy, it is not enough to gather considerable data about his or her physical attributes. Once we have those data, we must still appeal to some ideal value of what set of physical characteristics count as healthy and what deviations from that ideal can be described as sick and in need of medical attention.

In human medicine, value judgments informing the concepts of health and disease have largely been made by physicians, who—ironically—generally believe that they are making judgments of fact. Thus physicians have declared obesity to be a disease—not a cause of disease, but itself a disease—while failing to note that the notion of obesity itself that they employ is based on actuarial tables projecting longevity. This, of course, neglects the point that a person might rationally wish to live 3.2 months less on the average than someone at the "ideal weight" for their age, height, and frame, on the grounds that they would rather eat more over their lifetime and lose the 3.2 months!

Medical authority, increased medical specialization, and insurance coverage have combined to create more and more "illness." Positive readings on skin tests—notoriously inaccurate indicators, for example—often serve to brand a child as "an allergic," subject to endless desensitization injections and constraints on his or her lifestyle. Given what has been called the "Aesculapian authority" of physicians, the fact that the vast majority of people in our society never question a physician's diagnosis or therapeutic regimen, and the fact that in many cases costs of diagnosis and therapy are primarily covered by insurance or Medicare, the situation allows physicians to serve as the primary source of our cultural views of health and illness. Small wonder, then, that physicians often are insensitive to the human side of medicine. The demand for what they sell is inelastic. They are genuinely convinced that what they are dispensing is scientific truth, unencumbered by any social or value dimensions. Illness is a fact to be discovered by utilizing the tools of modern reductionistic biology and, once discovered, presented to the public as a fait accompli. Few in our society will challenge the pronouncements of the medical community on illness and treatment, though this is changing in virtue of the "wellness" movement, the rise of alternative medicine, and, in a more sinister vein, the rise of HMOs and "managed care."

Veterinary medicine has followed the lead of human medicine in research, veterinary education, and practice. Indeed, if anything, veterinary medical education actually has outdone human medical education in its emphasis on a reductive and mechanistic approach to disease. Whereas human medical education at least pays lip service to the study of social science, humanities, and ethics, veterinary medical education and even preveterinary education deal with these subjects in a very limited way. Even if physicians fail to realize that there is a social and valuational dimension to health and illness, they at least realize that they must operate in society and deal with human beings, and that it is easier to do this if one knows something besides hard science. Veterinarians, on the other hand, sometimes seem to think that they do not even have to pay lip service to such peripheral areas that are irrelevant to the scientific pursuit of medicine. Veterinary medicine, they believe, is in a better scientific position than human medicine, because it is free of these annoyances. One need not converse with one's patients, one need not worry about hypochondria or psychosomatic dimensions of illness: In veterinary medicine one deals directly and purely with a broken or impaired biological machine. Hence the veterinary curriculum has a far more mechanistic and reductionistic approach than the human medical curriculum.

Although many veterinarians and veterinary educators do stress the importance of dealing with people, pointing out that veterinary medicine is a "people profession," they typically mean something like the following: A veterinarian, in order to make a successful living, must be liked by his or her clients. To be (economically) successful, it is not enough to know one's (mechanistic) medicine cold. One must also be liked by people, be able to convince people to spend the money to follow one's suggestions, be able to get oneself in a position where people will allow you to practice the mechanistic truths only you as a scientist are trained to recognize. In other words, even when veterinarians acknowledge that they must be able to deal with people effectively, they generally view people as a hurdle that stands between them and financial success, not as a factor essentially involved in what counts as illness.

It is precisely this latter point that differentiates veterinary from human medicine and makes it impossible for veterinary medicine to be compared with human medicine, or to follow its lead. As suggested earlier, physicians are the source of what counts as illness and health, in virtue of the esteem in which they are held, their Aesculapian authority, the fact that most medical bills are covered by insurance, and the fact that we value health more than money. Most people do not question regular expensive checkups, expensive tests, referrals, and drugs: Either these things are paid for by insurance, or the patient will get the money somewhere—no one plays games with their bodies. And almost no one will place a monetary value on the health of a human being. But veterinarians typically do not have the same kind of Aesculapian authority. Those people who would never dream of challenging a physician about anything will often argue with a veterinarian about everything. Furthermore, the cost of veterinary care is not socially guaranteed. Many people do not value animals over money and do assign them a monetary value, with the exception of certain segments of the pet-owning population. In addition, people usually bring their animals to veterinarians when they think that there is something wrong—routine checkups are not sought on a wide scale in veterinary medicine. Finally, the percentage of the population that uses veterinary services is far smaller than the percentage that visits physicians. As a result, veterinarians simply cannot declare a certain physical condition an illness and expect that the client will be willing to treat it. In veterinary medicine *people* decide what counts as healthy and sick for their animals, and this decision is made not by reference to biological facts but to such things as economic considerations, the role the animal plays in a client's values, and the subculture the client comes from. Every veterinarian is aware of these facts in day-to-day practice. In many cases diagnostic and therapeutic decisions are made not on the basis of scientific considerations but by appeal to economic factors.

In our society, veterinarians do not have the Aesculapian authority to determine what set of physical conditions counts as healthy, sick, or worthy of treatment. This is the fault neither of veterinary medicine nor of a general lack of veterinary credibility. The truth is, rather, that the objects of veterinary attention—animals—are not in many cases prized above their market value. Animal life is cheap—it is no accident that, in the eyes of the law, animals are property. Thus, in a real sense the veterinarian is forced to practice his or her art in keeping with the client's conception of health and illness, a view shaped not to any significant extent by scientific considerations but, rather, by economic and cultural attitudes toward animals. The concept of animal health derives not from a scientifically based ideal of proper function, but instead from the client's idea of what state the animal needs to be in to function properly in the client's life.

Let us consider one extreme. A farmer employing intensive animal-agricultural methods will think of health not in terms of the individual animal, but in terms of herds, or in terms of the whole operation. Furthermore, health will be defined by reference to economic productivity of the operation, not by reference to biological parameters. The animal is healthy when its physical (or mental) state is consonant with its humanly designated function, and ill when it is not. As another example, consider purebred dogs or cats. Conditions that in human medicine might be considered illnesses or diseases—dwarfism, breathing difficulties, cross-eyes—that the physician should treat or help to forestall by genetic counseling, become ideals to be sought after by certain breeders, or at least acceptable consequences of the standards sought. Again, human extramedical considerations determine what counts as an ideal physical state for the animal. The fact that the animal suffers physical difficulties is accepted as an unfortunate corollary that, if it becomes too extreme, is "treated" by euthanasia.

In this way the veterinarian is placed in an uncomfortable position never faced by the physician. Whereas for a physician diagnosis of a treatable syndrome is tantamount to a go-ahead for applying a good therapeutic regimen, in veterinary medicine the veterinarian's diagnosis is often greeted with a "go ahead and put him to sleep." The diagnosis of sickness, rather than being a step to restoring health, is too often a death sentence. On the other hand, as is often noted, the veterinarian does at least have an appeal to "good death" when the best of scientific medicine fails, whereas the human patient tends to be kept alive at all costs.

Not all clients, of course, base their concept of health on the function of the animal in their business. There are those to whom the animal is essentially a person, and in these cases the veterinarian is free to call upon his or her scientifically based notions of health and illness. But even here the client is the final arbiter, for a reverse problem may arise. Every veterinarian has encountered the client who insists that the animal is ill despite the veterinarian's protestations to the contrary. In human medicine such a patient probably would receive a psychiatric referral. In veterinary medicine the veterinarian must either lose the client, cater to his or her demands, or as is so often the case, end up serving as the client's mental health professional—in essence, treating the client. In fact, many clients declare their animal sick just so they have a person with whom to consult. The significant degree to which veterinarians serve as counselors is invariably overlooked.

The moral of all this is that the concepts of health and illness germane to veterinary medicine derive not so much from mechanistic biology as interpreted by the veterinary medical community as from the values and concerns of clients. Given this reality, one would expect that veterinary medicine, and especially veterinary medical education, would reflect this human-centered dimension. In fact, this is not the case. If anything, veterinary education is far more reductionistic, mechanistic, and scientifically oriented than human medical education. Human medicine, despite the fact that it essentially mandates what counts as health and illness, nonetheless includes a good deal of nonscientific material in its curriculum. Medical schools have relatively few curriculum requirements for admission, and many premedical students study liberal arts, social sciences, and humanities. Indeed, many medical schools themselves allow room for such courses and often require specific courses in medical ethics, sociology, and psychology. Veterinary and preveterinary education, on the other hand, are almost totally mechanistic and grow increasingly more so. In essence, veterinary medical education needs to be more human centered than does human medical education, and yet is less so. And this need, as we have seen, is not merely window dressing, for the clients determine what counts as illness in veterinary medicine, not science, unless the veterinarian is skillful enough to sell his or her scientific view to the client.

The point should now be clear: As the moral status, and moral worth, of animals in society increase, there will be ever greater social pressure and expectations to treat animals—at least companion animals. In my view it is no accident that veterinary oncology in the United States has risen roughly contemporaneously with new moral concern for animals. (This is not to deny that many people in places highly sensitive to the moral status of animals— Sweden, for example—reject oncology, in favor of euthanasia, as causing too much suffering for animals, even as some people reject oncology for humans for the same reason.) As the value of animals rises in society, so will the value of those who treat animals, and so too will the opportunities to actualize the scientific medicine veterinarians have evolved. Health insurance for companion animals will doubtless increase, as will the subspecialties of veterinary medicine if people are willing to pay for the relevant expertise.

Shortly we will discuss one area wherein the growing public concern for animals has increased society's expectations of what veterinarians can and should manage, yet wherein scientific ideology has prevented veterinarians both from fully responding to these expectations and from benefiting therefrom—the area of pain management and control.

The Changing Role of Companion Animals and Their Value

The relatively recent rise of deep, love-based relationships with animals as a regular and increasingly accepted social phenomenon came from a variety of converging and mutually reinforcing social conditions. In the first place, probably beginning with the widespread use of the automobile, extended nuclear families with multi-generations living in one location or under one roof began to vanish. At the beginning of the twentieth century, when roughly half of the public produced food for themselves and the other half of the public, significant numbers of large extended families lived together on farms. The safety net for older people was their family, rather than society as a whole. The concept of easy mobility made preserving the nuclear family less of a necessity, as did the rise of the new idea that society as a whole, rather than the family, was responsible for assuring retirement, medical attention, and facilities for elderly people.

With the concentration of agriculture in fewer and fewer hands, the rise of industrialization, and as the post–Depression Dust Bowl and World War II introduced migration to cities, the nuclear family notion was further eroded. The tendency of urban life to erode community, to create what the Germans called "Gesellshaft" rather than "Gemeinschaft"—mixtures rather than compounds, as it were—further created solitude and loneliness as widespread modes of being. Correlatively, as selfishness and self-actualization were established as positive values beginning in the highly individualistic 1960s, the divorce rate began to climb, and the traditional stigma attached to divorce was erased. As biomedicine prolonged our life spans, more and more people outlived their spouses and were thrown into a loneliness mode of existence, with the loss of the extended family removing a possible remedy.

In effect, we have lonely old people, lonely divorced people, and most tragically, lonely children whose single parent often works. With the best jobs being urban or quasi-urban, many people live in cities or peripherally urban developments such as condos. In New York City, for example, where I lived for twenty-six years, one can be lonelier than in rural Wyoming. The cowboy craving camaraderie can find a neighbor from whom he is separated only by physical distance; the urban person may know no one, and have no one in striking distance who cares. Shorn of physical space, people create psychic distances between themselves and others. People may (and usually do) for years live 6 inches away from neighbors in apartment buildings and never exchange a sentence. Watch New Yorkers on an elevator: The rule is stand as far away from others as you can, and study the ceiling. Making eye contact on a street can be taken as a challenge or a sexual invitation, so people do not. One minds one's own business, one steps over and around drunks on the street, and "Don't get involved" is a mantra for survival.

Yet humans need love, companionship, emotional support, and need to be needed. In such a world, a companion animal can be one's psychic and spiritual salvation. Divorce lawyers repeatedly tell me that custody of the dog can be a greater source of conflict in a divorce than is custody of the children! An animal is someone to hug, and hug you back—someone to play with, to laugh with, to exercise with, to walk with, to share beautiful days with, and to cry with. For a child, the dog is a playmate, a friend—someone to talk to. The dog is a protector; one of the most unforgettable photos I have ever seen shows a child of six in an apartment answering the door at night while clutching the collar of a two-hundred-pound Great Dane, protected.

But a dog is more than that. In New York and other big, cold, tough cities, it is a social lubricant. One does not talk to strangers in cities unless he or she—or preferably both of you—are walking a dog. Then the barriers crumble. One of the most extraordinary social phenomena I have ever participated in was the "dog people" in the Upper West Side of Manhattan. These were people who walked their dogs at roughly the same time—morning and evening—in Riverside Park. United by a common and legitimate purpose, having dogs in common and thereby being above suspicion, conversations would begin spontaneously. To be sure, we usually did not know each other's names—we were "Red's owner," "Helga's person," "Fluffy's mistress." But names didn't matter. What mattered was we began to care for each other through the magic of sharing a bond with an animal and the animals not knowing New York etiquette and playing with one another. And we cared for each other's animals.

Red was a huge German shepherd owned by Phil (I don't know his last name), a former British commando. Though aggressive with male dogs (Phil put him in a pen alone to run or let him run with females), he was an obedient angel with people. When Phil had surgery, we all took turns walking Red for the two weeks Phil was in the hospital. We had a key we passed around; though Phil did not know our last names or addresses, he seemed to assume we were worthy of trust. Through the animals, Gesellshaft was replaced by Gemeinschaft.

Perhaps two years after Phil's operation, I was suffering from chronic asthma, experiencing attacks every night and sometimes multiple times in a night. My physician was preparing to hospitalize me indefinitely until the cycle was broken. I mentioned this to Phil one evening. He nodded and said nothing. The next evening he handed me an envelope. "What is this?" I asked. "The key to my cabin in Thunder Bay, Ontario, and a map. Stay there until you can breathe. The air is clean and there is no stress. It beats a hospital."

For more old people than I care to recall, the dog or cat was a reason to get up in the morning, to go out, to bundle up and go to the park ("Fluffy misses her friends, you know!") to shop, to fuss, to feel responsible for a life, and to be needed.

I used to walk my Great Dane very late at night feeling safe and incidentally other people spoke to me: A black woman who had gotten off at the wrong subway station while heading for Harlem and was terrified. With no hesitation, she asked me to walk her a mile to Harlem, where she felt safe. "I'm okay with you and that big dog," she said, never even conjecturing that I could be a monster with a dog!

Most memorably, I recall walking miles to the theater district at 4:00 A.M. At one all-night cafeteria, the prostitutes used to assemble after a night's work. "Helga!" they would shout with delight when my dog approached. I was simply attached to the leash and was addressed only when they asked permission to buy her a doughnut. These guarded, cynical women would get on their knees and hug and kiss the dog, with a genuine warmth and pleasure, letting the child in them show through in these rare and priceless moments. I cannot recall these incidents without emotion.

These companion animals then, in today's world, provide us with love and someone to love, and do so unfailingly, with loyalty, grace, and boundless devotion. In a book that should be required reading for all who work with animals, author Jon Katz has chronicled what he calls *The New Work of Dogs* (Katz, 2003), all based on his personal experiences in a New Jersey suburban community. Here we read of the dog that a woman credits with shepherding her through a losing battle with cancer, as her emotional bedrock. Katz tells of the Divorced Women's Dog Club, a group of divorced women united only by divorce and reliance on their dogs. He tells the tale of a dog who provides an outlet for a ghetto youth's insecurity and rage, and who is beaten daily. He relates the story of a successful executive with a family and friends, who in the end deals with stress in his life only by long walks with his Labrador, totaling many hours in a day. While raising the question of whether we are entitled to expect this of our animals, Katz explains that we do, and that they perform heroically.

Given this changing role of companion animals, it is inevitable that people will see greater value to them, and that this will ramify in changing social ethics. We argued earlier that the vast majority of the public does not use the new social ethic to illuminate the ethical problems in our treatment of companion animals. Even my veterinary students tend to think that companion animals receive the best possible treatment commensurate with their use, and ignore the mass euthanasia, the perpetuation of genetic defects by breed standards, the large-scale ignorance of dog and cat behavior that leads to bad treatment of companion animals and their relinquishment.

But, there is a gradually emerging feeling in society that the traditional market value of an animal (say, fifty dollars for a mixed breed), essentially replacement value, is out of synch with the role they ever-increasingly play in people's lives. This has led to a growing demand that those who kill a companion animal, whether out of animal cruelty or veterinary malpractice, ought to be liable for more than fifty dollars! This in turn has led to some social movement for raising the economic value of companion animals.

For decades, judges and juries have award large judgments to pet owners for loss of companion animals, but these have occurred *ad hoc*. In a prescient case in 1979 in New York, *Corso v. Crawford Dog and Cat Hospital*, the judge declared that "this court now overrules prior precedent and holds that a pet is not just a thing, but occupies a special place somewhere in between a person and a piece of personal property."

The first legislative attempt to provide for more than market value occurred in Tennessee in 2000, when the legislature granted pet owners the right to sue for pain and suffering incurred in virtue of a wrongful death of a pet, as well as punitive damage with a limit of four thousand dollars. A similar law was passed in Illinois in 2002, pertaining to animals killed by virtue of an act of cruelty. Similar legislative efforts are being attempted in other states. In some cases, the laws exempt veterinary malpractice, in others they do not.

These new laws and court decisions create a fertile field for malpractice lawsuits, with larger amounts of money at stake. The veterinary profession, fearing such lawsuits and escalation of malpractice insurance premiums, has vigorously resisted such legislation.

Advocates, on the other hand, argue that market value fails to reflect the value of animals to people. Also, they affirm that increasing the money at stake in veterinary malpractice will make veterinarians a lot more medically careful in their practice.

Thus far, organized veterinary medicine has utilized its political clout to deflect this trend. I believe that this is a serious error. As we remarked earlier, veterinary medicine has spent over thirty years extolling the value of pets in human life: It is unseemly and mean-spirited to kill efforts that attempt to articulate this insight in economic terms. Instead of fighting this tendency, veterinarians should help direct and lead it along rational pathways, forthrightly representing the view to advocates that neither clients, animals, nor society as a whole can afford to price malpractice insurance for veterinarians so high as to put them out of business, as has occurred in some branches of human medicine. I believe that a veterinary presence complete with veterinary credibility can help assure that emerging legislation does not lead to Frankensteinian results.

It is clear that a compromise position can be crafted. It is necessary to recognize increased animal value to people in monetary terms, but also to do everything possible to avoid demented multimillion-dollar lawsuits that have proliferated in other areas of society. One possible tack is that taken by the Tennessee law: Put a legislated ceiling on awards. Though not legally cast in concrete, and subject to being challenged by slick lawyers, ceilings are nonetheless valuable as indicative of social acceptability.

On the other hand, veterinarians have a reason to be wary. There are some alarming trends emerging in social ethics that put such a rational approach in peril. I am referring to the abrogation of personal responsibility that has been growing in society over more than a quarter of a century, wherein more and more people see themselves as victims and fail to take responsibility, and are encouraged in such stances by such diverse institutions as the courts and the medical community. Things that were paradigm cases of evil action when I was a child—alcoholism, child abuse, gambling—have moved from being seen as morally blameworthy actions to disease, that is, things that can happen to you for which you are not responsible. Obesity too, is now a disease, not a result of weakness of the will.

Correlatively, the courts have begun to support this sort of "victimology." When I was a youth, if I slipped and fell and broke my arm in an icy parking lot, my mother would have berated me to "be more careful, and watch how you walk on ice!" Today's response is to gleefully assert that "this should pay for your college education," and to sue whoever owns the lot!

We all know about frivolous lawsuits; who has not heard of the infamous case of the lady who sued McDonalds because she spilled coffee in her lap and won, at least at the first judicial level? Such lawsuits in the medical malpractice area, and the predatory lawyers who solicit "victims" on television, are in part responsible for the outrageous costs of health care. Who can forget such real headline gems as

> Teen hit by train while asleep on track sues railroad
> Woman who drove drunk gets $300,000
> "All you can drink" winner sues over fall
> Robber sues clerk who shot him during hold-up
> Florida DUI teen sues police (should have arrested him he argues)
> Crime does pay (Denver burglar shot by police gets $1.2 million)
> Toffee maker sued for tooth irritation
> Pitcher, hit by line drive, sues maker of baseball bat

This sort of thing leads to my favorite warning label:

Never iron clothes while they are being worn

We can laugh at these, but we should also cry. For, in essence, this sort of tendency makes mockery of any traditional sense of moral responsibility. Thus, the moral analysis we have given, rational though it may be, could be subverted if this tendency to disclaim responsibility continues unabated.

Education is once again the key. When veterinarians are involved in preparing legislation recognizing the increased value of animals, they also need to point up the dire consequences of creating yet another path to "let's get rich by lawsuits." Animal well-being is a reasonable place to draw the social line that should have been drawn before now.

Critics of increased economic value for pets have cogently pointed out that such awards benefit owners, but not animals, whose legal/ moral status needs desperately to be raised from property (or "chattel," which etymologically derives from "cattle"). There is some truth in this claim—the abused or killed animal does not (or may not) benefit from money channeled to the owner. So such critics have argued for raising the legal status of animals in themselves beyond property, so that they have legal standing in themselves. (I have discussed this at length in *Animal Rights and Human Morality* [Rollin, 1992].) One major impediment is that to truly grant animals such a status would require a constitutional amendment, not likely to be forthcoming in a society reluctant to approve an Equal Rights Amendment for women!

Some largely symbolic moves have been made in this direction by using the legal concepts of "guardian" and "ward." Boulder, Colorado; San Francisco; and Rhode Island have all adopted resolutions (or in the case of Rhode Island, legislation) that affirm that citizens who have animals are "guardians" not owners, as children have guardians, who can sue on their behalf! These are of course subject to constitutional challenge, on the grounds that animals are property. Rhode Island's law, in fact, simply says that henceforth "guardian" shall be a synonym for "owners"; otherwise nothing substantive is changed! Even more conceptually damaging to exporting the concept of "ward" to animals is that, according to legal tradition, a guardian must always act in the "best interests" of the ward. When it comes to animals, we don't know how to answer questions regarding an animal's "best interests." For example, is it in the best interests of a horse to be ridden? To be jumped? To be used in dressage? To be shown? Is it in the interest of a Labrador to jump into icy water to retrieve a duck? The case can be argued both ways but the key point is we have no decision procedures for answering these sorts of questions!

In the short run, the best hope for augmented legal protection for animals and their welfare is indeed the legal system, but probably in terms of restricting how they may be used as property! The U.S. laboratory animal laws of 1985 blaze the trail in this area, making plain that though animals may be property, people cannot use them as they see fit even in putatively socially important areas like health research. Restrictions on how one may use one's own property are well established in law regarding motor vehicles, guns, and art works. (In the latter area, laws prevent owners of major art works from having them burned on their funeral pyre.) The net effect of such laws restricting animal use is to provide animals with what amount to rights, as when the research laws guarantee the animals' right to proper anesthesia and analgesia if they are used in research. If social concern for animals continues to proliferate in all areas of animal use, we will correlatively see increasing protections for animals encoded in the legal system. Again, veterinarians should lead in crafting such protections.

Pain in Veterinary (and Human) Scientific Medicine

A layperson naively approaching human and veterinary medicine would probably expect that the control of pain and suffering—the aspect of disease most feared by humans, at least—would be the central thrust of scientific medicine. Surprisingly, as a function of the scientific ideology that has been as agnostic about subjective mental states and feelings as it has been about value judgments, this is far from the case. It is a sad truth that pain management is, in fact, one of the most neglected areas in all scientific medicine, human or veterinary.

The dismissal of pain as an issue of concern in veterinary medicine has historical roots antedating the development of scientific ideology in the twentieth century. Though people with ordinary common sense—or folk psychology, as it is sometimes called—never denied the existence of pain and suffering in animals, they never worried much about it either. The ethics and pragmatics of husbandry assured that by and large animal life was congenial to animal nature in order to assure productivity. Much as with ranchers today, agriculturalists were aware that management procedures such as castration, branding, dehorning, and so on caused pain, but they were considered necessary, and animals seemed to recover from them with no lasting harm. In any case, there were no modalities for controlling pain in humans or in animals. Anesthesia was not discovered until the mid–nineteenth century, and farmers did not embrace it; for that matter, neither did physicians. In addition to adding expense, anesthesia added risk to procedures; it is, after all, selective poisoning. If one could achieve the desired result without it, why add complications? In an age of child labor, slavery, devastating epidemics, and so on, social sensitivity to suffering was not particularly high. In veterinary medicine the sense of responsibility for controlling pain reflected that of society in general, as a quotation from a 1906 surgery textbook attests:

> In veterinary surgery, anesthesia has no history. It is used in a kind of desultory fashion that reflects no great credit to the present generation of veterinarians. . . . Many veterinarians of rather wide experience have never in a whole lifetime administered a general anesthetic in performing their operations. It reflects greatly to the credit of the canine specialist, however, that he alone has adopted anesthesia to any considerable extent. . . . Anesthesia in veterinary surgery today is a means of restraint and not an expedient to relieve pain. So long as an operation can be performed by forcible restraint . . . the thought of anesthesia does not enter into the proposition. (Merillat, 1906)

These traditional reasons for ignoring pain in veterinary medicine were potentiated by two components of the scientific ideology discussed earlier. The first is the claim that animal consciousness—what an animal thinks and experiences—is outside the purview of scientific inquiry. At the turn of the century the assumption was radically different. Darwinian theory dictated that if morphological and physiological traits were phylogenetically continuous, so too were mental ones, a position that fit beautifully with the ordinary commonsense attribution of thought and feeling to animals.

But by the late 1920s few scientists were prepared to talk scientifically of mental states in animals. Positivism in tandem with a new movement in psychology called behaviorism, launched in 1913 by J. B. Watson, banished consciousness from the scientific arena. In its pure form behaviorism denied the knowability and reality of consciousness in human beings or in animals. We do not really have thoughts, we only think we do, said the behaviorists in essence. And so psychology became the study of behavior, specifically of learning, not of mentation. The scientific acknowledgment of mental states in animals was dealt a deathblow. By the 1940s virtually all psychologists in the United States were behaviorists.

So strong was the positivist flame that it consumed talk of consciousness in animals even in Europe, where Lorenz and Tinbergen were opposing behaviorism with the fledgling science of ethology, on the grounds that behaviorism ignored genetic and evolutionary determinants of behavior. Nonetheless, ethologists too denied the legitimacy of talking about consciousness in animals, the one point in which they stressed their agreement with behaviorists. Lorenz spoke of appetite-behavior in animals, not of appetite, to stress the need for eschewing mentalism; behavioral psychologists spoke of aversive behavior and negative reinforcers, not of felt pain; biologists were carried along by the same current.

The denial of the legitimacy of discussing consciousness—in humans or in animals—worked synergistically with the idea that science was value-free. Had scientists been willing to confront the moral questions occasioned by the invasive use of animals, the notion that animals feel pain and suffer might have been unavoidable. But because science declared itself value-free, these questions did not emerge as moral concerns. In fact, these two components of scientific ideology, the denial of values in science and the methodological elimination of talk about consciousness, naturally reinforced each other and were in turn buttressed by other factors. In particular, the denial of the existence of thought and feeling in animals helped allay reservations that scientists might have had about hurting animals in the pursuit of scientific goals. Interestingly enough, the same thing occurred in the seventeenth century when Descartes declared that animals were machines with no souls, minds, or feelings, thereby reconciling in one masterstroke the Catholic theological demands that animals not have souls with his belief that biology was part of physics. This idea also met the demands of a growing science of physiology that, in its quest for knowledge, was forced to perform procedures on animals that common sense could only call painful. No need to control the pain, said Cartesian physiologists, because it is not really experienced pain, merely mechanical response. And so too, in the twentieth century, the study of animal pain became the study of mechanical responses, not of felt hurt. Similarly, "stress" became a catchall for what ordinary common sense would call suffering and misery in a variety of forms; and stress was described purely mechanistically, in terms of activation of the hypophysis (pituitary)-adrenal axis and its effects. Any notion of experienced suffering was suppressed as scientifically illegitimate (Rollin, 1998).

The upshot of all this was that veterinary medicine did not consider pain control an issue. In the 1960s, for example, students were taught to perform horse castrations using curariform—or paralytic—drugs such as succinylcholine chloride, with no thought about what the animal was experiencing. I learned this very dramatically when I was lecturing on pain to veterinary students in the mid-1960s. My co-teacher, a prominent surgeon, leaped from his seat. "Oh my God," he shouted. "It just dawned on me what the animals must have felt when we did horse castrations! I never thought about it before!" He went on to explain that succinyl was in fact an advance over knocking the horse down, tying it up, and performing the surgery under physical restraint, a method that created danger of injury for both surgeon and animal. Not surprisingly, the phrase "chemical restraint" was used synonymously with "anesthesia," as the primary concern was keeping the animal still. (Older veterinarians will still use the two terms interchangeably.) In Lumb and Jones's early textbook of anesthesia (1973), a variety of reasons are given for a veterinarian's having knowledge of anesthesia, but the control of felt pain is not mentioned!

Given this view of anesthesia, it is not surprising that analgesia for animals was virtually nonexistent. The late Dr. Harry Gorman, a brilliant and forward-looking man, who in 1978 began the teaching of veterinary ethics with me at Colorado State University, was an experimental surgeon of great renown. When he arrived at CSU in the mid-1960s, he went to the veterinary hospital pharmacy to get a supply of narcotics to provide analgesia for his experimental animals, something he had done throughout his career. Much to his surprise, he was told that the hospital did not stock these controlled drugs and, if he was concerned about pain in his animals, to "give them an aspirin."

In both the veterinary and scientific communities, ideological blinders made felt pain invisible. The role of ideology is evidenced by early efforts of the scientific community to address animal pain in the face of the increasing social concern about animals that led to the passage of the 1985 federal laws. In 1982 the research community held a conference on animal pain the proceedings of which were published as *Animal Pain: Perception and Alleviation* (Kitchell and Erickson, 1983). Despite the motivation behind the conference, clearly stated in the title, the overwhelming majority of papers were highly reductionistic, examining the chemistry and "plumbing" of pain and, with only a few exceptions, never mentioning pain as a negative subjective experience. In exactly the same vein, other forms of animal misery—fear, boredom, anxiety, distress; discomfort resulting from heat, cold, or crowding; the isolation of a social animal—were traditionally equated with the objective physiological stress response of the pituitary-adrenal axis. The widespread use of ketamine for ovariohysterectomies and other visceral procedures, especially in research—despite ketamine's total failure as a visceral analgesic—again bespeaks this conceptual conflation. And no one, to my knowledge, has yet formally addressed the residual flashbacks and "bad trips" ketamine can create in some animals.

The responses of many veterinarians trained before the late 1980s to concerns about animal pain and analgesia are telling. Such practitioners will sometimes argue that what an uninformed observer considers signs of pain is merely "reaction to anesthesia." Or they may claim that ruminants do not really suffer postsurgical pain because they eat immediately after surgery, although they surely know that animals that behave abnormally while in pain will be too easy targets for predators. Or they will argue that an animal that acts normally after a putatively painful procedure can't possibly be in pain, forgetting that the animal's behavior may well be skewed by the presence of humans. Or they will say that an injection of anesthetic hurts more than a biopsy, and so on. Dr. Bernie Hansen of the North Carolina State veterinary school has done much to dispel such ideologically inspired and dogmatically held myths in veterinary medicine, for example, by videotaping postsurgical dogs without humans present. Some laboratory animal veterinarians have argued that a postsurgical rodent behaves no differently from a normal rodent—both animals just lie around in the cage! As Dr. David Morton once snapped to a veterinarian who made this point: "Then take the two animals out of the cage; you'll quickly see a difference."

In the early 1980s I served on a panel with a group of laboratory animal veterinarians at an AALAS (American Association for Laboratory Animal Science) meeting. In the course of the discussion I asked them to tell me the analgesic of choice if one were using a rat for a crush experiment. None could respond; some even invoked scientific ideology and said, "We don't even know that the rat feels pain." I will return to this case shortly.

The role of positivistic ideology is equally pronounced, at times, in the human medical community's attitude toward pain in humans. To physicians trained to view medicine as applied biology, and thus to value that which is replicable, objective, and verifiable, pain experiences are likely seen as medically irrelevant, because they are "subjective." One cannot measure a person's subjective experiences; one cannot even be sure they are there—thus it is easy for scientific medicine (in a narrow positivistic sense) to discount their importance or even their "reality." This problem is further potentiated by scientific medicine's well-known tendency to treat the disease—"the kidney in room 306"—rather than the person, which in turn leads to a tendency to see patients, especially patients with cancer and other life-threatening diseases, in a bimodal way—as either "cured" or "lost." Palliation, especially of subjective symptoms like pain, suffering, and fear, is often invisible to highly scientifically oriented physicians. Like a patient's income, subjective experiences like pain are not the concern of the reductionistic physician. As one nursing dean said to me about the difference between medicine and nursing: "They worry about *cure*, we worry about *care*." Indeed, hospices are essentially not physician dominated; and it was and is, of course, physicians, not nurses, who prescribe medication to modulate pain and suffering. A 1991 article argued that although pain can be controlled effectively in 90 percent of cancer patients, it is in fact not controlled in 80 percent of such patients (Ferrell and Rhiner, 1991).

The traditional practice when performing open heart and other major surgery on neonatal humans was to use curariform drugs. When this practice was challenged in the 1980s, neonatal surgeons often responded in a manner based in ideology. Infants, they said, did not feel pain; their central nervous system was insufficiently myelinated. Or they claimed infants didn't remember pain (despite testimony from nurses that babies who did experience surgical procedures would grow extremely agitated if brought back to a surgery suite). Or they argued that anesthesia is dangerous, forgetting that it is equally dangerous to ill and frail adults. Indeed, one former student of mine working on these issues sent an old paper I had published about the denial of felt pain in animals to a prominent neonatologist. "Take Rollin's paper, substitute the word 'infant' for 'animal,' and you have an accurate picture of neonatology today," he replied. Even as we entered the twenty-first century, the official definition of pain accepted by the International Society for the Study of Pain affirmed that one can only be sure of pain in a fully linguistic being, thus relegating animal, infant, and neonatal pain to scientific limbo (Rollin, 1999).

For many years physicians often withheld analgesia from postsurgical and other patients in pain. Many orthopedic specialists, some of them ex-athletes, would scold patients who asked for analgesia, declaring that "pain builds character." A paper in the *New England Journal of Medicine* demonstrated that infants and children (who are powerless) receive less analgesia for the same procedures than do adults undergoing those procedures (Walco et al., 1994). And though ketamine is typically no longer used on adults because of the "bad trips" and "flashbacks" it can cause, it is still (or until very recently was) employed on "the very young and the very old" because, as one anesthesiologist told me, "they can't sue."

Further evidence of the same mind-set about pain can be found in the medical community's steadfast opposition to the use of marijuana and narcotics for terminally ill patients on the grounds that such people might become addicted.

The emergence of the new ethic for animals——as well as the coincidental emergence of social-ethical concern for disenfranchised humans, such as infants and children——made the ideological denial of felt pain in veterinary and human medicine less tenable. (Indeed, such denial has probably catalyzed the growth of alternative medicine in society.) In writing the current laws for laboratory animals, one of our CSU group's primary objectives was to force the scientific community to "reappropriate common sense" and deal with felt pain in animals. We believed that science was on a collision course with society if it continued to remain agnostic about felt pain in animals and failed to manage it. Thus we essentially declared in the law that animals feel pain, and that such pain needs to be controlled.

The result of the passage of the law was gratifying. Science and veterinary medicine began to concern themselves with animal pain and its control. Articles on animal pain and its detection, control, and alleviation proliferated. The AVMA Panel on Pain and Distress in Animals, which was chartered by Congress to help scientists respond to the law and on which I was privileged to serve, pointed out that if we can conduct pain research on animals, it is reasonable to assume that they feel pain (Panel Report, 1987). One prominent anesthesiologist told me of being invited to address groups of hitherto agnostic medical researchers on the detection of pain in animals. Although he was reluctant to belabor what to him was obvious, he dutifully recorded such signs of pain as tenderness at the point of injury, or the guarding of a limb, and embarrassedly read the paper. It turned out to be the most requested paper he ever wrote!

After the law went into effect, I phoned one of the laboratory animal veterinarians who had sat on the aforementioned AALAS panel with me, where I had challenged the panel to provide an analgesic regimen for a rat. "Now," I said, "you must control that rat's pain. What would you use?" He surprised me by rattling off three or four analgesic regimens. "When I asked you this question on the panel," I said, "you were agnostic about animal pain. How did you find these regimens?"

"Oh, that's easy," he replied. "We simply went to the drug companies. All analgesics for humans are tested on rats!"

Although he knew that at the time we were on the panel, he did not see it as relevant to rat pain until the law forced a change in gestalt!

Perhaps the most profound comment on the effects of this new law on veterinary medicine came from the late Hiram Kitchen, chairman of the AVMA Pain Panel. Kitchen pointed out that because federal law now mandates the control of pain and distress in laboratory animals, controlling pain has ipso facto become the standard of practice for all veterinarians. This further means that veterinarians must rethink even such routine and time-honored procedures as castration and dehorning in the beef industry. Though his claim stirred vigorous debate among the panel, in the end it was incorporated into the report, with even representatives of food animal practice recognizing the validity of the point and the inevitability of change.

The laws have certainly been a goad to stimulating veterinary concern about felt pain and analgesia. The impact on researchers reverberates through their students and into practice. And veterinary researchers have themselves been sensitized to be aware of pain and its control. For example, a committee of veterinary faculty at CSU has issued a report for researchers on the control of long-term (as opposed to short-term) acute pain (for example, orthopedic pain).

The laws, however, are only the tip of the iceberg. They do not themselves reflect the ethical changes this society has experienced—people do genuinely care now about animal pain and suffering. Clients, for example, are increasingly asking for postsurgical analgesia for their animals, speaking from empathetic identification with their pets. And as one veterinary leader told me, pain control is the one thing people will gladly pay for! Drug companies understand this and are actively promoting animal pain control in seminars, publications, and even in advertisements directed toward the general public. In one case the company that produces carprofen (used for arthritis in older dogs) cannot keep up with the demand.

Furthermore, it is now known in both human and veterinary medicine that pain is more than just a "ghost in the machine"; it is in fact biologically active. Pain is a significant stressor, leading to all the pernicious consequences of stress, such as immunosuppression, slowing of the healing process, acceleration of disease, and so on (Thurman et al., 1996). It has been demonstrated that failure to control pain contributes to neoplastic metastases, for example (Page et al., 1993). Conversely, the mitigation of pain accelerates healing and surgical recovery. And recent research has demonstrated that when infants undergoing open heart surgery are deeply anesthetized with high doses of sufentanil and also given high doses of opiates for twenty-four hours postoperatively, they have a significantly better recovery and significantly fewer postoperative deaths than a group receiving a lighter anesthesic regimen (halothane and morphine) followed postoperatively by intermittent morphine and diazepam for analgesia. The group that received deep anesthesia and profound analgesia "had a decreased incidence of sepsis, metabolic acidosis, and disseminated intravascular coagulation and fewer postoperative deaths (none of the thirty given sufentanil vs. four of fifteen given halothane plus morphine)" (Anand and Hickey, 1992).

We are thus in the midst of another scientific revolution, wherein the reductionistic, positivistic, mechanistic medicine, human and animal, tied to an ideology that denies the relevance of subjective experience and affirms that science is "value-free" and "ethics-free" is being replaced by a more comprehensive and socially acceptable medicine. Though such a medicine (and such a science) is far more difficult to conceptualize and implement, it is socially and morally necessary, and in the end more true to the reality it must deal with. And no issue is more fundamental to such a medicine, human or animal, than the management of pain and suffering. Surely nothing is more satisfying to a healer than to be able to free a patient from the clutches of pain and its attendant fear and distress.

Animal Distress and Animal Happiness

The "reappropriation of common sense" with regard to animal pain has been of direct and singular importance to animal welfare and has been of inestimable value not only to laboratory animals, but also to companion animals and, at least in Europe, to farm animals. We can expect that both recognition of pain and modalities for its amelioration will continue to grow exponentially.

There have also been less direct salubrious consequences of breaching the ideological barrier historically blocking scientific and veterinary concern with animal consciousness. In the 1985 laboratory animal laws described earlier, provisions were made for environments that "enhance the psychological well-being of primates." This, of course, represented a major blow to ideological agnosticism about animal consciousness. In fact, a very amusing anecdote illustrates this point beautifully.

I heard this story from Dr. Robert Rissler, the veterinarian charged with overseeing the guidelines interpreting the 1985 laboratory animal laws. Dr. Rissler recounted being extremely perplexed about how to deal with "primate psychological well-being," since he was a veterinarian who had never dealt with primates or animal minds. In desperation, he approached the primatology division of the American Psychological Association to ask for help in clarifying the concept. "Don't worry," he was told. "There is no such thing." He responded with great sagacity: "Well, there will be after January 1, 1987 [the date the laws go into effect], whether you help me or not." And lo and behold, the research community has stepped up to the plate on psychological well-being when forced to do so, even as they did with pain!

Recall that the laws mandate control of pain *and* distress in laboratory animals. From about 1985 to 2000, the USDA wisely focused exclusively on pain, presumably realizing that overcoming ideological barriers on physical pain was a big enough challenge, without adding something as putatively amorphous as "distress." But as soon as pain control was well established with thousands of papers in the scientific literature, USDA announced in 2000 that they would soon be focusing on distress.

In 2004, the Humane Society of the United States (HSUS) sponsored a conference on distress, inviting key regulators, scientists, veterinarians and others. I was asked to give the keynote address. I found myself surrounded by extremely bright people many of whom were nonetheless extremely skeptical of being able to define distress. In my speech, I pointed out that almost exactly twenty-five years earlier, I had given a speech for HSUS arguing for the scientific legitimacy of talking about physical pain to a similar audience. So unsettling was the idea to the scientists present that one high ranking NIH official actually phoned the CSU veterinary school Dean and affirmed that I was "a viper in the bosom of biomedicine, to whom veterinary students should not be exposed!" (To his credit, he recanted five years later, and became a close ally.)

Earlier, I explained that we perceive not only with our eyes, and ears, but also with our theories, beliefs, and expectations. In 1979, the idea of animal pain was precluded by a comparable group of people for ideological reasons. Today animal pain was fully accepted and well researched, with few if any people skeptical about its reality and knowability. I pointed out that current doubts about the knowability of distress followed exactly the same logic. Twenty-five years hence, I affirmed, we would gather together again to discuss the latest advances in research on distress, and have totally forgotten that we ever expressed doubts about its knowability.

The identification of other modes of animal misery follows precisely the same logic inherent in the revolution about pain. Suddenly, the blinders are off, and we can realize that boredom, fear, loneliness, and all other noxious states in animals are part of ordinary common sense's way of looking at the world, and that both ordinary common sense and Darwinian biology militate in favor of such mental states being phylogenetically continuous. This is not to say that ordinary common sense is always right about what it attributes to animal mentation; it does suffer from exaggerated anthropomorphism and gullibility in imputing such states to other creatures. But the *conceptual* impediments to such imputation have indeed been removed, and this has opened the door to the sort of splendid and careful scientific study of noxious mental experiences in animals pioneered by Marian Dawkins and Ian Duncan.

An editorial in *Nature* affirmed, in essence, that the scientific community now *must* study animal consciousness, in a world where social moral concern for animals is indelibly established:

> Whether or not animals have "rights," we should learn more about their capacity for suffering. In Germany, the right of freedom to research is enshrined in the nation's constitution. But that may soon have to be balanced against a new constitutional right of animals to

> be treated as fellow creatures, and sheltered from avoidable pain. Not surprisingly, biomedical researchers fear that their work will be mired in legal challenges.
>
> The latest moves in Germany are the product of political circumstances. . . . But attempts to give animal rights a legal foundation are quietly gathering momentum worldwide. Three years ago, New Zealand's parliament considered and ultimately rejected a plan to extend basic human rights to the great apes. And at a growing number of law schools in the United States, courses in animal law are popular. . . .
>
> Some commentators have already countered that "rights" are only created by beings capable of asserting themselves, therefore very young children, and animals, are properly accorded protection, not rights. . . .
>
> Nevertheless, most experts would agree that we have barely started to understand animal cognition. Even our knowledge of animal welfare is still rudimentary. We can measure levels of hormones that correlate with stress in people. But is a rat with high levels of corticosteroids suffering? We just don't know.
>
> Given the passions raised by animal experimentation, and the importance of biomedical research to human health, the science of animal suffering and cognition should be given a higher priority. We owe it to ourselves, as much as to our fellow creatures, not simply to leave the lawyers to battle it out. (Rights, wrongs, and ignorance, 2002)

For those who continue to doubt the studiability of distress or suffering or misery in all of its forms in animals, consider the following thought experiment: If the government were to come up with a billion dollars in research funding for animal distress, would that money go a-begging? We can study these states just as we studied pain: An excellent work on boredom by Franciose Wemelsfelder in a volume on laboratory animal welfare I coedited made the methodology for such study quite explicit (Wemelsfelder, 1989). And when the ideological scales fall from our eyes, we realize that the works of scientists like John Mason and Seymour Levine, and even the odious work of Harry Harlow on maternal deprivation in infant monkeys do provide clear ingression into animal unhappiness. Even more promising, it has recently became legitimate to talk of animal happiness, a notion we shall discuss shortly, and which I have in fact argued is clearer than that of human happiness!

What does all of this have to do with veterinary medicine, aside from its clear relevance to the laboratory animal veterinarians who must assure the control of distress in laboratory animals? A great deal! One can argue, as Dr. Franklin McMillan has done in a brilliant series of articles and books, that veterinary medicine, in historically ignoring animal consciousness in general and negative mental states, such as fear, loneliness, anxiety, boredom, apprehension, has ignored a host of considerations directly relevant to physical health of animals, as well as to mental health.

Indeed, in the early 1980s, Ian Duncan, Marian Dawkins, and I all argued that the concept of animal welfare traditionally defined in the agriculture community in terms of productivity (a human-oriented economic notion!) in fact needed to be primarily defined in terms of what the animal experiences and how it feels. An animal that suffers, be it pain or fear or boredom, cannot be said to be enjoying good welfare.

As society becomes more and more concerned with animal treatment and well-being, it becomes increasingly necessary to talk in terms of the animals' subjective experiences. Thus animal experience becomes a major focus for veterinarians working to improve welfare of animals in our charge, be they horses or zoo animals or farm animals. Similarly, handling animals, as Temple Grandin has shown, must be rooted in knowledge of how animals experience the world.

Consider farm animals. Arguably, there is more suffering among farm animals than anywhere else in animal use, if only because we produce such vast numbers of them. And there is increasing demand that systems such as sow stalls be changed. Elsewhere in the world, veterinarians have led in such reform. Similarly with zoos as prisons, the state of the art in my youth.

While giving a captive lion an acre instead of a cage is certainly an improvement, mere increase in space is not enough. We must take cognizance of the animal's biological *and* psychological needs and natures, what I have called their *telos*: the pigness of the pig, the cowness of the cow, the lionness of the lion. For example, the burying of food treats in litter for monkeys, allowing them to root and pick as they might in nature, is an ingenious improvement in these animals' well-being.

Hal Markowitz has been a pioneer in enriching environments for zoo animals. In one famous case, he was asked by the Portland (Oregon) Zoo, which had just built a new enclosure for cervals (South African bobcats) that looked just like the Kalahari, their native range, why the animals were depressed and languishing. After much study, Markowitz concluded that though to us the enclosure looked natural, to the animals their basic needs were unmet. In particular, in nature, these animals spend much time predating low-flying birds. Markowitz advised the zoo to give the animals their food in the form of meatballs shot across their enclosure randomly by an air cannon. This instantly alleviated their depression (Markowitz, 1989).

It is important in reforming confinement agriculture that what matters to the animals be considered, not just or primarily what looks good to us. For example, just mindlessly throwing sows outdoors regardless of terrain, forage, or climate would not necessarily create positive welfare. If veterinarians are to lead in such reform as society expects them to, they must understand the animal mind. And this is true wherever we keep animals.

We are leading up to the point that proper treatment of animals is not simply a matter of controlling physical pain or even of mitigating "distress." Ideally, we need to think in terms of creating a positive subjective life for animals, in short, a state of animal *happiness*, or if one prefers, positive welfare.

Historically, as mentioned, an animal was considered well-off if it was productive, and that in turn meant, in essence, fed and watered—a very physicalistic view of welfare. A moment's reflection on the concepts of welfare and happiness reveals that these judgments are bound up with value judgments in general, and ethical judgments in particular. The concepts of welfare, like the concepts of health and happiness, admit of gradations.

Thus the ethical question that arises is this: Given a spectrum of animal feeling running from abject misery to total euphoria, at what point have we fulfilled our moral obligation to the animal? Suppose we are talking about a horse, whose interests include running, or a pig, whose interests include foraging. It has been demonstrated that under extensive conditions, sows would cover about a mile a day foraging (Wood-Gush and Stolba, 1981). Clearly a horse would be better off (subjectively) given a vast pasture to gallop in, as opposed to a relatively small corral, in which he can nonetheless run in circles. Are we fulfilling our obligations with the corral? If pigs prefer woodland loam, do we fulfill our obligations by letting them forage in desert terrain? We can certainly identify the ideal and the unacceptable extremes, but deciding where an acceptable mean is requires a moral judgment based on balancing expense, terrain availability, management considerations, and so on.

A similar point holds of health, which is clearly part of welfare. If we take seriously the World Health Organization definition of health (for humans) as "a complete state of mental, physical, and social well-being," very few if any of us are fully healthy. Furthermore, social policy must decide what degree of health society *ought* to guarantee to its members. This is a fortiori true of animal health, where the social use of the animals, and society's view of their value, determine what counts as health and acceptable degrees of pain and suffering allowed to go untreated in animals.

As I have shown elsewhere, what counts as worthy of being treated in animals is not only what science deems it to be, but what society considers significant. When the role and value of animals in society is overwhelmingly economic, symptoms, syndromes, discomfort or abnormality that have no apparent relevance to animal productivity, marketability, or other human uses do not become of concern medically. Conditions not cost-effective to treat lead to euthanasia. Hence the ignoring of animal pain by science and veterinary medicine during most of the twentieth century we have discussed. The only time animal pain was implicitly recognized in science was when it served human ends, as when pain was induced in animals to test analgesics in humans. No one ever thought to worry about animal pain per se and its control, and it was common to deny its reality. As mentioned, anesthesia was called "chemical restraint." Food animal veterinarians typically didn't (and still don't) worry about the pain associated with cattle castration, dehorning, branding or other procedures; such worry was not perceived as economically viable.

In an agricultural context, and in the society in general to whom agriculturalists are accountable, the role and value of animals was traditionally defined in terms of their productivity and the prices for their products. In this valuational context, animals' welfare (and its study) is restricted to what has an effect on production and price. This is graphically illustrated in a letter I once saw from a government agricultural official supporting the principle of establishing a chair in animal welfare at a university. The official wrote that he viewed the job of the chairholder to be "the development of definitive criteria in assessing the amount of stress that animals are undergoing and the compatibility of the stress with the animal's productive life."

Thus, the traditional view of animal welfare was purely physicalistic, and animal happiness was not discussed. If pressed, proponents of that view would probably say that an animal that is productive is happy, equating happiness with welfare. A more sophisticated view places the focus of welfare in animal consciousness, and would presumably equate happiness with positive mental states in animals, and absence of negative ones. A yet more sophisticated view acknowledges the presence of value judgments, particularly ethical judgments in animal welfare, and admits that such judgments are necessary even if one is talking about welfare in terms of animal experience.

It is this third view of welfare I wish to defend, and from which I hope to deduce an explication of animal happiness. Clearly the meaning of welfare changes with development of social ethics for animals. In today's world, where the companion animal is the paradigm for all animals, the old production view of welfare is as socially unacceptable as the rejection of animal feelings. Thus welfare today must be cast in terms of consciousness, and animals experiencing pain, suffering, distress, loneliness, boredom grows increasingly morally unacceptable.

I have stressed the nature of the emerging social ethic for animals. In my view, as buttressed by our Western cultural history over the last three decades, society has moved well beyond the traditional concern for deliberate, sadistic, intentional, willful cruelty to animals to concern about all animal suffering whether it be the result of cruelty or decent, legitimate motives such as providing cheap and plentiful food or curing disease (which most people see as accounting for 99 percent of animal suffering). Society demands that animals' needs and natures be protected even as we use animals. The basic interests protected are thus derived from a reasonable view of animal nature or, to use Aristotles' phrase, *telos*, that generates interests for the animal as important to it as speech, religion, and holding on to one's property are to us. Since modern uses of animals such as factory farming or research often fail to respect such basic animal interests, society is increasingly demanding that the legal system protect animal *telos*. The Swedish law of 1980, demanding environments for food animals that suit their natures, is a paradigm case of the legalization of animal rights based on *telos*.

The concept of animal welfare, therefore, in today's moral world, rests on legally protecting animal *telos* from the negative experiences occasioned by its violation. Correlatively, animal happiness, at least as an ideal, is presumed to be allowing the animal to actualize the interests dictated by its *telos*, where thwarting of those interests causes some form of suffering. The *degree* to which those who use animals in various ways must respect *telos* is still evolving, hence the move we mentioned from zoos as prisons fifty years ago to animal quarters that at least attempt to respect animal interests.

One more important point must be noted. Virtually no one denies that animal mentation is far less sophisticated than human—indeed, various versions of the Cartesian claim that animals are machines are still flourishing today. But the consensus seems to have emerged that animals do experience morally relevant states of awareness such as pain, pleasure, fear, boredom, loneliness, anxiety, and so on. (Ordinary common sense never denied this, and science seems to be "reappropriating common sense," as I have elsewhere characterized the situation.) In the area we are discussing, animal happiness, the relative simplicity of animal awareness seems to lead to the startling conclusion that we can be more certain of animal happiness than we can of human happiness, despite the presence of language in humans. If we observe animals in ideal conditions allowing them to fully actualize their *telos*, it is hard to deny that these animals are happy—well-fed dogs frolicking in the park; groups of horses let out into lush green pastures kicking up their heels. This is even recognized in ordinary language by the phrase "Happy as a pig in shit."

With humans, on the other hand, in part *because* of the enormous complexity of human consciousness, it is more difficult to affirm with certitude that an individual is happy. Recall the poem "Richard Corey" by Edwin Arlington Robinson (1921) where, despite all outward appearances of happiness, the protagonist goes home and commits suicide:

> Whenever Richard Cory went down town
> We people on the pavement looked at him:
> He was a gentleman from sole to crown,
> Clean favored, and imperially slim.
>
> And he was always quietly arrayed,
> And he was always human when he talked;
> But still he fluttered pulses when he said,
> "Good-morning," and he glittered when he walked.
>
> And he was rich—yes, richer than a king,
> And admirably schooled in every grace:
> In fine, we thought that he was everything
> To make us wish that we were in his place.
>
> So on we worked, and waited for the light,
> And went without the meat, and cursed the bread;
> And Richard Cory, one calm summer night,
> Went home and put a bullet through his head.

Human consciousness allows for an infinite series of reflexivity creating unhappiness. I may have everything I need or desire and yet be unhappy because I don't think I deserve it, or worry about what might change or have some sort of survivor's guilt. Woody Allen and *Seinfeld* have made fortunes capitalizing on this sort of neurosis. It seems clear that animals do not fret at the meta-levels we do. We may be morally certain that the horse gamboling on lush pastures is not feeling guilty that he is doing well while other horses are starving somewhere across the world.

Historically, veterinarians were faced with the problem of clients not wishing to spend a significant amount of money on an animal, electing euthanasia for treatable disease or reparable fracture. The veterinarian was thrust into an advocacy role, convincing the client not to trash a salvageable life, even drastically cutting fees to save the animal.

In today's world, the opposite problem presents itself—clients willing to spend any amount of money to save the companion animal, without regard to the animal's suffering, for essentially emotionally selfish reasons. Thus, ironically, veterinarians remain advocates for animals, only now on behalf of timely euthanasia, the great gift veterinary medicine has for ending suffering. Although traditional wisdom says that a veterinarian should never answer the question as to when it is time for euthanasia or respond to the query, "What would you do if it were your animal, Doc?" on the grounds that "people will later blame you for killing their animal," I strongly disagree. The responsibility for helping with such decisions is part of one's Aesculapian authority. Oftentimes, a client is too blinded by selfish need for keeping the animal alive to notice that the animal is suffering, and needs a reality check from a medical professional. Sometimes guilt at ordering a death needs to be checked by a gentle, "It is time."

I was once speaking at a veterinary conference on this issue when a veterinarian leapt up. "I knew you were just another patriarchal, chauvinistic, dominionistic pig," she shouted. "That may be," I replied, "but what does that have to do with what we are discussing"? "Only a dominionistic pig would deign to decide for another life form when it should die," she retorted. "Regardless of suffering?" I said. "Absolutely!" she said. "I have a client that has an eighteen-year-old cat with a spinal tumor who brings it in every day for hydration and IV feeding, since it has stopped eating or drinking." "That's crazy!" I said. "Not at all!" she replied. "She is just very bonded." "Let me get this straight," I said. "If the client asked you to stabilize the animal so she could take it to Lourdes for the holy water cure, no matter how much suffering was involved, you would do it?" I queried. "Absolutely," she replied. My response, I'm afraid, confirmed her opinion of me: "Then you have no business being a veterinarian." I fear too that "Pawspice"—hospice for dying animals—could turn into a cash cow for unscrupulous practitioners taking advantage of neurotic clients.

With the huge medical armamentarian at the disposal of veterinarians, how does one assure that the client does not go too far at the expense of great suffering? According to my colleague, Dr. Steve Withrow, pioneer in modern animal oncology, the key lies in establishing a proper rapport with the client from the beginning, and engaging in open and candid communication. It also behooves all practitioners to start thinking about criteria for judging quality of life. In addition to obvious ones such as eating, drinking, movement, the practitioner should elicit others from the client unique to that animal; for example, "Fluffy never fails to play tug of war even when she doesn't feel well." Invoking the clients' own criteria when treatment begins to fail and the animal deteriorates can work wonders against denial and force clients to face unpleasant reality. I once did such an exercise with a colleague and he phoned me six months later to let me know that it had helped him realize when it was time to let go. "Thanks," he said. "By setting up my own criteria for quality of life, I was able to recognize its absence."

Animal Quality of Life

All of this leads us to a new area of ethical concern in veterinary medicine—animal quality of life, of particular importance to companion animal practice.

We live in an era dominated by quantitative assessment. University promotions are based upon number of publications, which can be objectively counted, not quality, a fact that drives the production of mediocre work. Teachers are judged by student credit hours produced, not by quality of teaching. Agriculture has become assimilated to business, with values such as husbandry, way of life, and sustainability completely subordinated to efficiency and productivity. And, in human medicine, physician success is often judged by how much more life has been garnered by treatment, regardless of the subjective cost to the patient. Care is subordinated to cure, and modes of awareness crucial to the patient, such as pain and suffering, are too often treated as epiphenomena, as we discussed earlier.

As pets have increasingly become "members of the family," new treatment modalities developed in human medicine have been transferred to veterinary medicine. Animal oncology, dialysis, and transplantation provide salient examples of such transfer. Though insurance for animals has not kept pace with veterinary medical progress, many clients are financially willing and able to assume the burden of new, sophisticated, and extended treatment. Unfortunately, medical agnosticism, ignorance, and lack of care about quality of life in patients have also been exported to veterinary medicine. It is exigent that veterinarians address these issues while learning from the mistakes of human medicine: It is patent that fear of pain, suffering, loss of dignity, and distress have driven terminally ill human patients to demand the right to die. And it is clear that people fear pain and degradation and helplessness far more than they fear death.

If human medicine pays little attention to human suffering, veterinary medicine is even more culpable regarding its patients, though such neglect is somewhat mitigated by the presence of euthanasia as a treatment modality for ending pain. Since animals lack language, we know relatively little of animal mentation; it is only recently that veterinary medicine has even acknowledged felt pain in animals, or studied its control. From what we do know of animals' minds, it seems clear that animals are incapable of conceiving, let alone valuing, increases in duration of life. Whereas humans may willingly trade considerable suffering for extensions of life (though they aren't always willing to do so!), this is not a choice for animals. While a human being may wish to see his or her children graduate from college, visit Ireland again, or finish a book and thus value extended life over suffering, an animal's life is not defined by completion of such projects; animals are much more trapped in the now. Longer life at the expense of suffering is not a value for an animal.

Thus in exporting human treatment modalities of veterinary medicine, we must be cognizant of the degree of suffering which extension of life may exact as a price. Even if we don't always ask humans if they wish to continue to fight, we can in principle ask them. This is not the case with animals! And owners may be so emotionally dependent on the animals that they wish to forge ahead with treatment regardless of the degree of suffering incurred by the animal. For this reason, it is imperative that veterinarians working in fields like oncology constantly monitor animal quality of life, and advocate for the animal in terms of not extending length of life at the expense of suffering. For this reason, serious studies of objective criteria for assessing quality of life must be developed, while at the same time not neglecting what experienced clinical judgment dictates. Widely disseminated criteria of this sort will help veterinarians confute self-centered wishful thinking on the part of owners inattentive to suffering because of an unwillingness to let go. Clinicians should involve owners early in their relationship in setting up such criteria, since the owner knows the animal best, and since they are likelier to respect criteria they have helped to develop, and must now "recollect."

The Ethics of Critical Care

The past two decades have witnessed a major proliferation of veterinary specialties. Among these specialties is critical care and emergency medicine. Though some of the ethical issues faced by critical care practitioners are amplifications of issues faced by general practitioners, the critical care veterinarian is in some ways in a special position to address these issues, as we shall see. And, as we shall also see, the core of these issues involves pain and distress.

In critical care medicine, as in veterinary medicine in general, the most problematic moral/conceptual dimension one confronts is the issue of whether veterinarians owe primary moral obligation to the animal and its interests, or to the client. It is that question which underlies virtually all of the pressing moral issues one encounters in the field. Consider, for example, the problem of how long a clinician should keep a suffering animal alive, given our ever-increasing capacity to do so, and the client's lack of cognizance of, or lack of concern with, the degree to which the animal is suffering. Many clients want the animal kept alive at all costs for selfish reasons and simply refuse to acknowledge the terrible price paid by the animal. In the same vein, in CCUs maintained in veterinary schools or other research institutions, the animal may be a research animal and the owner a zealous researcher interested primarily in milking every drop of data from that animal, again at considerable costs in pain and suffering to the animal. Another issue is the unowned animal brought to a CCU by a Good Samaritan who cares about the animal but is not willing to assume financial responsibility. Additionally, there is the issue of a reasonable owner who wishes to have the animal treated not excessively but enough to return the animal to relatively pain-free normalcy, but cannot afford the ever-burgeoning expenses of critical care. The issue of "cure" versus "care," with the latter often taking a back seat to the former in veterinary as well as human medicine, is also central. Fixing the patient is given significant precedence over patient comfort. The measure of winning the battle against disease or injury is keeping the animal alive.

How one responds to these questions will almost certainly in large part depend upon how one answers what we have called "the fundamental question of veterinary ethics": To whom does a veterinarian owe primary obligation: owner or animal? If one adopts the *pediatrician model*, one serves the animal, with the client's interests shunted to the side if they are inimical to the animal's, as when the client won't spend money on a fixable animal, or, conversely, when a client spares no expense to keeping an animal in misery alive. On the other hand, if one adopts the *garage mechanic model*, the veterinarian basically pursues the satisfaction of client interests or desires, with animal interests shunted to the side.

As we have said, the key feature of what we have called the New Social Ethic for animals and the laws following in its wake is control of pain and distress. In all of these emerging laws, little attention is paid to preserving animal life per se—the emphasis is on limiting pain and suffering. In fact, to my knowledge, nowhere do laws address the most senseless waste of animal life, the euthanasia of healthy pet animals for convenience!

The taking of animal lives for research, testing, or food is not addressed; the quality of that life is very seriously addressed.

As we discussed, the most momentous of these new laws in the United States are the 1985 laws regulating the use of animals in research. As we have already mentioned, at an AVMA conference on the legal mandate to control pain held in 1987, Hyram Kitchen pointed out that, being embodied in federal law, the mandate for control of pain in research animals sets the standard of practice which veterinarians must live up to or be (theoretically at least) legally actionable. This is directly relevant to a number of the issues we raised in critical care medicine. The first problem we raised is keeping a suffering animal alive: How long should one do this for an owner? For a researcher? How much suffering is justified by a cure? Are owner demands sacrosanct?

The issue is clear from the dictates of the social ethic with regard to a research animal in critical care: If euthanasia is the only way to control suffering, the animal should be euthanized. Intractable and prolonged suffering is not permitted under these laws. If the purpose of the experiment is realized, the animal must be terminated immediately, and no Animal Care Committee would ever permit a protocol requiring prolonged, uncontrolled pain.

The same logic, in my view, applies *mutatis mutandis* to an animal owned by a private individual. If society will not accept prolonged suffering in an animal for biomedical reasons (that is, reasons that benefit humanity in general), it will surely condemn the owner who keeps a suffering animal alive for egoistic (or egotistic) reasons, because he or she cannot bear to let go. Similarly, it would clearly be wrong to the consensus ethic to keep an animal alive heroically, and at considerable suffering cost, if the animal will never be capable of a decent (not perfect!) quality of life, for example, if the animal will be unable to move or dramatically be wracked by pain.

I have already indicated that part of the emerging consensus social ethic is a respect for—and increasing demand for legal protection of—animal natures, what I call, after Aristotle, *telos*—the "pigness" of the pig, the "dogness" of the dog (Rollin, 1992). The fact is that the U.S. laboratory animal laws mandate "exercise for dogs" and "environments for primates that enhance their psychological well-being," that the Swedish agricultural law of 1988 demands environments for animals that suit their psychological and biological needs and natures, and that U.S. zoos now try to create *functionally* naturalistic environments for their charges, rather than aesthetically naturalistic environments that look good to us—all attest to the extent to which society worries about animal nature. In that light, a dog (or any other animal) suffering constant significant pain is no longer a dog—its normal life is subordinated to the pain, even as humans tell us that extreme pain leaves little else to focus on in life. And animals in pain may well suffer more than people in pain; at least we are capable of hope and anticipation of pain's end (Rollin, 2000).

Thus I am arguing that whether the CCU client is a researcher or a pet owner, the emerging social ethic militates in the direction of the veterinarian acting as a pediatrician, not as a garage mechanic, at least as far as pain and suffering is concerned. In the case of a research animal, the clinician has explicit law on his or her side; in the case of a private owner, though the law is not explicit, it certainly sets the standard of practice on the side of stopping pain. Thus, a CCU clinician could say to a client, "We've gone far enough; keeping the animal alive at any cost involves too much suffering; going any further would not be allowed in research and, in addition, in my view violates my understanding of the Veterinariarian's Oath"—and they would have the moral force of federal law and society behind them.

Technically, though, the animal is still property, and a client could be intransigent. In this case, there are three options for the clinician:

1. *Capitulate*. You have done what you can.
2. *Persuade*. Utilize your Aesculapian authority (which is considerable and which we shall shortly discuss) to move the client to a different place, for example, by explaining the suffering, making the client watch, visit, and so on.
3. *Extract a commitment allowing you to keep the animal comfortable*. Even if you truly believe that the animal should be euthanized, it is almost as reasonable to gain client support for keeping the animal unaware. In the first place, you forestall suffering. Second, there is a fine line between keeping an animal comfortable with increased analgesia and moving toward euthanasia. The former can well entail the latter.

Obviously some combination of options 2 and 3 is probably optimal. Resorting to option 1 on a regular basis would probably generate what I have elsewhere called "moral stress"—the tension between what one is doing and what one believes one *ought* to be doing—which ultimately erodes both personal health and job satisfaction (Rollin, 1986).

Thus, although the social ethic clearly determines the path a critical care veterinarian is obliged to take regarding a suffering research animal, it merely suggests, without compelling, the decision regarding a suffering companion animal. For even though federal law sets the standard of practice in theory, *de facto* there is no one to impose it upon a private owner. At best it provides a powerful argument for the critical care clinician who must, in the end, appeal to his or her personal ethic in adjudicating such a situation. If the veterinarian holds strongly to the pediatrician model, he or she will strongly object to prolonging life at all costs. I believe, as we will shortly discuss, that veterinarians, like physicians, enjoy a great deal of what is called *Aesculapian authority*, the powerful, almost mystical authority that healers enjoy in all cultures. Deploying this authority by first of all convincing the client that you have the animal's best interest at heart and second by demonstrating your considerable experience with situations like the one in question, both go a long way towards securing client trust.

A special case, midway between research and private ownership, is the case of a client animal being used in an experimental research protocol for therapeutic purposes. In some ways, the use of animals with naturally occurring disease for research obviously represents a moral advance over creating the disease in experimental animals. But this sort of activity, for example in oncology, creates its own moral problems. In particular, the clinician-researcher usually has a vested interest in keeping the animal alive as long as possible for the understandable purpose of garnering data. The animal owner may be subtly (or not so subtly) swayed by the Aesculapian authority of the researcher-clinician to keep the animal alive for longer than he or she would be inclined to do. (Such researchers often build close emotional bonds with clients after many months or even years of therapy.) Thus the client may decide to take the animal home after a very dramatic invasive experimental therapy, say, radical intestinal resection, amputation of the tongue, or removal of the mandible. The animal may have been stabilized in the research institution's CCU but is by no means normal. While at home, the animal crashes, sometimes far away from the research institution, and the animal is brought to a local CCU. Since the local veterinarians may not be familiar with the intricacies of the protocol, they are faced with a suffering, failing animal about whose situation they may know very little. With the client-researcher complex strongly leaning toward keeping the animal alive, the CCU veterinarian is faced with controlling pain and suffering in an area in which he or she lacks familiarity. Although endpoints for ordinary research animals are generally set by researchers in consultations with Institutional Animal Care and Use Committees, the euthanasia decision for client-owned research animals in the sort of situation we described is left to the client!

In my view, the CCU clinician should address his or her moral problem very directly and honestly. If he or she believes that saving the animal or even keeping it comfortable requires specialized knowledge or facilities lacking in the practice, or believes that the animal cannot in fact be made comfortable, he or she should say so directly. He or she should explain to the client that, while perhaps CCU clinicians at the research institution may have the specialized knowledge necessary to manage the suffering adequately, he or she is uncomfortable with the responsibility. In my view, by no means should this private clinician trade extra data for animal suffering, particularly if he or she embraces the pediatrician model. Once again, the spirit of current social ethics supports this decision.

While typically a critical care clinician does not enjoy the long-term relationship with a client that allows you to put your arm around the client and say, "It's time to let go," the lack of such a relationship can also be a boon. Many oncologists who treat animals over a long period of time warn that directing the client towards euthanasia may well lead them to later blame the veterinarian for "killing my dog." The very fact that the critical care clinician steps into the picture only *in extremis*, for a relatively brief and dramatic moment, militates against long-term resentment and increases the power of your advice. If the client later resents you, it won't have the same effect on you professionally or emotionally as it does on a primary care clinician or oncologist. To put it crudely, you are able to focus more on the animal.

Our analysis is buttressed by looking at professional ethics. It is manifest that society expects veterinarians to champion animal welfare and lead in welfare reform (Rollin, 2000). This is clearly evidenced by the laboratory animal welfare laws in the United States and Britain designating veterinarians as responsible for assuring research animal well-being. It is also something any veterinarian can confirm through ordinary experience. Though U.S. organized veterinarian medicine has been slow to shoulder this burden, society expects veterinarians to perform the same role with regard to all animals, including agricultural animals, race horses, zoo animals, wild animals, and companion animals. And once again, except for endangered species, the area of concern is animal suffering rather than animal life. We all know from personal experience that society unequivocally condemns people who won't euthanize a suffering animal (though we are split on suffering humans). It would therefore behoove organized veterinary medicine as a whole—and certainly the specialty of emergency/critical care veterinarians—to adopt as a principle of professional ethics that they are committed to not prolonging the life of an animal when suffering is uncontrollable or when the prognosis is permanent suffering, pain, distress, or disability. The details of such a professional ethical position should of course be worked out by the professionals involved. This leaves room for professional judgment and flexibility, but some such principle would be of great social value both in setting out the ground rules regarding uncontrolled suffering, and in preempting eventual loss of professional autonomy to legislation.

On the basis of the analysis we have hitherto developed, we can generate a response to the problem of pain control, the third ethical question we raised in our introductory paragraph—what we may call "care" versus "cure."

It is manifest that twentieth-century scientific medicine, human or animal, was captured by the ideology outlined above and, desirous of eschewing talk of unverifiable subjective states, has schematized the battle against disease, injury, or death as won or lost. If a disease is cured or life is prolonged, medicine wins; if not, it loses. Little emphasis is placed on patient *comfort*—that is one reason the voluntary euthanasia issue has become so pronounced. Physicians routinely argue against morphine and marijuana for terminally ill patients. As one nursing dean said to me, "Physicians worry about *cure*, we worry about *care*." Patients whose situations are perceived as hopeless end up cared for by nurses, and it is all too revealing that the hospice movement, aimed at keeping patients comfortable and as pain-free as possible, is almost totally a creation of and staffed by nurses, not doctors.

Veterinary medicine too, has been guilty of ignoring patient comfort (McMillen, 1998). For much of the twentieth century, anesthesia was confused with chemical restraint both in nomenclature and in practice. Surgical procedures such as spays, castrations, dehorning, wound repair, and others were performed with "bruticaine" on small and large animals or with paralytic, curariform drugs, or visceral procedures were performed with drugs like ketamine, which provide virtually no visceral analgesia but do immobilize. Killing of animals was often done with these paralyzing drugs via asphyxiation—a far cry from the "good death" entailed by the term "euthanasia." Early textbooks of veterinary anesthesia do not even mention pain control as a justification for anesthesia, and routine rationalizations for not using anesthesia or analgesia were rife: "The anesthetic bothers the animal more than the pain," "The analgesia will allow the animal to reinjure itself," and so on.

In today's society, enduring pain is not seen as a virtue or as building strength or character. And indeed, pain is a major biological stressor that, if unalleviated, can retard healing and even promote morbidity and mortality. One can argue that one of the major causes of the movement in society toward scientifically unproven alternative medicine is that alternative practitioners openly address and sympathize with human and animal pain, suffering, and distress.

Our earlier discussions of the question of keeping animals alive are directly relevant to the issue of controlling pain and suffering. As detailed in our earlier reasoning, social ethics values control of animal suffering more than it values animal life, as do owners not blinded by selfish concerns. Thus the moral imperative for CCU veterinarians to keep animals as pain-free as possible seems to rule, and in some cases can be used to trump the selfish owner's willingness to keep the animal alive at all costs, since death can be a serendipitous *sequela* to controlling pain.

Obviously, not all pain can be controlled all the time. In some cases, like physical therapy, some pain must be accepted in order to return the animal to normalcy. There are no hard and fast rules for such situations; common sense and common decency should suffice. As a general moral principle, it is only reasonable not to control pain and suffering when controlling pain interferes with a clear and pressing health demand that leads directly to rapid return to normalcy (as in physical therapy).

When, however, one is tempted to withhold pain control, one should bear in mind that, contrary to old Shibboleths, animals may actually suffer pain more intensely than humans. It used to be said that, lacking language and future concepts, animal pain is limited to the now, as opposed to human pain, which can be potentiated by fear and anxiety. (Thus part of the suffering of going to the dentist may be fear that he is Josef Mengele.) In response to that claim, I would argue that, lacking such concepts, animals have no *hope* of pain cessation or anticipation of a future without pain, and thus they *are* their pain.

In the same vein, Ralph Kitchell has pointed out that the experience of pain has two elements, a sensory discriminative dimension and a motivational dimension (Kitchell and Guinan, 1989). Since animals lack the intellectual power humans have to reason out the source of pain and how to stop it, the motivational aspect may be stronger and thus animals may well suffer more than we do.

Thus keeping the animals comfortable should be a top moral priority for the CCU clinician. The social consensus ethic points in that direction, and the professional ethics of such clinicians should be developed to be in accord with that ethic. Control of animal pain, suffering, and distress should be a primary and articulated ethical imperative across all of veterinary medicine and should be made an unequivocal top priority in the Veterinarian's Oath.

The issue of clients who cannot afford to pay for CCU fees is one that leads to pervasive problems across veterinary medicine. Unlike human medicine, there is no social guarantee in veterinary medicine that a patient will get the requisite care. There is little animal health insurance in society, and what there is favors upper-middle-class animal owners. Unlike the situation for children, society does not yet see fit to guarantee medical care for animals, especially the costly sort of care entailed by CCU modalities. So euthanasia for animals belonging to poor people often presents itself as the only option.

In some cases, veterinary schools may run a clinic for indigent clients, both as a public service and as a way of educating veterinary students, but this sort of operation is relatively rare and is not found in all (or even most) veterinary schools. Given that society is increasingly reluctant to allow veterinary students to practice surgery and other skills on unwanted companion animals slated for euthanasia, such clinics may well proliferate. But given that there are only about thirty veterinary colleges in the United States, even creating such clinics at every veterinary college would only deal with a very tiny percentage of such cases.

In large measure, then, solutions to this problem will emerge from the personal ethics of veterinarians engaged in critical care. If a veterinarian strongly adheres to the pediatrician model, or strongly values the strength of the human-animal bond in at least some cases, such as where the animal in question is all that gives meaning to the life of an elderly, lonely person, he or she may choose to do the requisite work at cost. But in many such instances, the owner in question can still not afford to pay. The veterinarian is then left with a dilemma—either euthanize the animal or do the work gratis. While idealistic students are often inclined to work for free, they soon realize that they simply cannot afford to do this very often, particularly in critical care cases that are extremely consumptive of time and resources.

One solution that was quite prevalent in veterinary medicine in general during hard times earlier this century was barter. Oftentimes cash-poor clients may have a good deal to trade for veterinary services. I have heard of veterinarians trading their services for farm products such as eggs, milk, vegetables, or meat. I have also heard of barter for client labor, skilled or unskilled. Clients can trade house painting, fence building, lawn maintenance, snow removal, mechanical work, trash hauling, or general cleanup for care given to their animals. Alternatively, some veterinarians allow clients to pay a small amount each month, in effect extending long-term, low-interest credit to poor people.

In the end, however, there is only a limited amount that a critical care veterinarian can do, as he or she will always encounter more hardship cases than can be managed by the approaches mentioned. State-of-the-art critical care is expensive, and it is likely to become even more expensive as new cutting-edge technology is incorporated.

A final related issue concerns the unowned animal requiring critical care, say, a trauma victim brought in by a Good Samaritan or public servant such as a policeman, fireman, or animal control officer. The owner is unknown, and the animal rescuer is unwilling to assume financial responsibility. Obviously, as we saw earlier, even the most morally concerned veterinarian cannot do many such treatments without pay. What does one do?

Many of the considerations relevant to the indigent owner clearly apply here. But there are some new aspects worthy of note. Once again, the key to resolving the problem lies in the veterinarian's personal ethic. If one holds a Garage Mechanic view, the choice is simple—euthanize the animal. But if one leans towards Pediatrician, the old difficulties arise.

One of my veterinarian colleagues has found a very Solomonic solution to such cases. Unlike most veterinarians, he welcomes these situations. He first of all sees them as "continuing education from God," helpful in sharpening his clinical skills. Secondly, he has a unique agreement with the local newspaper. When such an animal is brought in, he photographically documents the animal's condition. He then proceeds to treat the animal to the full extent of his ability. When the animal returns to normalcy, he takes a new set of photographs. He then presents both sets of photos to the newspaper. The paper devotes a page to the "before" and "after" and offers the public the chance to adopt the animal if the owner does not claim the animal. In some cases, grateful new owners will pay my colleague. Even if this does not happen, my veterinarian friend argues that he has acquired, relatively cheaply, priceless publicity and advertising that he could not have bought for any amount of money!

Another option is for the local humane society to develop a fund covering unowned injured animals. Such funding drives are often quite successful and in some areas come close to covering all the requisite expenses. Finally, some fortunate veterinarians have their own funding from rich clients precisely earmarked to cover such situations. In my view, rather than being unethical, it is laudable for a veterinarian to solicit such funding and thereby perform a public service that furthers the social plausibility of the Pediatrician model.

In sum, then, as long as society is in flux regarding the social ethic for animals, the ethical issues in critical care medicine will be solved by reference to reasonable implications from extant social ethics, collective professional ethical decisions, and the veterinarian's personal ethic. In the latter case, I would suggest that what we have called the Pediatrician Model can well serve as a practical moral beacon.

Aesculapian Authority in Veterinary Medicine

Although the concept of Aesculapian authority—the unique authority that accrues to medical professionals—has long been implicitly recognized in human medicine, and explicitly articulated since the 1950s (Siegler and Osmond, 1974), it has not been similarly applied to veterinary medicine. This is in part a function of the fact that, until relatively recently, veterinary medicine was primarily and overwhelmingly focused upon the economic value of animals, usually in agriculture, and that value defined and circumscribed the degree to which treatment was accorded to a sick animal. It is only since companion animal medicine has come to dominate veterinary medicine (and society has, to a much lesser extent, expressed concern about laboratory animals) that economic value of the animal as a constraint on expenditure for diagnosis and treatment has been superseded, and companion animals have come to be seen more as persons, valued for their uniqueness. Fewer and fewer pet owners would be inclined to trash Fifi, their pet beagle, because it is cheaper to buy a new beagle than fix the old one, though such a mind-set would certainly be prevalent in areas like agriculture, where animals bear primarily economic value. Since the early 1980s, for example, it is quite common for pet owners to spend over six figures at our veterinary hospital for cancer treatment.

And society, during that period, has begun to acknowledge in judicial decisions granting emotional damages for losses of animals, and in explicit legislation, that companion animals possess more than market value. Municipal resolutions in San Francisco and in Boulder, Colorado, have affirmed the (currently legally indefensible) notion that humans are *guardians*, not owners, of companion animals, and numerous legal scholars are exploring various strategies for raising the legal status of animals from property.

Thus, as society moves away from an economic conception of companion animals to something closer to a notion of personhood, veterinarians serving that population are forced (or, in most cases, given their personal predilections, are allowed to move) out of what we have called a *garage mechanic model* of treating animals, toward a pediatrician model. (There is also good evidence that horses are being increasingly viewed as companion animals—for example, California legislation making it a felony to ship a horse to slaughter—so our discussion is also relevant to equine practice.) And with that new model of treating the animal as a direct object of moral and medical concern, as opposed to a utilitarian object whose value is overwhelmingly economic, comes increasing relevance of the concept of Aesculapian authority to companion animal practice, and correlative relevance of potential abuse of that authority.

What is Aesculapian authority? The locus classicus where the concept is most carefully analyzed is Siegler and Osmond's *Models of Madness, Models of Medicine* (1974), where it is discussed in the context of human physicians. According to their discussion, Aesculapian authority is the uniquely powerful authority vested in those that society perceives as healers, historically traceable to the time when medicine was inseparable from magic and religion. It is Aesculapian authority that licenses a medical practitioner to handle a patient with greater intimacy than a sexual partner does. Physicians may probe all parts of the body of patients of either gender with barely a "by your leave"—they tell a patient they must enter an otherwise forbidden area rather than ask for permission. Aesculapian authority confers the sick role, allowing patients escape from responsibilities of work, school, or family. Such authority also compels patients to ingest vile nostrums and medications; surrender spinal fluid to painful procedures; change one's eating or sleeping habits; submit to moral lectures on child rearing; surrender blood, urine, or fecal material; be immobilized; undergo surgery preceded by imposed loss of consciousness; even change one's temperament. What would be dismissed as "torture" in the absence of Aesculapian authority is meekly accepted by even the most powerful in its presence. As one physician once told me, "As a physician, I can get almost anyone to do whatever I tell him or her. If a captain of industry or a general or a senator comes to me with an illness, I can order them, as a therapeutic modality, to dangle their naked butt out of a window on the top floor of the Empire State Building, and they will do so."

In fact, argue Siegler and Osmond, Aesculapian authority is far and away the most powerful authority in society. Even kings, politicians, and dictators submit to medical authority they don't understand and can be scolded and ordered about by physicians.

According to these authors, this authority derives from a combination of traits: sapiential (that is, special wisdom and knowledge); moral (deriving from the overwhelming moral imperative to heal, relieve suffering, and retard death); and charismatic (derived from the fact that medicine is still related to magic in the eyes of the scientifically and medically naive, that is, most people). (The latter explains why physicians are often threatened by dealing with medical students, veterinary students, or veterinarians: They know too much!)

Aesculapian authority is further reinforced by other members of the medical community; for example, in never calling each other by first names around a patient and almost never directly challenging the pronouncements of peers.

There are, however, strict limits to such authority. For example, it must be deployed to further the best interests of the patient; pursuit of any other end, such as extracting sexual favors from a patient, represent a clear-cut case of abuse of that authority. This creates ever-present moral problems of abuse of authority for physician/researchers. As one prominent physician/researcher told me: "Informed consent is a joke. I can extract informed consent for questionable experimental procedures not in their best interest from damn near any patient by deploying my authority!"

Virtually everything we have said of physicians increasingly holds true of veterinarians; indeed many human patients seek medical advice and even assistance from their veterinarians, who are in fact often held in higher esteem in society than are human medical doctors (A. P. Knight, personal communication, 2004)! They too confer a sick role on animals and absolve them of tasks and responsibilities (particularly companion animals but also working animals like horses), approach animals with great intimacy, perform operations otherwise deemed tortuous outside of a medical context, and so on. The only difference, in fact, is that a veterinarian almost always works through a third party, the client and owner, whereas physicians usually work directly with patients. But this is certainly not always true; consider pediatricians or those who practice gerontology or psychiatry—they too must often deal with a third party. But the key point is that, morally speaking, neither the pediatrician nor the companion animal veterinarian owes primary allegiance to the third party. Their moral duty is to the patient: They are obliged by the nature of their profession to act in the best interest of the patient, and they consequently need to avoid orders or requests from the third party that are not in the best interest of the patient.

The major difference, of course, between pediatric physicians and veterinarians is the fact that the consensus social ethic will back the pediatrician in circumventing the obstructive third party, as when a parent refuses to allow a child to receive requisite medical care, courts will order it done. We have not yet reached that stage with animals. But insofar as the animal owner claims to be interested first and foremost in the health of the animal, the situation is logically the same for a pediatrician and (at least) the companion animal veterinarian.

Plato made a highly relevant point in *The Republic* (Book I, Chapter 3) when he pointed out that, conceptually, the primary obligation of a shepherd is to further the well-being of the sheep in his purview. The money he makes accrues to him in his capacity as wage earner and does not take precedence over his primary obligation. Indeed, this analogy helps us to understand why we are so morally horrified at a shepherd who accepts a bribe to hurt or kill his sheep. (Compare this with the monsters who allowed or arranged for the killing or crippling of the horses in their charge for insurance money. It is no surprise that law enforcement officers—who have seen everything—pronounced these crimes as "the worst they had ever seen.") By the same token, the veterinarian, or at the very least the veterinarian treating companion-animal owners view as "persons" or family members, are obliged to give primacy to the animal, with the owner being certainly someone who should not be antagonized but ultimately, as one successful and prominent veterinarian said to me, as someone "to be gotten around in pursuit of my real job, helping to heal the animal or alleviate its suffering."

This is not to deny that veterinary medicine is a "people profession," for "getting around the owner for the benefit of the animal" can be a major problem. It is here that full Aesculapian authority can and should be invoked *for the benefit of the animal.* This may involve all of the elements of Aesculapian authority mentioned earlier: appeal to knowledge, wisdom, and experience; appeal to moral authority; and appeal to healer's charisma. The key point is that veterinary medicine can indeed require great "people skills" and more time spent in dealing with owners than with actual diagnostic and therapeutic modalities performed on the animal, yet, conceptually, the ultimate function and goal of veterinary medicine can still be the best interests of the animal.

One aspect of Aesculapian authority that has never been discussed in either human or veterinary medical contexts derives from concepts developed in the philosophy of language. During the mid–twentieth century, Oxford philosopher J.L. Austin (as well as numerous other linguistically oriented philosophers, including Wittgenstein), called attention to hitherto unnoticed dimensions of language beyond the descriptive, that is, beyond the uttering of descriptive statements that are true or false (Austin, 1965). In particular, Austin stressed the concept of *performative utterances*, whereby a speaker, by virtue of his or her social role, performs an action beyond the linguistic when saying certain words. Examples abound: When an umpire says, "You're out," you *are* out, even if later examination of videotapes shows that you are factually safe. When a king says you are banished, you'd best be out of the kingdom forthwith. When a minister says, "I now pronounce you man and wife," only complex legal machinations can cancel the resulting state.

The ability to create powerful performative utterances accrues naturally to those possessed of Aesculapian authority. A doctor or a veterinarian is required to declare one sick and thereby create the sick role, with all its attendant removal of responsibility for person or animal. A psychiatrist who declares a person "a possible danger to himself or others" thereby creates indefinite commitment for a person without appeal, something even judges cannot do. A declaration from a public health veterinarian regarding foot and mouth disease or rabies or BSE can effectively doom thousands of animals to death with no appeal.

Even outside the complex tissue of social regulations presupposed in the examples in the previous paragraphs, a physician or veterinarian can create uniquely powerful performative utterances. We have all heard of people who, when told by a physician that "you have only six months to live," will obligingly die during that period (whereas others, less trustful of physicians, will make it a point to confute that prognosis). The same holds true of "You will never walk again" or "Your animal will never walk again." To put it simply, for at least some people, a pronouncement made from a base of Aesculapian authority by a physician or a veterinarian becomes a self-fulfilling prophecy. Even if the veterinarian is physiologically wrong, the client will not, after that pronouncement, attempt to have the animal walk, thereby, through lack of attempt or through subsequent muscle atrophy, validate the prognostication!

It follows from this discussion that Aesculapian authority is an extremely powerful notion and, like any other power, is subject to abuse. We are not interested here in deliberate, self-conscious, intentional abuse, such as using that authority to extract sexual favors or money from patients or, in the case of veterinary medicine, from clients. Rather, we are concerned with the unconscious, non-deliberate abuse of this most powerful of authorities in virtue of lack of reflection on it, the obliviousness to its full extent or influence, the failure to recognize it is being deployed where it shouldn't be, or equally pernicious, not being deployed when it should. In our ensuing discussion, we shall chronicle some examples of this sort of non-deliberate abuse of Aesculapian authority in the hope of making veterinarians more aware of this neglected notion and its dangers.

Probably the most common issues surrounding Aesculapian authority in veterinary medicine devolve around euthanasia, both medical euthanasia and convenience euthanasia. These issues come from two opposite problems: clients who demand euthanasia for trivial reasons, and clients who refuse euthanasia despite its being medically indicated to end suffering. Historically, the issue of greatest concern to veterinarians related to euthanasia has been being assailed with regular requests to perform convenience euthanasia for reasons that the veterinarian perceives as morally unacceptable. Discussions with veterinarians and humane society workers reveal that clients may request euthanasia for appalling reasons: The animal no longer matches the color scheme; we are going on vacation and it is cheaper to get a new animal than to board it; the animal is getting old and can no longer run with me.

Veterinarians who morally lean toward the pediatrician model report that being asked to euthanize healthy—or potentially healthy—animals is one of the most odious aspects of their job. Indeed, constantly performing such euthanasias is highly erosive of both physical and mental health by virtue of the stress it engenders. As I have discussed elsewhere in detail, the stress in question is far worse than the ordinary stresses of too much to do, whining clients, financial pressures, and so on. It is *moral stress* (Rollin, 1986), based in a fundamental and inescapable belief that what you are doing is totally inimical to your professional raison d'être, as you are being asked to destroy healthy functional beings, many of whom you may have worked furiously to save in the past.

Ordinary stress management techniques do not touch such stress. And, if you are morally conscientious, it does not help much to send these clients packing, for you know well that *someone* will kill the animal for them. I have argued that the only escape from moral stress in the context of demands for convenience euthanasia is to do everything in one's power to save that animal, including exerting one's Aesculapian authority as forcefully as possible. Unfortunately, too many veterinarians, having been trained in a context where the mechanic model was prevalent, however much they may personally lean toward the moral primacy of animal interests, will perform the euthanasia and swallow their moral stress. This in turn leads not only to spirally escalating moral stress but helps perpetuate client expectations regarding the viability and moral acceptability of convenience euthanasia.

In short, I am arguing that failure to wield one's Aesculapian authority to save the life (= healthy functioning!) of an animal by acquiescing to requests for convenience euthanasia represents a significant moral problem in veterinary medicine. This in turn cheapens animal life in the eyes of the public and validates irresponsibility—"The vet sees nothing wrong with killing the animal"—and erodes job satisfaction. In this case, as in many others, failing to act *is* a form of acting, generating bad consequences for animals, society, individual veterinarians, and veterinary medicine in general.

Ironically, in many cases of convenience euthanasia, the veterinarian can save the animal if he or she does use the authority inherent in his or her healer role: If the euthanasia is for behavior problems, the veterinarian can recommend retraining, behavior modification, or in extreme cases, pharmacological intervention. If euthanasia is requested for the sort of bad reasons cited above, the veterinarian can forthrightly indicate that he or she did not struggle to acquire and pay for a veterinary education in order to destroy healthy animals, and should suggest other options—fostering, adoption, and so on. And, in my view, there is nothing wrong with a veterinarian morally educating a client regarding the clinician's view of the ethical unacceptability of convenience euthanasia anymore than there is anything wrong with pediatricians counseling against child abuse. Veterinarians need not eat the sins of clients.

To accomplish these goals requires that veterinarians become consciously aware of their Aesculapian authority and learn to consciously deploy it. (Obviously, good clinicians do so intuitively, but, like natural athletes, they can benefit from "coaching.") This in turn requires recognition and discussion of that authority by the veterinary community, and the incorporation of these issues into veterinary school curricula and continuing education.

It is likely that, as society continues to evolve in the direction of what I have called the "new ethic for animals" (Rollin, 1995), the issue of convenience euthanasia will gradually be mitigated, for societal disapproval of such euthanasia will help shape behavior and education will influence subsequent generations. It is also conceivable that legislation growing out of this new ethic will make it more difficult to "trash an animal." There is an analogy here with the rapid and revolutionary changes in social thought and behavior with regard to despoliation and preservation of the environment. In the 1960s, environmental concern was not a social issue; by 1970, we had experienced the first Earth Day.

Meanwhile, as more and more people in society profess to view their animals as "members of the family," another and opposite problem for veterinarians has emerged (Rollin, 2001). Now ever-increasing numbers of people are unwilling to surrender their animals to disease and sometimes are unwilling to authorize medical euthanasia despite the animal's dismal prognosis and high degree of suffering. Since the late 1970s, people have been spending enormous amounts of money on their companion animals' health, which has in turn driven the development of lucrative practices in oncology, surgery, cardiology, and other specialty fields. Such commitment to one's animals, although often laudable, sometimes is pathological and selfish, as when owners refuse to accept that the animal is in such a state of suffering that euthanasia is the moral course of choice, yet are unwilling to let go for their own emotional needs. Thus, in a given day, a morally aware veterinarian may face one client who wants a perfectly healthy dog killed and another who will not consider euthanasia of an irreversibly damaged painful animal.

This new attachment to animals is quite understandable. As divorces increase, as people live longer and longer, and as our culture gets increasingly urban, loneliness grows epidemic and the love and reciprocal care once provided in extended families has vanished. An animal may be the only "person" in the world who can fill the human need for giving and receiving love, or it may be the only reason an elderly person has to wake up in the morning. Under such circumstances, it is easy to understand the temptation to keep the animal alive at all costs. Nonetheless, this raises a major problem for the veterinarian who sees his or her primary responsibility as serving the best interests of the animal.

It is true that reasons once thought definitive for justifying euthanasia have now been supplanted. Whereas, for example, amputation of a limb was believed to cause sufficient suffering and inadequacy for the animal to justify euthanasia for the sake of the animal's welfare, we now realize that this is not the case. In fact, films exist showing an animal with both foreleg and rear leg amputated happily catching a frisbee in mid-air. Such advances notwithstanding, however, it is well to remember that an animal totally consumed by unalleviable pain is incapable of fulfilling its nature and of being happy. Humans tell us that when they are in chronic, unalleviable pain, they *are* the pain; their other roles—parent, professional, friend, lover—are subordinated to the pain. How much more so, then, for an animal, who, lacking *hope*, cannot even imagine an end to the pain (Rollin, 2000)?

It is commonly taught to students in veterinary school that they are not to direct clients towards euthanasia. A clinician who does so, or even answers the question "what would you do?" it is claimed, is being paternalistic and directive and will likely be rejected by the client later—"You made me kill my dog." The client must make his or her own decision.

In my view, this is a grievous and mischievous error. One would not ask a client's opinion on what antibiotic or surgical approach to use. The same logic holds for euthanasia, which is, for the veterinarian adopting the pediatrician model, the ultimate treatment for otherwise unalleviable suffering. One would hope that veterinary education prepares a professional to judge when that situation is the case better than a layperson can. Thus, if one is committed to the best interests of the animal, one should not surrender deployment of the ultimate treatment for suffering to the clients, especially when they are focused on their own interests, that is, fear of loss of the animal on which they emotionally depend.

Once again, veterinarians should not hesitate to utilize their Aesculapian authority to treat suffering, even if that means countering the client's desire. This is a logical consequence of focusing on the interests of the animal. The same moral concern that drives veterinarian resistance to convenience euthanasia should drive veterinarian resistance to allowing the animal to suffer; failure to end the animal's pain and suffering is as much a source of potential moral stress as is capitulating to a client's desire to destroy a healthy animal for frivolous reasons.

In sum, it is well within the role of a veterinarian as a healing professional to deploy one's Aesculapian authority to keep a healthy animal alive; medicine aims at restoring *or* maintaining healthy living. Similarly, it is also conceptually part of the veterinarian's duty to end suffering totally erosive of quality of life for the animal. By no means should one be insensitive to the client's putative reasons for wanting to kill a healthy animal or keep alive a suffering one. But being sensitive to these reasons and using one's Aesculapian authority to do so does not mean that one should abrogate serving the best interests of the animal. It simply means learning to communicate that requirement to a client in a way that helps ease the pain of thwarting their desires. In the event that even Aesculapian authority cannot move the client to euthanasia, it should be deployed to convince the client to acquiesce to heroic pain control, which may in the end be tantamount to euthanasia, yet easier to accomplish.

In our discussion thus far we have presupposed a long-term relationship between client and clinician, which sometimes makes it easier for the doctor to exert Aesculapian authority over the client. But such a long-term relationship is not essential for such authority, or presuppositional to it. A surgeon one sees for moments before and after an operation may enjoy greater Aesculapian authority over a patient or client than a medical professional who is also a family friend. Thus a critical care veterinarian, encountering a client he or she does not know, and unsullied by intimate knowledge of client emotional reliance on the animal, can say, "It is time to stop trying" with greater lack of ambiguity and ambivalence than can the veterinarian whose attention is focused in part on the human, and who thus may be more sympathetic towards resolution of the situation not in the best interests of the animal.

Another significant problem relating to improper use of Aesculapian authority can arise when the clinician is also a researcher, as is the case with some oncologists whose research is performed on client animals. This is a laudable approach to making progress in biomedicine, for it is far less morally problematic to utilize naturally existing disease than to create it in healthy animals. Yet such research runs the risk of the clinician's confusing roles.

As a clinician, the veterinarian's primary obligation is to the best interests of the animal. As a researcher, however, the veterinarian's primary obligation is to extract the most data possible from the experiment. These two functions may inevitably conflict when, qua researcher, the veterinarian is tempted to keep the suffering animal alive as long as possible to glean additional knowledge form the case. Yet qua clinician, the veterinarian knows that his or her obligation is to end the suffering. (The same conflict is evident in the Veterinarian's Oath, when one is asked to commit to advancing medical knowledge yet also alleviating animal suffering.) Grave danger exists of the veterinarian utilizing his or her Aesculapian authority with clients to move them toward prolonging life when suffering is present. This is clearly wrong, since, as we know, the very basis of Aesculapian authority is managing the patient for *his or her own benefit*, not for the benefit of science. Indeed, if the clinician is acting for any other reason than the direct benefit of the patient, Aesculapian authority is not present or at least is being exercised illegitimately.

Similar problems arise in human and veterinary medical research with regard to enrolling research subjects in clinical protocols, as we mentioned briefly earlier. A human experimental surgeon once told me that, in his view, there is often no real informed consent in such research: "Oh I go through the motions of garnering consent, warning subjects of dangers, and so on. But the bottom line is that I rely on the patients' reverence for me as a healer. When they sign up for my research projects, they do so because they trust me to be working in their best interests, which is not always the case when I am doing research. They enroll willingly because of my [Aesculapian] authority. They don't believe that I would ever do anything that could harm them, *even when I detail the risks*." The same holds true in veterinary research.

Guarding against this abuse of Aesculapian authority is extremely difficult—more difficult, ironically enough, for a client's companion animal being used in clinical research than for a research animal owned by the researcher. In the latter case, Animal Care and Use Committees demand endpoints for the research in order to control animal suffering. Such endpoints are almost always set before the advent of major pain or distress. Yet, in the case of clinical research, the endpoint is left to the animal owner who, unlike the committee, may well confound the veterinarian/researcher's separate and distinct role as healer and experimenter.

We mentioned earlier Plato's point that one's role as a healer should be kept separate from one's role as a wage earner, with the interests of the patient taking precedence. This distinction is easier to maintain, however, in theory than in practice and may well become blurred, leading to pecuniary abuse of Aesculapian authority. One of the veterinarians I most admire has told me how this may occur: "You recommend an expensive diet that you stock to a client for a temporary usage; for example, for a young puppy or for a temporary nutritional problem. The animal is no longer a puppy or no longer needs the low or high calorie diet. Yet you never explicitly tell the client that a cheaper diet will work just as well, so he or she continues to pay far more than they need to because of the authority behind your initial suggestion." You are certainly not getting rich by virtue of your authority, but you are prolonging unnecessary expenditure. A similar point can be made with regard to recommending or even raising the issue of heartworm medicaments in an area where heartworm is as likely as cobra bite!

An emerging issue of Aesculapian authority is the degree to which that authority can be used to foist unproven therapies upon clients or, more subtly, to validate their demands for such therapies. We are all familiar with the paranoid fantasy we sometimes have as patients that the physician is holding something back that will cure us or alleviate our symptoms. (Unfortunately, given the history of twentieth-century medicine's ideological denial and/or ignoring of felt pain, and its parsimony in managing pain, there is an element of truth here. Too often physicians and veterinarians do hold back pain control for reasons growing out of ideology.) That paranoia seems to have run wild in society, and people are gravitating toward all sorts of scientifically baseless, clinically unproven "therapeutic" regimens coming from "alternative" approaches—homeopathy, colored lights, crystals, laying on of hands, Bach flower essences, magnets, and so on, with new approaches emerging rapidly (Schoen and Wynn, 1998).

Billions of dollars are spent annually on such nostrums, despite the fact that many were empirically discredited a century or more ago. And, as discussed elsewhere, there are good reasons for public disaffection with science-based medicine: neglect by that tradition of psychological dimensions of sickness; failure of science-based medical professionals to focus on unique elements of disease embodied in a unique individual in favor of focusing on what follows repeatable laws; iatrogenic problems coming out of medicine; the high cost of medication and medical care; the emphasis on cure over care, prolongation of life without regard to its quality; and so on. Such problems lead some of us to a search for simple solutions to medical problems. A sort of good-old-days, noble-savage mentality seizes some people's imaginations, and they yearn for "natural" or "spiritual" remedies, forgetting that arsenic, prions, and snake venom are all "natural" without thereby being healthful or even innocuous.

In any case, client demands for such daydreams have increased to fevered pitch and client pressure for veterinarians to supply them is overwhelming—and clients are willing to pay! Further, in some cases the "disease" you are called upon to treat is in the client's imagination: They come to you for companionship, advice, counseling, friendship, and so on under the aegis of having a sick animal. So what is the harm in prescribing alternative therapies for clients that (a) provide hope for clients, (b) give them what they want, (c) may have a positive placebo effect (at least in human medicine!), provided such remedies do no harm? Why shouldn't we place our Aesculapian authority behind these unproven remedies?

Many clinicians have begun to provide such therapies for a variety of reasons. These include "The clients demand them," "They will get them from somewhere; it might as well be me," "We need to keep chiropractors and other phonies from getting a foothold in treating animals." Yet the concept of Aesculapian authority is seriously imperiled by such reasoning, for one of the sources of that authority is one's medical expertise, based in the best knowledge one can garner. If one prostitutes that authority to endorse non-remedies posing as remedies, it can well lead to erosion of that authority, particularly when the social pendulum swings, as it inevitably will, away from faddish fascination with therapies that have no basis in proof of efficacy and are, in many cases, incompatible with what we know of nature. Like one's reputation for veracity, medical credibility, once lost, is difficult to regain.

We shall discuss alternative medicine in detail in relation to veterinary ethics in our next section. Here we are concerned with a subset of such issues: the relationship between Aesculapian authority and prescribing or condoning alternative therapies.

We may seek some guidance from a highly relevant group of professionals who have examined this issue—the American Academy of Pediatrics—and whose results are clearly highly significant for veterinarians who embrace the pediatrician model. The American Academy of Pediatrics Committee on Children with Disabilities has developed guidelines for "Counseling Families Who Choose Complementary and Alternative Medicine for Their Child With Chronic Illness or Disability" (American Academy of Pediatrics, 2001). These guidelines are quite reasonable, and conceptually address many often-neglected aspects of disease and treatment. While acknowledging that all medical therapies, conventional or alternative, should be science-based and evidence-based, the guidelines wrestle sympathetically with the mind-set leading desperate people to seek such therapies. In particular, they address some of the reasons we cited above both explicitly and implicitly.

The guidelines stress the need for medical professionals not to relinquish their ability to influence treatment and serve the best interests of the child, that is, to retain their Aesculapian authority in their relationship with parents. That does not mean endorsing therapies that might be dangerous, but it does mean not relinquishing one's medical purview over the child. That in turn means being extremely sensitive to parental frustration, desperation, and overwhelming desire to do something. The practitioner should study the alternative modality sought by the client and, in a sympathetic way, critically evaluate the scientific basis of and evidence for the therapy, and forthrightly explain the likelihood of success as he or she sees it. This is likely to entail a discussion of types of evidence, the weakness of anecdote, the compatibility with known laws of nature, and so on. Even more important, he or she should communicate possible dangers of these therapies:

> Alternative therapies may be directly harmful by causing direct toxic effects, compromising adequate nutrition, interrupting beneficial medications or therapies, or postponing biomedical therapies of proven effectiveness. Indirect harm may be caused by the financial burden of the alternative therapy, other unanticipated costs (e.g., the time investment required to administer therapy), and feelings of guilt associated with inability to adhere to rigorous treatment demands. If a child receiving alternative therapy is at direct or indirect risk of harm, the pediatrician should advise against the therapy. In some circumstances, it may be necessary for the pediatrician to seek an ethics consultation or to refer to child welfare agencies. If there is no risk of direct or indirect harm, a pediatrician should be neutral. (American Academy of Pediatrics, 2001)

To assure that the animal comes to no harm, the veterinarian must be even more skillful than the pediatrician in displaying sensitivity to the client and in deploying Aesculapian authority, as animals do not have the legal protection children do.

The guidelines also suggest Aesculapian authority–based discussions of improving quality of life for the patient. This can mitigate the hopelessness that leads people to "try anything." Directing the family to support and advocacy groups relevant to the disease in question can be of value. In addition, the practitioner should not be cavalier in dismissing the alternatives, but empathetic and open, not defensive. If the client insists on adopting an alternative modality, the practitioner should not disengage, but "offer to assist in monitoring and evaluating the response" in a critical but sympathetic way.

In sum, while one should be careful about using one's Aesculapian authority in support of baseless therapies, it is perfectly appropriate to deploy it vigorously to address the reasons people turn toward alternatives. Empathetic concern with the uniqueness of the patient and client situation; reassurance; careful, sensitive communication; and discussion of quality of life—all conveyed with Aesculapian authority in an unhurried, personal way—can help alleviate the client's powerful need to seek these elsewhere. More empathy in human dimensions of medicine may well help to end people's desperate (and fruitless and expensive, financially and emotionally) search for magic cures.

As Siegler and Osmond point out, Aesculapian authority is the most powerful authority one can have in society. As animals become increasingly personally and morally important in society, veterinary Aesculapian authority will increase. Indeed, as disaffection about human health care increases, veterinary Aesculapian authority will probably be augmented, with veterinarians serving as trusted authorities about medical matters.

Such authority is invaluable in furthering health but, as we have seen, is subject to inadvertent abuse. We may hope that increasing practitioner awareness of Aesculapian authority will help in avoiding such pitfalls.

The Ethics of Alternative Veterinary Medicine

The lure of alternative or non-evidence-based medicine is undeniable, and I, at least, must confess that I have succumbed to it on occasion. During a period when my energy flagged, I popped ginseng, chugged awful-tasting but expensive tonics, and probably would have aligned my bed with the earth's electrical impulses or Feng-Shui lines if I had known how to do so! Did it work? I have no idea! How could I test it? If I felt more energetic, how could I know that I was not experiencing wishful thinking or falling victim to observer bias, in the well-known manner of the Rosenthal effect or Dumbo's feather?

Nonetheless, we continue to succumb, thinking "What harm does it do?" "Stranger things have happened!" And we are not so civilized or sophisticated that we have lost the lifeline to magic thinking: witness perennial fascination with alien abductions, yeti, and the Bermuda Triangle.

In their nonprofessional moments (that is, most of the time), scientists are as vulnerable to the lure of the non-science-based as anyone else. (I vividly recall the Society of Orthodox Jewish Scientists at CCNY; colleagues in the biological sciences who are creationists in their private lives; or all reductionistic physicists and philosophers who are very Aristotelian in their daily lives.) I witnessed this very dramatically more than thirty years ago, when I first arrived at Colorado State University, and was placed on a committee to award small "seed money" grants to worthy researchers. All the other committee members were senior scientists; I was the token humanist representing the College of Liberal Arts to meet a legal requirement. Twice a year, we would meet and receive our assignments of submitted protocols, which we would review for a month and then reconvene to make the awards. The committee did not know what to do with me, and finally gave me two protocols, one on mycorhyzoids, since mycorhyzoids are important for food production, food production was an ethical issue, and I was in philosophy! The other was on music therapy, which was the only submission from my college. I recall spending an inordinate amount of time mastering the protocols so as not to disgrace myself or my field. When we came to the music therapy protocol, which involved a request to fund an organ to try to teach autistic children to speak, I was very critical of it, as no evidence had been cited to support any connection between organ music and acquisition of language, nor was there even a reasonable hypothesis regarding a connection. Clearly, the researcher wanted money for an organ! I articulated my objections and concluded by saying this proposal, though from my college, was neither conceptually nor empirically well-founded and should not be funded.

I was shocked when the committee chairman looked directly into my eyes and intoned, "Well I don't know about you, but I for one want to leave no stone unturned to try to help those poor children, and I'm surprised you don't." Worse still, all the other members were nodding and looking at me as though I were Scrooge. They unanimously voted to fund it and ignored my rejoinder about "Why don't you hire a witch doctor?" *Mirabile dictu*, all but myself were accomplished scientists!

All of us, and particularly those of us whose vocation is healing, want to help the afflicted. So it is understandable that we are drawn to untested modalities and "alternative" modalities sanctified by public demand and by anecdotal testimonials. After all, where is the harm? In my ensuing discussion, I will argue that there is indeed considerable ethical mischief in such an attitude and that in fact every major ethical vector relevant to veterinary medicine is actually or potentially compromised by failing to hold to a demand for a scientific evidentiary base for treatment modalities.

Earlier in this book, I have outlined the sorts of ethical vectors confronting veterinarians and creating the complex skein that is veterinary ethics. Veterinarians, like physicians, have obligations to clients, society, peers and their profession, and to themselves. What makes veterinary ethics in some ways more difficult and complex than human medical ethics is that veterinarians also have an obligation to their patients, the animals, which are not the same as their clients, and where, unlike the case of pediatricians, society is relatively silent about codifying our moral obligations to those patients. So we need to look at pressing forward non-evidence-based medicine (be it accepted or alternative) in terms of the moral categories relevant to veterinary decision making.

Veterinarians, like all other professionals, have obligations to society in general. Society grants professionals special privileges (such as writing prescriptions and doing surgery) in virtue of the function they are expected to perform. In addition, society gives a considerable degree of autonomy to professionals and is loath to regulate professions to any considerable extent, since legislators lack the requisite familiarity with the nature of veterinary practice. Instead, society, in essence, says to veterinarians, "You regulate yourselves the way we would regulate you if we understood in detail what you do (which we don't), but if you violate this charge and trust we will know and hammer you with Draconian rules."

We have already mentioned an example of this occurring when it became clear that some veterinarians were over-prescribing antibiotics for growth promotion in livestock and thereby also promoting the development of antibiotic-resistant pathogens, which in turn created a danger to human health. Congress reacted by considering legislation that would have eliminated extralabel drug use for veterinarians, a move that would, in essence, have hamstrung veterinary medicine. So if veterinary medicine wishes to preserve its autonomy, it has a prudential as well as moral reason to respect society's demands and conditions.

In any event, it is evident that among society's expectations of veterinarians (and, for that matter, of all medical professionals) is that they be solidly rooted in science and a scientific approach. This is clearly illustrated in myriad ways. The first line of the Veterinary Oath commits a veterinarian "to use my *scientific knowledge* [emphasis mine] and skills for the benefit of society." Again, presuppositional to the accreditation of veterinary schools (graduation from which is in turn presuppositional to licensure) is instruction in *biomedical sciences*, as well as substantial research activities in the sciences. And, whereas the defense against malpractice used to be consonance with the practices of one's peers, more and more one must refer to veterinary textbooks, which are of course science-based.

In other words, veterinary practitioners are chartered by society to be scientifically and evidentially based. One cannot open a veterinary school based in voodoo and expect accreditation, that is, social acceptance. Plainly, society expects veterinary medicine to base what it does, diagnostically and therapeutically, in science. The fact that some "non-alternative" or mainstream therapies are not scientifically and evidentially validated does not falsify or negate this claim. It simply means that medicine needs to do better in that area. Alternative practitioners who point out that some mainstream therapies are not scientifically based, therefore they themselves do not need to be scientifically based, are in essence guilty of a classic logical fallacy known as a *tu quoque*, "you too": If I accuse you of beating your wife, and you attempt to justify that beating by saying you have seen me beat my child, that is clearly irrelevant. At most, critics may say that science-based medicine is not living up to its commitment, not that its commitment is wrong. It no more disproves the ideal of evidence-based medicine than the fact of a philandering minister disproves the validity of Christian ethics! And there is certainly much to criticize as non-evidence-based in standard veterinary practice—firing and freeze-firing of horses leaps to mind.

What, in essence, is science-based or evidence-based medicine? Are not anecdotal reports of cures evidence? Don't positive results count as evidence? Unfortunately not. Think of all the people who prayed for a leukemia cure for a member of their family and, lo and behold, the person was cured. Do we count these stories? If we do, we must count the stories of all those who prayed for a cure and there was no cure! There are myriad forms of observer bias, from the Rosenthal effect (Rosenthal, 1966), where people have been shown to find what they are told to expect, to wishful thinking. And physicians and veterinarians are not exempt from these human frailties, and they are as prone to them as anyone else.

It is for these reasons that the notion of objective, randomized, double-blind clinical trials was developed: To get results that are as objective as humans can get; to remove bias, self-interest, expectations and other deforming variables; to put medicine on a firm and repeatable foundation. Such trials are the "gold standard" of proof. Clearly, suspected clinical advances often occur prior to such trials (else we wouldn't know what to test!), but we should always aim at gold standard confirmation before we put a therapeutic modality into general use. This is not a way of singling out so-called alternative medicine; it is a rule that should be applied to all therapies that remain untested even in mainstream medicine. This is in fact a major component of what it *means* for medicine to be science- and evidence-based.

Another component is equally important. To be taken seriously, a therapeutic modality needs to be logically compatible with empirical verification and, ideally, compatible with scientific knowledge we currently have. An example of a modality that is excluded by the former is talking to the souls of animals to learn how to treat them (which some people profess to be able to do). This is logically unverifiable, for what would count as evidence for such a claim, our not even knowing what a soul is or if there are any! An example of a modality excluded by the latter is homeopathy, wherein substances are diluted to the point that they cannot be biologically active according to the known laws of biochemistry. It is, of course, always possible that we are wrong about the laws, but not terribly likely. Thus it should not take Herculean experimental efforts to disprove something like homeopathy.

In sum, if for no other reason than that society expects medicine to be science- and evidence-based, and charters veterinary medicine accordingly, it is a violation of veterinary medicine's moral obligation to society to do otherwise. This principle holds equally for unproven "accepted" treatment modalities as for "alternative" ones, and should not be seen or used as a cudgel to preferentially assault putative therapies coming from any given source, unless those therapies are fundamentally untestable or totally incompatible with what we consider certain in modern science, though even in the latter case we should keep a bit of an open mind (vide the Michelson-Morley experiment).

Thus, with regard to veterinary moral obligations to society, it is wrong to promulgate unverified, non-evidence-based therapies. Let us now consider the veterinarian's obligation to his or her peers and the profession, and address the issue of unverified therapies in terms of that question.

We have seen that society expects medical professionals to base their activities on science-based, empirically validated modalities. But perhaps society is in the process of changing its mind, or is inconsistent in its demands. After all, the American Medical Association reports that consumers are spending billions of dollars on alternative modalities, the NIH is mandated to explore alternative medicine, the Canadian government allotted $100 million (Cd.) to the study of alternatives, so why shouldn't veterinary practitioners cash in on this trend, given that clients request it?

I see no moral problem in studying, in a controlled double blind way, putative modalities, so I applaud NIH and Canada's approach. Indeed, I would like to see more money allocated to the testing of conventional therapies taken for granted but not empirically verified as well as more novel "alternatives." After all, pharmaceutical companies have for decades used ethno-pharmacologists to search for empirical treatments deployed in primitive cultures. There is good evidence that animals seek out therapeutic (and even intoxicating!) biologicals, and "primitive" people are as intelligent as (and more observant!) than we are. Furthermore, there are bound to be some excellent insights and nuggets in a society like China, with a sophisticated cultural history and a five thousand-year-old history of medicine. By all means, test these modalities. My only objection is to accepting them uncritically because they are old or "natural" (so is cyanide!) or Asian.

The problem is that veterinary practitioners are not equipped to test effectively modalities of any sort, so they must rely on research institutions to do so. All most practitioners ideally can do is prescribe on the basis of solid scientific evidence, which is of course not always or yet there. So one can argue that veterinarians should wait until the evidence is in before prescribing unproven modalities. But the question arises again, why not rely on clinical judgment, anecdote, and so on if no harm is done and if a modality seems plausible?

The answer is that all these can be wrong, unrealized harm may be done, and what seems plausible may not be. It seems plausible that acupuncture is likelier to have some effect on lower back pain rather than on nausea, but the opposite is the case! Using an untested modality may have unsuspected side or long-term effects, and it has the immediate effect of precluding a tested one.

The real problem with a "What the hell, let's try it without evidence" approach is that it opens the floodgates to anyone taking that approach, from Christian faith healers to voodoo priests to purveyors of snake oil. The only way of demarcating unproven from proven, as we have seen, is controlled study. If veterinarians abandon controlled study, why should they enjoy a special position in treating animals? If veterinarians use acupuncture in an unverified way, to which science is irrelevant, why not have "acupuncture specialists" treating animals; why not witch doctors; why not chiropractors (who already have demonstrated designs on treating animals); why not anyone who has an anecdote about any sort of modality, including the power of prayer!

The point is that it is wrong vis-à-vis a veterinarian's obligation to the profession to use or advocate unproven therapies because such use or advocacy implicitly erodes the special status of veterinarians in society. To abandon scientific proof and evidence and replace it with anecdote, attestations, and clinical judgment is to create a situation of medical anarchy, and invite a world in which solid empirical verification has no pride of place, and a DVM degree is nothing special, as there are then no rational grounds for excluding Doctors of Voodoo Medicine from treating animals, or even spiritual healers who treat damaged souls. And this works against the hard battle for scientific credibility and respectability that veterinarians have fought (and largely won) in the twentieth century.

It is important to realize that medical anarchy is not in and of itself absurd. One could argue that we should let everyone practice whatever they wish without constraint and let the market decide. Such a situation was in fact obtained in human medicine during the nineteenth and early twentieth centuries. The problem is that most veterinarians do not realize this anarchism is the logical outcome of freewheeling use of unproven modalities, and they would not in fact endorse that outcome, since it denigrates veterinary medicine to just one voice in a cacophony of competing hucksters. More to the point, most veterinarians do in fact believe that scientific medicine is in the end superior and would reject anarchism not only because it harms veterinary medicine, but also—and primarily—because of the incalculable harm and suffering anarchism would bring the unfortunate animals treated by unproven—and nonfunctional—modalities!

Thus, we are forced to say, as regards veterinarians' obligations to their peers and to the profession, that the use and advocacy of unproven therapies is largely morally unacceptable, as it plays into the hands of those who would undermine the hard-won authority and credibility of veterinary medicine in society and inexorably leads to a loss of quality control in medicine. I am morally certain that even many clients who demand alternative therapies from a veterinarian would see the power in the medical anarchy argument and would not want to see science-based veterinary medicine in free competition with every conceivable outrageous approach to treating animals. Thus, one should approach the dispensing of non-proven and non-evidence-based therapies with clear understanding of its implications for the status (and well-being) of the profession, and should realize that, if one universalizes using unproven therapies whenever one feels like it, the inevitable outcome is totally unfettered relativism, for we have ignored and debased the hard-edged criterion separating scientific medicine from unconfirmed speculation.

The next set of morally relevant considerations we must deploy in assessing the morality of medical practice not based in hard evidence is the effect of such practice on animals, the direct object of the veterinary art. Ultimately, in my view, the primary moral obligation of a veterinarian is to the animal. And, in my experience, the overwhelming majority of veterinarians would affirm that obligation. While the client legally "owns" the animal, charters the veterinarian's services, and pays the bills (society not yet seeing fit to guarantee animal health), the veterinarian's duty is to do his or her best to heal the animal or to relieve its suffering; dealing with the client, keeping the client happy, is a "necessary evil," to put it harshly. As Plato says, and we quoted earlier, the fundamental function of a shepherd is to protect and improve the sheep under his aegis; his role of wage earner is secondary to that mission. Hence our shock and revulsion at equine caretakers who hurt the animals for insurance money.

Ultimately, when I have asked veterinarians whether they perceive their role as being *ideally* more like a garage mechanic, doing whatever the car owner wishes, or more like a pediatrician, working for the child's well-being regardless, in the end, of what the parents want, the answer is overwhelmingly pediatrician for pet practitioners, and, in many cases, even for food animal practitioners working for husbandry agriculturalists such as western ranchers when dealing with sick calves.

So what issues does using unproven therapies on a sick or suffering animal raise? The most obvious issue is the following: Should one use an unproven therapeutic modality when there is a modality available that is safe and efficacious? The answer is simple —one obviously uses what is known to work! As one of my veterinary pain specialist friends put it to me bluntly: "If a client demands some unproven alternative for pain control, for example, post-surgically, when there is a known effective treatment, such as an opiate analgesic, it is grossly immoral to use something unproven that might not work." He might have added "no matter what the client wants." After all, the client is coming to you for your expertise, not to tell you what to do. It is as absurd for the client to dictate therapy as it is for a family member of a sick baby to tell an internist, "Why don't you try Dr. Sleaze's Snake Oil."

While it is neither necessary nor desirable to antagonize a client, there is nothing wrong with firmly explaining the difference between proven and unproven therapy and what the distinction is based on. In fact, the more clients understand about this difference, the more they comprehend scientific validation, the more likely they are not to pester you with anecdotes of the form, "So and so said her dog had cancer and mudpacks fixed it." But in any such discussion, you need to make clear that the fundamental principle of all medical ethics is "Do no harm"; that you operate always with the best interest of the animal in mind and following a given unsubstantiated rumor about miracle therapy is not in the best interests of the animal.

What if the client says, "What harm will it do to try this anecdotally based therapy?" The answer depends on the circumstances. Most obviously, we need to know that the treatment does indeed do no harm. Sprinkling holy water into the dog's water dish is unlikely to do any damage. But stopping antibiotic therapy for an animal with a major infection where the pathogen is susceptible to antibiotics in favor of holy water or untested herbs is clearly harmful and thus wrong. But what if no one knows the effect and the client is willing to use the alternative modality she heard about as an adjunct to what you are doing, that is, to established therapy, or when there is nothing left to treat with that is evidence-based? There I believe the veterinarian should look into possible dangers of the therapy, and discourage trying it if there is any possible risk and no known benefit. If I am reasonably certain the therapy will do no harm, I would continue to work with the client to help monitor the animal's condition and make sure that "wishful thinking" on the client's part is not selectively ignoring untoward effects.

It is important not to lose oversight over the animal so that you can be vigilant for negative changes. I would personally be careful not to profit directly from an unproven therapy, but it is legitimate to charge for one's time monitoring the animal. Whatever one decides to do, it is usually wisest to tell the client the truth as you see it, including making the point that the animal may get better after treatment without the treatment having had anything to do with it! We should help the client understand the *post hoc, ergo proctor hoc* fallacy, namely that just because B follows A, it does not mean that A caused B. Many conditions just resolve, and only well-controlled double blind studies can conclusively demonstrate causality.

For the animal's sake, one should not sever a working relationship with a client. As mentioned, the problem of medical professionals monitoring therapies that are unproven has arisen for the pediatric community, who are often faced with situations where clients are (understandably) desperate to try anything after all conventional therapies have failed. To assure that the animal comes to no harm, the veterinarian must be even more skillful than the pediatrician in displaying sensitivity to the client and in deploying Aesculapian authority, as animals do not have the legal protection children do. In our last section, we referred to the American Academy of Pediatrics guidelines on dealing with parents who choose alternative therapies. As we saw, these provide suggestions for helping desperate clients and for clinician action when people do choose alternative modalities.

By following these suggestions, the veterinary clinician can give primacy to the well-being of the animal, yet avoid alienating the client who ultimately captains the animal's fate.

The next category of moral problems we must address concerning unproven therapies relates to the veterinarian's moral obligations to the client. In the end this is probably the most difficult moral area to deal with, as clients can well stand in the way of effective treatment for animals, however much they "love" them. Ultimately, in the eyes of the law the owners have virtually complete control over their animals, with the exception of the laws barring overt cruelty and outrageous neglect. Owners may choose not to treat sick animals, may choose to euthanize a sick animal, may opt for any bizarre therapy they choose including—I have actually seen this—a veterinarian who allegedly talks to animals' souls asking when they wish to be euthanized. This creates, of course, a major problem for veterinarians embracing the pediatrician model we mentioned earlier, because the clinician does not have the power of law behind him or her in the way a pediatrician does. The pediatrician can go to court to force treatment, prevent demented treatment not in the interest of the child, and, of course, parents cannot elect euthanasia.

So, although veterinarians may see their role as analogous to pediatricians, society (that is, the legal system) has not yet caught up with the ethic underlying that view, though many if not most members of society would probably agree with it. It is for this reason that veterinary medicine is even more of a "people profession" than human medicine—one's power to act as an animal advocate depends on the power of persuasion and the ability to deploy one's Aesculapian authority successfully.

Aesculapian authority is probably the veterinarian's most powerful tool for getting clients to act in the best interest of the animal. But there are two ways that this authority can fail. In the first place, a veterinarian can deploy it in favor of unproven therapies, where a proven therapy exists. In my view, this is clearly immoral, given what we have said about obligation to the animal and obligation to society to be science-based.

The harder case is when the client is imbued with an ideology refractory to a veterinarian's Aesculapian authority. To take a simple example, consider a suffering cancer animal where there are no options except euthanasia. Despite many veterinarians' opinion that euthanasia decisions should be left up to the client, there are cases where the client refuses to let go, preferring to try myriad unproven therapies. In such a case, as we have discussed earlier, I believe the veterinarian should do whatever it takes to end the animal's suffering, and pull out all stops to persuade the owner to euthanize, even exceeding the safe limit to pain control, if in your judgment the animal has no positive quality of life left.

The harder case is when the owner is fundamentally committed to alternative medicine as a world view that is "natural," "holistic," "new age," based in "the wisdom of the East," and so on. For example, when I published a paper with Dr. Dave Ramey defending evidence-based medicine (Ramey and Rollin, 2001), I received some nasty missives from animal rights-oriented colleagues, who were good solid scientists, castigating me for embracing science. "You of all people," wrote one such person, "who has criticized scientific ideology for ignoring ethics and animal pain, should not be embracing a view that requires scientific evidence for therapies, because that leads to more animal suffering in virtue of the need for experimentation." In my response, I pointed out that evidence can be achieved through clinical trials, and that not all evidence requires hurting animals or making them sick. Equally important, I pointed out that using unproven therapies can lead to enormous animal suffering *if they don't work*! In the 1980s, I saw "true believers" do surgical wet labs on animals using acupuncture (after sedating and strapping the animal down); they convinced themselves that anesthesia was adequate, yet to the rest of us it was clear that the animals were feeling pain! I also pointed out that criticizing bad aspects of science does not also entail rejecting the whole package.

I'm not sure how to deal with such ideologues (who often are highly intelligent and well educated), except to give them a quick primer on why evidence-based therapy is superior to speculation, and how your moral commitment to animals forces you to choose evidence-based medicine. If they insist on pursuing a path leading to harm to the animal, you should, I believe, resist this as forcefully as you can.

Equally problematic with such ideologues or even with ordinary clients is the situation where evidence-based medicine has been exhausted, the animal is not suffering, but clients refuse to give up because they have heard or read or seen on the Net that magnets or chiropractic or homeopathy work for this condition, and they want you to try it. Although you are convinced the therapy will do no harm, you are also convinced it will do no good.

We must recall that useless therapies often do harm by sapping resources, substituting for validated therapies, keeping up false hope, and so on. Further, claims that a therapy *may* work, if only as a placebo, may have some validity in human medicine, but are hard to believe about animals (though Dr. Frank McMillan has ingeniously argued that there are conceivable mechanisms by which placebos could sometimes be operative in veterinary medicine [McMillan 1999]). Interestingly enough, a recent paper on placebos in human medicine that appeared in the *New England Journal of Medicine* has argued, by looking at placebo-based studies, that there *is no placebo effect*, except in one area of pain, presumably because of the psychological dimension of pain (Hrobjartsson and Gotzsche, 2001)!

In any event, what does a veterinarian do if a client demands essentially harmless but probably worthless therapy? I think the best one can do is articulate one's reasons for rejecting the therapy in question, but, as the pediatric guidelines cited above suggest, one should not relinquish the client (and the animal) totally to the alternative therapist. The veterinarian should continue to work with the client, in part to help assure that they are not financially bled by unscrupulous practitioners of alternatives, and in part to keep the client focused on objective milestones that signify efficacy or lack thereof.

The final ethical category relevant to our discussions is the veterinarian's obligation to himself or herself. Here the issue is straightforward. A practitioner must vector into all such decisions his or her own comfort with a therapy. If he or she is uncomfortable in working with a non-evidence-based chiropractor or holistic healer in situations where it appears that little harm can be done, he or she should not do so but perhaps could refer the client to another practitioner who will monitor the therapy. On the other hand, if he or she is extremely persuaded of the safety and efficacy of a new but unproven modality, for which one can see a reasonable theoretical basis and has reasonable evidence that it will do no harm, he or she can proceed with it, provided one explains to the client that this attempt is experimental and unproven, obtains informed consent, and, most important, does not profit more than breaking even from the attempt. If one does this, however, one should be cognizant of the singular lack of power of such an experiment and should, if one does get encouraging results, do all one can to get the modality tested in a proper experimental setting.

In conclusion, we have seen that a variety of ethical vectors militate in favor of veterinarians depending on evidence-based medicine. It is what society has chartered you for; it provides the animal with the best chance of cure or control of pain and suffering; it best meets the client's ultimate desire for the animal to get better; it secures the profession's status as based in empirical verification. In limited cases, one can deviate from these prima facie moral commitments, but this should not be done cavalierly or for profit.

Part II

Cases

Introduction

By now the reader should have garnered a sense of the richness and complexity of theoretical moral issues found in veterinary medicine. I have devoted the most attention to issues of animal ethics, both because the moral status of animals represents the fundamental question of veterinary medical ethics and because so little ethics (both $ethics_1$ and $ethics_2$) is devoted to animal issues in ordinary life.

In Part II of this book, I present a compendium of real-life ethically charged situations that veterinary practioners in a variety of areas and fields have found challenging and have been kind enough to share with their colleagues through the ethics column in the *Canadian Veterinary Journal.* I hope these scenarios will help stir readers' moral thoughts about situations they may encounter, and I am very grateful to all the veterinarians who sent in these examples, as well as to those who have written to say that, like medical histories, these ethics cases are excellent practice for handling real-life situations.

Case

1

Cow with Cancer Eye

Question

You examine a cow in late pregnancy that has keratoconjunctivitis, blepharospasm, and photophobia due to an ocular squamous cell carcinoma. You recommend enucleation or immediate slaughter. The owner wants to allow the cow to calve, wean the calf, and then ship the cow. He does not want to invest in surgery for a cow that will soon calve.

Is it ethically correct for the cow to be left untreated for several months?

Response

For this case to represent a genuinely difficult challenge for a veterinarian, one must assume that it is not in the economic interest of the farmer to treat the cow, as, for example, it would be if the untreated eye were to eventuate in an aborted calf or if the cancer were to spread sufficiently to result in condemnation of the carcass. If the veterinarian can persuade the client that by doing good, he will also do well, the issue is resolved. With this understood, and assuming from the signs that the cow is experiencing significant pain and suffering, the case provides a classic example of what I have elsewhere called the Fundamental Question of Veterinary Medicine: Does the veterinarian have primary obligation to the animal or to the owner? Traditional consensus social ethics, being essentially silent on the treatment of animals save for proscribing overt cruelty, provides little help with this question. Similarly, traditional veterinary ethics, such as that embodied in the Veterinarian's Oath, gives no guidance in such a case, for it commits the veterinarian both to serving the client and to serving the animal, in this case two incompatible demands. Thus, for a veterinarian concerned with the animal's suffering, given these traditional approaches, the case devolves into a confrontation between the veterinarian's personal ethic and the client's personal ethic (or lack thereof) regarding one's obligation to an animal.

Currently, the social consensus ethic seems to be appropriating concern for animal pain and suffering, beyond cruelty, into its purview. Federal law in the United States, for example, now mandates control of pain and suffering in laboratory animals as part of the meaning of "adequate veterinary care," and one could argue that in virtue of such a law, amelioration of pain has become the new standard of practice. Indeed, a number of state anticruelty laws now specify adequate veterinary care as essential to proper animal husbandry. In other words, it appears that society is in the process of abandoning its laissez-faire attitude regarding animal pain, and encoding the demand for its control in public policy. Thus it is likely that, before too long, a requirement for controlling pain, and by implication, not allowing the cancer eye to go untreated, will be encoded in statute, thereby arming the concerned veterinarian with the force of law, or at least with the ability to use law as a rhetorical lever.

But what of the veterinarian currently facing this dilemma without legislative backing? Clearly he or she must attempt to find a third or middle way, a compromise, characteristic of how controversial ethical issues are resolved in a democracy. Unfortunately, the way this case is phrased deflects attention from the middle way, when it suggests that the cow must be "left untreated" if one fails to enucleate or euthanize. This is not necessarily the case. There are palliative treatments that are not as financially burdensome on the client, yet that may relieve the animal's suffering. One can simply debulk the tumor, for example, using a local block, and reduce fly irritation and attendant eye pain with a topical fly repellent. Alternatively, one can treat the animal with BCG or some other immunostimulator to cause tumor regression, again without imposing a major financial burden. One can also use one's Aesculapian authority and communication skills to attempt to persuade the client to spend the $120, perhaps suggesting extended payments if the client is indeed financially pressed. Perhaps the client is not aware of the extent to which the animal is suffering and, if made aware, will soften his position. Reminding the client of the profound nature of human ocular pain may shame him into concern. As a last resort, one can offer to do the surgery at cost.

If the veterinarian has indeed pursued all these avenues, then he or she is morally blameless, even if the client remains intransigent. As Kant pointed out, we are morally obligated to do only that which we are capable of doing. If the veterinarian has done everything possible short of donating the surgery, something veterinarians will often do but cannot be morally obliged to do, he or she has done all that could be morally demanded. The animal's owner, however, is patently blameworthy; one should not leave a suffering animal untreated. Thus veterinarians should embrace social and legal change mandating control of animal suffering, for only through this avenue can their authority be made commensurate with their responsibility.

Case

2

Substandard Husbandry for Sheep

Question

You examine a lamb for anorexia on a small farm you visit once or twice a year. It weighs 35 kg, is emaciated, covered in sheep keds, and pregnant. There are approximately twenty other sheep on the farm in a similar state of ill health. The owner wants you to treat only the "sick" lamb. Despite repeated suggestions over the years the quality of animal husbandry on the farm has not improved.

Is it ethically correct to do as the farmer wishes and leave this sheep flock to a substandard level of husbandry?

Response

This case illustrates an important point often neglected in discussions of ethics, namely, that every ethical decision need not involve a dilemma, with the morally conscientious agent being pulled in two incompatible directions. As has often been remarked, food animal practitioners frequently face dilemmas arising out of obligations to the client's economic interests conflicting with obligations to the animals. The cancer eye case already discussed contained elements of this sort of tension.

The present case, however, contains no such conflicting obligations. The veterinarian's duty to the client as business owner necessarily involves assuring that the health of the individual animal and the herd as a whole is sufficient to assure normal production. This of course entails proper nutrition, husbandry, hygiene, and management. The veterinarian's duty to the animals also entails doing everything in his or her power to assure at least the same level of health, and very probably an even higher one. But, in any event, the interests of the economically rational producer and the interests of the animals coincide regarding the health and welfare of the animals in this case. Furthermore, for a stockman to fail to provide proper care at least at this level is in violation of public policy (social morality) as embodied in the laws, as some readers have pointed out.

Thus the veterinarian's obligations to owner, animal, and society coincide in this case.

The only question that remains is whether or not to report the farmer to the appropriate agency. Such a course of action is certainly justified by the case. Alternatively, some veterinarians will use the threat of reporting cruelty (or neglect) as a lever to make the client provide proper care for the animals. Which tack to take would depend on the veterinarian's knowledge of and relationship to the client. If the client is irrational, the legal route may be the only recourse. If the client is simply sloppy, ignorant, or lazy, the threat alone, coupled with a list of remedial steps for the client to take, may be enough to rectify the situation, especially when the client eventually sees that he fares better economically by doing the right thing.

Case

3

Fracture Fixation

Question

You take a job in a high-quality small animal practice in a Toronto suburb; they perform internal fixation on all long-bone fractures. A father and his eight-year-old daughter bring you a kitten that they were given two months ago. The father accidentally stepped on the kitten, and you can palpate a fracture of the tibia. The kitten is bright and alert and seems in little pain but carries the leg. You advise the client of the condition and that the standard procedure for surgical correction of the fracture has a success rate of around 98 percent and will cost approximately $300. The father cannot afford such a bill. You have had moderate success (85 percent) with such fractures in your previous job using Thomas splints and charged only $75.

Is it ethically correct to offer only the internal fixation option to the client?

Response

Most veterinarians agree that it is not ethically acceptable to withhold an account of any viable option from a client, and an 85 percent success rate certainly represents a viable option. There are other elements of the case that are worth pursuing. We have been told that the father accidentally caused the injury by stepping on the animal. Let us further presume from the facts of the case that the kitten is, at least nominally, the child's animal. Does the father feel some guilt over his role in inflicting the injury? Though it was an accident, does he feel that he should have been more careful? Correlatively, does the child resent or blame the father? If either of these conditions obtains, it would presumably be very important to the family to provide the best possible treatment for the animal, and "settling" for the splinting might leave unresolved familial tension in the event the procedure was not totally successful. If the veterinarian sensed or determined that such a situation existed, it might behoove him or her to allow the client the option of extended payments—$75 to be paid now, the remainder over a period of some months. Many veterinarians of my acquaintance do make such financial arrangements in special circumstances. I would stress that a veterinarian is certainly not morally obliged to offer such an arrangement; rather, that in certain cases, it might provide an alternate route for choosing the highest-quality medical option. If, as the facts suggest, the veterinarian is working in an upscale practice, such cases should be relatively rare.

Case

4

Farmer Using Illegal Growth Promotant

Question

While examining calves in a veal unit, you find that the owner gives all calves in the room a hormone implant for beef cattle, which he grinds up, mixes with tetracycline, and injects subcutaneously in all calves. This procedure was recommended by a feed salesman several years ago and greatly improved rate of gain. You advise the farmer that this preparation is not approved for use in veal calves in any form, let alone by the method employed here. The farmer says he knows that, but everyone does it, no one has ever been caught, and without it he can't compete in the marketplace.

Is it ethically correct to ignore this situation?

Response

In order to comment sensibly on this case, one must make certain assumptions. I assume for the sake of discussion that the procedure in question causes no pain or suffering to the animals, nor does it otherwise compromise their welfare. Thus one can exclude any ethical component regarding obligations of the veterinarian to the animal. Furthermore, since the veterinarian neither recommended nor sanctioned, but merely happened to discover, this farmer's hormonal regimen, no issues arise regarding the veterinarian's engaging in extralabel drug use. The issue that remains seems to be one of "whistle-blowing," analogous to riding as a passenger in a friend's car when the friend sideswipes another car in a parking lot and simply drives on. In both cases, the problem is that an illegal act has occurred to which one is witness but not party. Is one then morally obliged to turn the perpetrator in to the authorities?

Cases wherein whistle-blowing may be called for are often highly ambivalent. In the first place, they may well involve conflicting moral principles. On the one hand, attempting to effect a cessation of illegal behavior is certainly a morally praiseworthy goal in general. On the other hand, "squealing" is also viewed as morally contemptible and may create a very uncomfortable situation for the informer—losing a friend, for example.

These antithetical pulls make for a difficult moral situation that most of us have experienced even in grade school—we know someone is cheating on a test and thus compromising the grading process, yet we are reluctant to be a "tattletale." Usually, this dilemma is resolved by appeal to how serious the consequences are likely to be if one does not blow the whistle. Thus few of us would feel any disapproval for someone who informs the authorities that a chemical factory is polluting a river or calls the police regarding a drunk driver. (Case 2 describes such a case, when a farmer is failing to provide minimal husbandry for his lambs.)

Thus, in this case, the first thing the veterinarian must decide is whether the illegal practice can have serious consequences that justify blowing the whistle and possibly compromising his own credibility with this and other farmers. (One would not, presumably, blow the whistle on a client who violated laws against posting billboards.) Here, however, the infraction is nontrivial, as no data exist on dangers to the humans consuming the meat produced by way of this illegal regimen. It is very possible—indeed likely—that subcutaneous administration of the hormone could greatly increase absorption by the animal and thus increase concentration of the hormone in the tissues. In a society morally committed to food safety, short-cutting safety checks for the sake of profit is unacceptable; thus the infraction is significant and should not be ignored.

The second important empirical question to be resolved by the veterinarian is whether this illegal and possibly dangerous shortcut is indeed widely or even universally used in the industry. If not, if the producer is an isolated exception, there will be less pressure on the veterinarian not to blow the whistle. Indeed, if the veterinarian does it with a minimum of fuss, other farmers are likely to be grateful to him or her for dealing with it quickly and quietly; the potential for scandal and bad publicity in an already besieged industry should be obvious to all.

The mere threat of exposure by the veterinarian, accompanied perhaps by peer pressure, may suffice to cause the farmer to stop if the practice is not widespread. If, however, the problem is industry wide and a farmer cannot compete without engaging in the same practice, the situation is more difficult. In such a case less pressure exists on the individual veterinarian to blow the whistle, but more accrues to organized veterinary medicine to educate and/or confront the veal industry on the issue of public health to which veterinarians are professionally committed. Unilaterally reporting the individual farmer will only create a scapegoat and not really address the major issue, and is likely to damage the veterinarian's effectiveness with the agricultural community. This is not to say that the veterinarian should simply shrug and walk away; rather, he or she should seek peer assistance in addressing the pervasive and unacceptable practice. The moral burden is then shared by the veterinary community.

I am grateful to the following veterinarians for dialogue regarding this case: Drs. Tony Knight, Bob Mortimer, and Ken Odde.

Case

5

Client Sells Known BVD Shedders

Question

You are working with a farmer to eradicate bovine virus diarrhea from his herd. You identify several chronic shedders among some of his better cows and recommend that these be shipped to slaughter. Several days later you find that he has sold these cows to another of your clients without advising him that the cows have been identified as significant risks for transmitting bovine virus diarrhea.

Is it ethically correct to maintain client confidentiality in such a case?

Response

This case represents a genuine dilemma. On the one hand, although there are no legal bases for confidentiality in veterinary medicine as there are in law or human medicine, the sort of trust that confidentiality assures is presuppositional to the very possibility of effective veterinary practice. If clients do not believe that what a veterinarian may see or hear in the course of a professional visit will remain confidential, they will naturally be reluctant to employ such an individual, to provide relevant information freely, or to trust that veterinarian. Thus, in the case at hand, if the veterinarian attempts to help the second client by informing him that the cows he bought are viral shedders and thus sources of potential infection to his other cattle, the veterinarian is revealing knowledge he or she acquired while in a position of trust with the first client. Even worse, that revelation will very likely harm the first client financially, in terms of reputation, or both.

On the other hand, failure to inform the second client of the fact that the animals are infected will likely have grave consequences for the remainder of his herd. Not only will the innocent client suffer economic damage, which can be controlled if he is informed expeditiously, the animals in his herd that are subject to the infection will suffer as well. So there is, upon examination, a question here of the veterinarian's obligation to the animals. There is also a public health or epidemiological dimension to this case; BVD is difficult enough to control when everyone is cooperating. Allowing people to salt other herds with infected animals negates the diligent efforts of the veterinarian and other veterinarians in the area who have judiciously worked toward its eradication and control.

It appears that in this case we have a general moral principle—respect confidentiality—at loggerheads with the fairly unique circumstances of a particular case. Thus we should recall that all moral principles are presumptive, not unconditional. To use a familiar example, those of us who believe strongly in freedom of speech would not use that principle to justify shouting "Fire!" in a crowded theater or to justify divulging troop movements that can endanger our soldiers during a war. To be sure, strong burden of proof is on one who wishes to abrogate the principle in a given case, but, as the previous examples indicate, we are all familiar with circumstances wherein this occurs.

Do the special circumstances of this case justify overriding the general principle of veterinarian-client confidentiality? I believe they do. In the first place, failure of the veterinarian to act is very likely to result in significant harm to innocents, that is, the second client and his herd. That in itself, of course, would not suffice to override the principle of confidentiality, for keeping of confidences often results in harm, as when a reporter refuses to divulge his sources on an issue like illegal drug traffic, even though disclosure might lead to curtailing the drug flow. But there is a second point operative here, which tips the scales: The first client has sold the cattle with full knowledge of the possible consequences, wantonly ignoring the veterinarian's advice. He has not made an honest mistake but callously disregarded the welfare of the buyer and his animals, the efforts of the veterinarian to limit the disease, the epidemiological consequences of his selfish action, and so on. In short, he has acted in a grossly immoral way.

In the face of the unequivocally immoral nature of these actions, the veterinarian's obligations to the second client, to animal welfare, and to public health seem to me to trump the confidentiality, for maintenance of confidentiality would be tantamount to collusion in gross immorality. If I were the veterinarian, I would therefore inform the second client of the fact that he had purchased shedders. Before doing so, however, I would contact the first client, explain my position, and give him the opportunity to rectify his misdeed. I would also point out that were I called upon to testify in a lawsuit, I would have to say that I had identified those animals to him as shedders. I would not worry about losing such a client, nor would I worry about my reputation in the community, as the majority of the public would support the disclosure. I do not think that the other clients would lose faith in my ability to keep a confidence, as the mitigating circumstances would accord with the general ethical intuition to protect the innocent from the predatory.

I thank Dr. A.P. Knight for stimulating dialogue.

Case

6

Client Requests Dog Euthanasia Because She Is Moving

Question

A woman brings you her five-year-old cocker spaniel for euthanasia. She is not a regular client of yours, and you ask why she wants the dog destroyed. She says she is moving into an apartment with her boyfriend, he doesn't like the dog, and pets aren't allowed in the apartment building. You ask if she has tried to put up the dog for adoption, but she replies it is none of your business. She simply wants the dog humanely destroyed, and if you don't euthanize it, her boyfriend will shoot it.

Is it ethically correct to euthanize the dog?

Response

This case represents one of the most profoundly disturbing and difficult problems that can confront the companion animal practitioner—the demand that he or she kill a healthy animal for trivial or no reasons. As one of the originators of the symposium on pet-owner grief held at the Columbia University College of Physicians and Surgeons in 1981, I was amazed to discover that most of the many veterinarians attending the conference were at least as interested in discussing their own grief, arising out of the incessant client demand for "convenience euthanasia," as they were in exploring approaches to client grief. A similar grief phenomenon occurs among humane society workers who perform regular euthanasia of unwanted healthy animals. The stress associated with such activity is profound and non-trivial and can result in mental and physical health problems, substance abuse, familial problems, and so on. Unlike other stresses, the stress associated with euthanasia is not easily dealt with by standard devices for "stress management," for it is a paradigm case of what I have elsewhere called "moral stress" (Rollin, 1986), that is, stress arising out of radical dissonance between what one finds oneself doing (killing healthy animals) and one's foundational reasons for entering veterinary medicine (or humane work)—caring for animals, preserving their health, lives, and well-being, treating them as objects of moral concern and not disposable personal property to be trashed at will.

I have further argued that the only viable mechanism for alleviating this moral stress is to be able to feel that one has done *everything possible* to resist or change this pernicious social tendency, and to save the animal's life—a position confirmed to me by many veterinarians and human workers. Only in this way can one check the stress-inducing guilt that inevitably accompanies doing that which one thinks is fundamentally wrong.

Thus, I would argue that most veterinarians find euthanizing a healthy animal for owner convenience contrary not only to their ethical view of a veterinarian's obligation to an animal, but also to their view of a veterinarian's obligation to society (veterinarians are significantly morally opposed to perpetuating the view of animals as disposable trash), and to their obligations to themselves (veterinarians are obliged to alleviate the destructive effects of stresses, and a fortiori *moral* stresses). Thus all of these moral considerations converge in the same direction—it is not, prima facie, ethically acceptable to euthanize the animal.

But what is the alternative? The client has already refused to discuss adoption and has further threatened to shoot the animal if the veterinarian refuses to euthanize it.

As most morally concerned veterinarians will attest, this sort of case exemplifies the need for the veterinarian to serve as an animal advocate, as a spokesperson for the animal, a role for which veterinary schools have not typically prepared them. Nonetheless, veterinarians often find themselves quite literally negotiating for the animal's life, and doing it with consummate skill. One veterinarian told me of a similar case in which she used a combination of Aesculapian authority (jargon for the profound authority that any physician or veterinarian possesses in virtue of being able to cure and heal), and shame and guilt to persuade the client to allow her to adopt the animal out. Though this was not a regular client, the veterinarian nonetheless responded to her impassioned and accusatory rhetoric: "I did not go to school for ten years and make great personal sacrifice and go many thousands of dollars in debt to murder healthy animals. How dare you make such a request! This animal could be a fine companion to some family. After all the love he gave you, don't you at least owe him a chance?" In a few moments she had used her skill as a natural psychologist, won over the client, and picked a strategy that worked. This would, of course, be a much easier task with a regular client, when the veterinarian knows the person, the animal, and what rhetorical ploy is likely to work.

Were I the veterinarian in this case, I would adopt a similar strategy: "What do you mean, it's not my business? I have spent my whole life trying to save animal life—of course it is my business. And it is my business if your boyfriend plans to shoot it, because such an action is very likely legally actionable under the cruelty laws." Correlative to their animal advocacy, many veterinarians maintain lists of people willing to adopt an animal, or to provide at least a foster home. Still others will offer to hold the animal in a clinic kennel for a day at no cost to let the client reconsider.

But what if the client is intransigent? Many veterinarians will simply refuse and tell the client to try another veterinarian, the humane society, or a pound. But, as my veterinary students are quick to point out, this is passing the buck. One student suggested that one must deal with evil, not fob it off on others. On the other hand, if one is truly convinced, on the basis of reasonable evidence, not rationalization, that the dog will suffer a far worse fate if one doesn't euthanize—if, for example, one genuinely believes that the demented owner would throw it out of a moving car or drown it—it would surely be morally justifiable vis-à-vis one's obligation to the animal to euthanize it, provided one can truly believe one has done everything possible to save it.

It is in the face of the latter proviso that many veterinarians choose a dangerous and controversial avenue—agreeing to euthanize the animal and then failing to do so. Although such a recourse is patently actionable, and renders one open to litigation, veterinarians who choose such an avenue often appeal to a legitimate moral principle—it is permissible to perpetrate a relatively minor wrong (breaking a contract) in order to prevent a greater wrong (killing a healthy animal). Such veterinarians of my acquaintance have literally perceived their actions as analogous to that of manning an Underground Railway for rescuing slaves, and they will go to great lengths to adopt the animal out in a remote location so as to minimize the chance of being caught. I do not view such "conscientious objection" as morally required of a veterinarian; on the other hand, I do not find such actions blameworthy, either.

Case

7

Farmer Requests a Fetotomy

Question

A registered Hereford heifer is having problems calving. The calf is too big for the heifer, and the calf is alive. When you tell the producer that a caesarean section will be required, he declines. He has had only one previous caesarean section and both the cow and the calf died. He is unwilling to try this option a second time. He has had two out of two heifers live following fetotomy, and he is firm in this viewpoint. It is 11:00 P.M., and he wants a fetotomy. Although you point out that the cost benefit leans in favor of a caesarean, the farmer does not wish to pursue this option.

Is it ethically correct to perform a fetotomy in this case?

Response

This case is, in some respects, similar to the case discussed earlier, wherein a farmer had failed to provide adequate husbandry for his lambs. The similarity lies in the fact that, in both cases, what the client is doing (or wishes to have done) is contrary both to his own interests and to the interests relevant to animal welfare. Thus the first point of attack for the veterinarian is to explain the economic and cost/benefit dimensions to the client in clear terms. The cost to the client of the caesarean section and the fetotomy are comparable, somewhere between \$85 and \$125 for both. (Note that all figures are based on Colorado prices.) Indeed, if the fetotomy requires many cuts, it may well be more expensive than the caesarean. At the same time, the fetotomy virtually assures a live cow and a dead calf (though fetotomies can also occasionally result in a dead cow). The caesarean, assuming the veterinarian intercedes at the correct time, virtually assures a live cow (I am told that only one in one thousand fail, assuming that the client has not waited too long), and also a live calf, worth several hundred dollars at weaning. Thus a negligible risk is significantly balanced by a substantial benefit in the caesarean option.

It would be important to know—and, unfortunately, the case does not relate—why the previous caesarean failed and if the same veterinarian was involved. (I assume that he or she was not.) If the timing was wrong, the veterinarian can assure the client that, in this case at least, the timing is correct. The veterinarian can further stress his or her own record for success in caesarean sections.

But suppose the client is adamant and will simply not accept the caesarean option. As a fallback, the veterinarian could, in the first place, articulate his or her reasons for not wishing to do a fetotomy—quite simply, that the calf is alive, that it is likely to experience significant pain, and the cutting up of a live, healthy animal is a frankly terrible experience both for the animal and for the veterinarian. Indeed, it is paradigmatically opposed to the mission of veterinarians to ameliorate pain and save lives, and to provide a good death when those goals cannot be realized. In tandem with making these points, the veterinarian could suggest a symphysiotomy, that is, the procedure whereby one splits the pelvic bone in order to provide more space for the calf. The cost of this procedure is comparable to the other options and will virtually assure a live cow and a live calf. The problematic dimension of this option, however, is that the cow should not be bred again, as the procedure results in callus formation around the pubic bone, making dystocia even more likely in subsequent pregnancies. Thus the producer would need to be willing to cull the cow following weaning of the calf.

But suppose the client finds this option unacceptable as well, for example, if he wishes to keep the cow as a breeder. The veterinarian is now faced with performing the fetotomy or refusing to do it. (I, like many of my clinician colleagues, would not do it.) If the veterinarian elects to perform the fetotomy, the overwhelming moral imperative becomes assuring that the calf does not suffer. Although some veterinarians argue that severing the jugular and, in essence, pithing the animal with the first cut will assure a "good death," one cannot depend on this option being practicable if the calf is awkwardly positioned, nor would I feel confident in any case that the calf was not suffering. Thus, in my view, the veterinarian would be obliged to anesthetize the calf deeply prior to performing the fetotomy. I do not believe that a proposal that the veterinarian inject some euthanol into the calf is a good one, as euthanol is caustic and would itself cause pain unless injected IV, something one could not assure. A more viable solution, I believe, would be to inject enough xylazine IM into the calf to produce anesthesia. The effect on the cow would be to generate some degree of sedation, which would not cause any problems, and indeed might make it easier to perform the fetotomy. In this way the veterinarian can at least protect the calf from suffering in this unfortunate, no-win situation.

I thank Drs. Frank Garry, Bruce Heath, and Bob Mortimer for dialogue regarding this case.

Case

8

Suspected Dogfighting

Question

A pit bull terrier is brought to you for suturing of several lacerations on its face and trunk. There are many other old scars also present on the dog. You have never seen this client before, and he claims to have owned the dog only a short time and has no idea how the present lacerations occurred nor how the old scars came to be. You suspect the dog has been used for fighting, but the owner denies this.

Is it ethically correct to report this man to the humane society?

Response

This case further explores a number of issues: animal abuse, confidentiality, cruelty laws, and so on. In this instance the relevant questions are fairly straightforward. First, the veterinarian needs to know if the current lacerations are a result of the client intentionally fighting the dog. The fact that the client claims to know nothing of the dog's history and claims to have no idea of the current cause of the lacerations certainly ought to ring alarm bells in all but the most credulous. His lack of responsiveness and apparent lack of curiosity about the dog's present wounds and past history certainly hint at an unwillingness to engage the issue—most clients would at least venture guesses and possibilities, and certainly most people would at least be interested in speculating. So the first thing the veterinarian ought to attempt is subtle conversational cross-examination of the client while treating the animal. Such a gambit is likely either to confirm one's suspicions about fighting or to underscore patently the client's evasiveness. Either way, the veterinarian will have presumptive grounds for assuming that the animal has been fought, especially if fighting is endemic to the area and the client fits a demographic profile for a dogfighter.

Let us assume, then, that the veterinarian emerges from the conversation with a reasonable prima facie belief that the animal has indeed been used for fighting. The fact that the client is not a regular client militates against the veterinarian having the sort of rapport with him that would enable the veterinarian to lever the threat of cruelty reporting into making him change his behavior (see the sheep case discussed earlier).

Indeed, even if a dogfighter is a regular client, it is very unlikely that he would be amenable to persuasion of this sort, since a dogfighter must surely be aware of the illegality of dogfighting, yet chooses to continue doing it. *Thus the only real choice for the veterinarian is either to do nothing or to report the man to the humane society.*

Buttressing the first option—doing nothing—is the fact that reporting such cases often results in many lost hours for the veterinarian with little to show for it. It is well known that courts do not take cruelty cases very seriously. The veterinarian must therefore lose time from practice or family, with the end result likely being that the perpetrator emerges with a slap on the wrist—or worse, with no penalty at all. On the other hand, not only is dogfighting a paradigm case of what society considers cruel, in most locales it has been deemed extreme enough to warrant separate legislation. Thus one could argue that the veterinarian, like the pediatrician confronted with good evidence of child abuse, is morally obliged to report his or her suspicions. (Ideally, the veterinarian should be *legally* obliged to report suspected animal abuse, just as the pediatrician is legally obliged to report suspected child abuse. Indeed in California, veterinarians, as health care professionals, are ironically legally obliged to report suspected child abuse, but not animal abuse.) (See Case 41.)

As to the frustration regarding cavalier court treatment of animal abuse cases, sometimes even including dogfighting, this can be remedied. I recently heard from a veterinarian in California who had spent weeks involved with a spectacular, well-evidenced cruelty case only to see the defendant released. The veterinarian's response, gratifyingly, was not to give up on cruelty cases, but rather to galvanize the local veterinary association into undertaking a major educational thrust about cruelty, aimed at attorneys, prosecutors, judges, and the general public. He was quite confident that such an educational blitzkrieg would be successful, given the ever-increasing social concern about animal welfare. I would therefore argue that it is not only ethically permissible to report this client, it is ethically obligatory. Society has taken a clear moral stand on dogfighting; veterinarians are guardians of animal welfare; the veterinarian has reasonable grounds for making the assumption that fighting has occurred. (Note that reporting is not the same as convicting; presumably the humane society and the court will examine the case in detail.) And if the veterinarian is concerned about the anticruelty or anti-fighting laws not being taken seriously, he or she can use this case to galvanize other members of the profession. If the practitioners are concerned about violating client confidentiality by reporting suspected cruelty, the local association can adopt (and publicize) a uniform policy of reporting suspected cruelty, as the Colorado State University Veterinary Teaching Hospital did in 1987. In this way all veterinarians are bound by the consensus, and notice is served that veterinarians are committed to reporting animal cruelty and abuse.

Confidentiality should not shield flagrant immorality.

Case

9

Docking and Cropping of Dobermans

Question

A breeder of Doberman pinscher dogs moves into your practice area and asks, *Do you*

1. *Dock tails?*
2. *Crop ears?*
3. *Remove dewclaws?*
4. *Castrate?*
5. *Spay?*
6. *Debark?*
7. *Remove canine teeth from fear biters?*
8. *Tattoo?*
9. *Euthanize the "poor doers" in a litter?*
10. *Euthanize an older breeding animal when her kennel is overcrowded?*

Response

This case again raises the fundamental question of veterinary medical ethics—to whom does the veterinarian owe primary allegiance, owner or animal? The question, and the conflict it bespeaks, is ubiquitous in food animal practice and other primarily economic uses of animals; unfortunately, it also arises in companion animal practice.

In my own writings I have argued that there are two opposite ideals toward which a veterinarian can strive when confronted with this sort of question. One is to see himself or herself as analogous to a garage mechanic, who is there to do what the customer wishes. Alternatively, a veterinarian may see his or her ideal role as analogous to that of a pediatrician: Though the parent pays the bill, the pediatrician is guided by concern for the child. These extremes are, of course, ideal types; in the real world most veterinarians function in the middle, though they do tend to gravitate toward one of the two poles. I have urged veterinarians to lean toward the pediatrician model, for I have long argued that veterinarians are the natural vanguard of animal welfare. Indeed, as the new U.S.

law regarding animal experimentation shows, the public looks to veterinarians to protect the interests of animals.

Many of the procedures mentioned in this situation—for example, docking and ear cropping—are patently of no benefit to Dobermans and, indeed, cause suffering. Further, they are based in purely aesthetic and arbitrary breed standards.

Kennel clubs seem unwilling to effect change in this area, despite increasing public concern. Thus, the veterinarian is a plausible person to press forcefully for the abolition of these practices, especially in urban areas, where the client is unlikely to undertake such procedures on a tabletop if the veterinarian demurs. And the best way to press for their abolition is to refuse to do them and try to get one's local association to concur, at all times explaining one's position to the public.

Castrations and spays are in a somewhat different category. Again, there is little advantage to an animal to being sterilized—indeed, it suffers the risk and trauma of major surgery—but these procedures can help to reduce the number of animals being euthanized. There are also some health advantages to spaying and neutering, notably the elimination of pyometra and mammary tumors in older females, and the prevention of prostatic disease in older males. On the other hand, spays and neuters represent a surgical solution to a social problem. Were people responsible about companion animals, one would not need to use these procedures. Unfortunately, far more money and effort have gone into spay-neuter programs than into the public education of pet owners, and in one sense spay-neuter programs help to perpetuate owner irresponsibility. In the end, I would spay and neuter, though with some unease.

Devocalization and removal of canine teeth are again surgical solutions to behavior problems, that is, to problems arising out of poor human tutelage and management. I would recommend consultation with an animal behaviorist, if the veterinarian is not well versed in animal behavior. I would consider devocalization only if all else had failed, and I was faced with either doing it or seeing the animal euthanized.

Fear biting may indeed involve a genetic component, and may be refractory to behavioral modification. If this were the case, I would be loath to remove the canine teeth, for the biting behavior would still exist, and the animal, though less dangerous, would still not be able to participate normally in the "social contact." Euthanasia or putting the animal in a highly truncated and restricted environment might be the only solution. Since fear biters clearly do not enjoy meeting new people, the latter solution may not be as onerous as it sounds.

Tattooing and removal of dewclaws in the neonate do not appear to me to present a major infringement on the animal, and can be justified in cost-benefit terms. Tattooing is minor at any age, and removal of dewclaws is minor if performed when the animals are newborn. Both should be performed under anesthesia (either a local or in concert with a general procedure, such as spay or castration). Equally important, there may be benefit to the animal, as the tattoo provides permanent identification and can thus help a lost animal get home. Similarly, at least for some dogs, such as those who run extensively in brush, removal of dewclaws protects against painful tearing and possible infection. On the other hand, for an urban apartment-dwelling older dog, removal of the dewclaws becomes analogous to ear cropping or tail docking, so the morally concerned veterinarian needs to determine what sort of life the animal is to live before making a decision. Removal of dewclaws is a good deal more arduous for older animals than for younger ones, and I would discourage it.

Finally, the questions about euthanizing "poor doers" and older breeding animals hark back to an earlier discussion of euthanasia for owner convenience. If the "poor doer" is ill, suffering, and untreatable, and euthanasia is the only indicated solution, I would consider it acceptable. If, however, the choice of euthanasia is dictated by owner convenience, I do not view it as moral. When one orchestrates a mating, one is morally responsible to care for the progeny. Similarly, euthanizing older breeders to create space smacks too much of the garage mechanic model, and I would not find it acceptable.

It is important to stress that I have just sketched a number of strategies in this discussion; a book could be written on subtle questions and sub-questions raised in this case. Furthermore, any veterinarian can adduce examples of variations on the case that would call for different responses. It is of paramount importance, however, to stress that ethical principles do not change as cases change. Rather, *which* principles apply and to what degree they apply are a function of the facts of the case. Different cases demand different principles, but the principles themselves, like the principles of surgery, remain constant across cases.

Case

10

Leaving a Sow Untreated

Question

You are called to a five-hundred-sow farrow-to-finish swine operation to examine a problem with vaginal discharges in sows. There are three full-time employees and one manager overseeing approximately five thousand animals. As you examine several sows in the crated gestation unit, you notice one with a hind leg at an unusual angle and inquire about her status. You are told, "She broke her leg yesterday and she's due to farrow next week. We'll let her farrow in here, and then we'll shoot her and foster off her pigs."

Is it ethically correct to leave the sow with a broken leg for one week while you await her farrowing?

Response

Society seems to be evolving a new ethic for animals that accords them greater concern than they have traditionally enjoyed. But even before the advent of this increased social awareness, certain principles were well established. As far back as biblical times, for example, the idea was unequivocally endorsed that whenever one owned an animal, one was responsible for its proper husbandry, such as provision of food, water, and rest. Implicit in this ethic was also the management of disease and injury, according to the medical knowledge of the time. Such requirements were a matter of prudence and self-interest, as much as ethics; failure to meet such needs meant loss of livelihood for the farmer as much as suffering for the animal.

This traditional accord between animal interests and human interests has been eroded by the application of industrial and technological methods to agriculture for the sake of efficiency and productivity. In modern, mechanized animal agriculture, animals are cheap, machinery is expensive, profits per animal are small, and economic benefit accrues to farmers through large-scale animal production. Animal husbandry has become animal science, and concern and care for individual animals have diminished. Whereas each animal was of significant economic value in traditional agriculture, confinement agriculture emphasizes the productivity of the operation as a whole. From a veterinary point of view, demand for herd health has replaced demand for care of individual animals.

Hence the issue described in this case. The cost of veterinary treatment, and the labor cost (or time) required to move the animal out of the gestation crate into a larger area where splinting or casting the leg would be effective, led the producer to leave the broken leg untreated. In such cases economic considerations systematically militate against animal welfare. The veterinarian is caught in the middle.

This case serves to explicate the growing social concern about confinement agriculture. For, while social moral concern for individual animals is increasing, mechanized agriculture is actually retreating from even traditional concerns for individual animals. Few people in society would endorse leaving the sow's broken leg untreated for a week, and if that is where the economics of confinement agriculture leads, a clash between its values and those of society is inevitable.

Veterinarians are chartered, trained, and bound by oath to relieve individual animal suffering. In this sense confinement agriculture has hurt veterinary medicine, in that fewer veterinarians are needed to treat ever-greater numbers of animals.

How, then, should a veterinarian deal with this case? Certainly, he or she cannot accept leaving the treatable animal untreated: This flies in the face of his or her professional raison d'être. On the other hand, he or she cannot long provide such service without pay, for the veterinarian is also a wage earner. Furthermore, such altruism shifts the responsibility away from its proper focus, the producer.

In economic terms the cost of minimally treating the animal, that is, splinting the leg, is not prohibitive, especially if the fracture is a lower-leg fracture. The producer's hesitancy grows out of the extra labor involved in moving and caring for the animal, which may leave the producer close to a bare break-even point.

The veterinarian must therefore serve as an animal advocate, indicating that, in terms of social morality and veterinary ethics, leaving the animal to suffer for a week is unacceptable. He or she should point out that such fractures are not a common occurrence, and that failure to treat the animal, if it became known, would inexorably bring down significant public ire, not just that of radical animal advocates. The producer would be wise and is morally obliged to undertake the requisite extra effort. The veterinarian should stress his or her willingness to keep costs down by doing only as much as it takes to keep the animal from suffering. If necessary, the veterinarian should accept less than usual for his or her time, thereby underscoring a willingness to "put one's money where one's mouth is."

Ultimately, the provision of adequate veterinary care and the control of pain and suffering in animals are as much the duty of anyone using animals as is the provision of food and water. In the United States and Britain, society has explicitly stated as much in national legislation governing the care of animals used in research. As the late Hiram Kitchen pointed out at the 1987 AVMA Symposium on Pain and Suffering of Animals, with the advent of such national laws, the standards for animals used in research become, ipso facto, the standards for the care of all animals. If such cases as the one described become known to the public as an inevitable consequence of industrialized agriculture, we will undoubtedly see the advent of legislation governing the treatment of farm animals, assuring that such treatment is consonant with social morality.

Case

11

Euthanasia of Cat Who Sprays

Question

A woman brings you a four-year-old castrated male domestic shorthaired cat that recently has begun "spraying" in the house. This behavior began shortly after the birth of her first child six months ago and has cost her over five hundred dollars in cleaning bills alone. She wants you to euthanize this cat. You recommend several behavioral specialists, but she is too busy with the new baby to spend any more time or money on the cat. You already have five stray cats in the back room that are, to the best of your knowledge, problem free and have been waiting for adoption for over two weeks. You are fairly certain the cat would do well in a childless home, but so would any of the other cats awaiting homes.

Is it ethically correct to euthanize the cat?

Response

This case is similar, in logical type, to Case 6, wherein a woman brings in a cocker spaniel for euthanasia. Both are clear cases of convenience euthanasia, and the reader should consult the earlier case discussion for some general comments on that weighty issue and its psychological toll on practitioners. In discussing the current case, I will presuppose the structure developed for the previous analysis.

There are a number of relevant features that distinguish this case. First, I assume that the cat owner is a regular client, rather than a walk-in. This is highly relevant, for it allows us to presuppose some sort of rapport between veterinarian and client, and some familiarity on the part of the veterinarian with the woman's psychological makeup. As we discussed earlier, these factors are extremely important when the veterinarian is forced to function as an advocate for the animal, essentially to negotiate for the animal's life.

Second, this is a classic situation with which most veterinarians are familiar. Presumably the woman has had the cat for most of the four years of its life and has lavished a good deal of attention upon it. Indeed, the cat has probably served as a child substitute for the woman, a role it has ceased to fill after the birth of the child. The emotions experienced by a client in such a situation are mixed and complex. On the one hand, there is often a sense of guilt at no longer lavishing time and attention on the animal after the birth of the child. On the other hand, there may be vague or pronounced unease at the realization that the animal was indeed a child substitute. These two emotions alone may create a mind-set oriented toward getting rid of the source of the discomfort—the animal. This tendency is in turn buttressed by the spraying, a genuine and expensive problem. Additionally, the woman clearly feels that now that she has a "real baby," there is no time to spend on the cat and she would just as soon be left with pleasant memories. Her underlying motives, then, converge to have the problem deleted from her life.

From the animal's point of view, the spraying is explicable. The cat has been used to a good deal of attention and affection, which has suddenly been cut off. The spraying is very likely a strategy for regaining the lost attention.

The veterinarian is correct in suggesting consultation with behavioral specialists, who would probably recommend that the woman devote more attention to the animal and attempt to achieve a relationship where she does not perceive an "either baby or pet" dilemma, but in fact realizes that caring for the two is not mutually exclusive, and that the presence of the cat may even be good for the baby. Given her unwillingness to complicate her life by consulting behavioral specialists and her related desire to have the problem vanish, the veterinarian ends up performing the behavioral counselor function. In addition, he or she can point out (correctly) that euthanasia will probably engender significant guilt in the woman at a future time, if she does not first exhaust all avenues for solving the problem, and may indeed cause friction with her husband, if he is at all bonded to the animal.

Ideally, the veterinarian should educate people in the woman's situation, a fairly common one, before the baby is born. When my wife was pregnant, she was alerted to the problem by a perceptive physician and was also warned to expect some possible "sibling rivalry" between cat and child. Conscious of these factors, she ended up with a happy cat and a happy baby, who enjoyed an excellent relationship.

At any rate, in this case preventive medicine is impossible. So I would explain the situation to the client as I perceived it and try to get her to realize that she was burying the problem, not attempting to solve it. I would use my Aesculapian authority to get her to visit the behaviorist at least once. Failing that, I would press upon her the suggestions already mentioned and attempt to get her to see that concern for the child and for the animal are compatible and even complementary.

As part of my discussion with her, I would emphasize my inability to take the cat, because I was trying to save five others, and my firm belief that the animal would do well in a childless home. I would impress on her that if she was unwilling to assay behavioral treatment, she was certainly obliged to do everything possible to place the cat in another home. I would underscore my abhorrence to killing as a solution by telling her, forthrightly, that I could not, in good conscience, even consider euthanasia until all other possible avenues had been exhausted. Thus, if she persisted in seeking an easy way out, I would suggest she find another practitioner or that she take the animal to a humane society, where at least it would have a chance (albeit a slim one) of a decent life. In the end, for my own peace of mind, I would have to tell her that as a veterinarian, I am not in the business of killing animals for convenience, and that she has a responsibility for a life that does not cease just because she has now taken on responsibility for another life.

Case

12

Euthanasia of Treatable Horse for Insurance

Question

A valuable yearling Thoroughbred horse is found at pasture with its left fore fetlock joint extending laterally at a forty-five-degree angle from the metacarpus. After phoning you, the farm manager contacts the insurance broker, and their adjuster gives permission for euthanasia on humane grounds based on a presumed fracture with a poor prognosis. You radiograph the limb and diagnose a fetlock luxation. In your experience such injuries respond well to reduction and cast application, although subsequent racing performance may be impaired by periarticular fibrosis that may (or may not) ensue. The owner requests that you euthanize the horse because the insurance broker has promised payment (thirty thousand dollars). You phone the insurance broker and advise him that the condition is treatable. You are advised that the insurance broker has decided to make an ex gratia payment to the owner because the farm has not had a claim for several years.

Is it ethically correct to euthanize this colt?

Response

This case raises once again, as we have seen in numerous earlier cases dealing with both companion animals and farm animals, the fundamental question of veterinary ethics—to whom does the veterinarian have primary allegiance in cases of competing interests: owner or animal? Clearly, it is in the owner's interest that the animal be euthanized, else he or she cannot collect the thirty thousand dollars and has lost a functional racehorse. Equally clearly, it is in the animal's interest to have the injury repaired, since it will then be capable of a decent quality of life under the appropriate circumstances and will not be consigned to extensive pain and suffering, either during treatment and rehabilitation, or during the remainder of its life.

As in the case of euthanizing a healthy pet, the veterinarian's options are limited. He or she may flatly refuse to perform the euthanasia, arguing that it is wrong to destroy a healthy animal, which could enjoy a decent life, were the veterinarian permitted to practice the medicine for which he or she is trained. Such a refusal would be largely a noble but empty gesture, as the client would inevitably find another practitioner willing to effect the euthanasia. Indeed, such a course would almost certainly prolong the untreated animal's suffering. In addition, the veterinarian would probably lose some authority and credibility with many clients in the equine industry. Is there a more satisfactory alternative, a third way that respects the interests of both animal and owner?

The key to this situation lies in the nature of racehorse insurance. The simplest policy covering a racehorse is a mortality policy, with the animal insured against death due to illness or accident. Such a policy, presumably the policy in this case, forces the owner's demand for euthanasia. Indeed, it is in the interest of the insurance company to opt for all possible treatment rather than pay off. This fact alone militates in favor of the extreme rarity of such cases as this one. It is very odd that the broker agreed to pay the thirty thousand dollars on what the veterinarian describes as a treatable condition; this goes against the insurance company's interest—namely, not making the payment—and is therefore highly unusual. Nonetheless, the case has arisen, and the veterinarian must deal with it.

A far better insurance policy, from an ethical point of view, involves extending a simple mortality policy to include "loss of use," so the company pays if, for *any* reason, the horse can no longer race. Thus, there would be no owner incentive to seek death in this case. Such policies, however, are significantly more expensive. Obviously, concerned veterinarians should, whenever possible, educate clients toward the purchase of loss-of-use policies.

In any event, how does one deal with this deviant case? Presumably the insurance company has adopted its unusual stance because of some special relationship with the client, else it would eagerly embrace the veterinarian's information that the condition is treatable. Therefore, the veterinarian should approach the client with whom he or she presumably has a good rapport, and, acting as animal advocate, see if the client can be persuaded to spend one thousand dollars out of the thirty thousand dollars he or she will collect to save the animal (the approximate cost of successfully treating the injury to the point of relative normalcy). Presumably, anyone who owns such a valuable animal could spare such a sum without hardship. If so, the veterinarian could approach the insurance company and attempt to garner permission to save, and place, the horse. Because they have already agreed to pay the client, they do not lose anything by doing so. The veterinarian could then place the animal in a suitable, nonracing home, where the horse could be used for pleasure riding or for breeding and live a decent life. Indeed, one might even be able to recoup the thousand dollars from the person with whom the animal is placed. On rare occasions insurance companies have done this themselves. In this way no one, including the animal, loses, and one has structured a "win-win" situation.

Case

13

Euthanasia of Grieving Dog

Question

A man brings you a thirteen-year-old cocker spaniel, which appears on cursory physical exam to be lively and seeking affection. The man requests that the dog be euthanized. The dog is old but has no obvious medical problems. You inquire regarding the reason for euthanasia, and he replies that the dog belonged primarily to his wife, who died six weeks ago. He says the dog just lies around the house all day "grieving" over its recently deceased mistress. The man says the dog is suffering. You feel the man is suffering and that the dog is a reminder of his recent loss. You suggest he give the decision more time. He says that he has been thinking about it for six weeks, and that's long enough. You ask him to consider adoption knowing full well you seldom find homes for aged dogs. He replies that he knows the dog better than anyone, it will never be happy without his wife, and, besides, his wife would have wanted it this way.

Is it ethically correct to euthanize the dog?

Response

Boiled down to its bare bones, this case is yet another example of a client asking a veterinarian to perform convenience euthanasia. We know that the animal is physically healthy but seeking affection. Presumably, the attention previously lavished on the animal by the man's wife is no longer forthcoming, and the dog misses it. For whatever psychological reason, the man cannot provide the dog with affection or attention. Thus the dog probably lies around the house because no one is willing to give it the attention to which it is accustomed, and there is nothing else for it to do. The husband perceives the dog as "grieving" as a projection of his own grief, which projection reinforces his desire to rid himself of a painful reminder of his dead wife. Thus he has constructed a series of rationalizations to justify his expunging this reminder of his loss—the dog is unhappy, would not be happy with anyone else, and his wife would have wanted the animal euthanized.

As the late Dr. Leo Bustad and other experts have noted, animals are by and large far more resilient than the "Greyfriars Bobby" mythology would suggest. Most animals can live happily with a new owner; the veterinarian's noting that the animal is seeking affection confirms the relevance of that generalization to this case. Furthermore, the veterinarian has no reason to believe that the husband is indeed respecting the dead wife's wishes by suggesting euthanasia.

Is it correct to kill the animal because the husband's perception is distorted by grief? I think not. Nor can the veterinarian be expected to serve as a therapist treating that grief. So what can be done? Presumably the veterinarian has established connections in the community with psychiatrists or psychologists or social workers who are trained to deal with grief, as veterinarians not uncommonly face such situations. (Indeed, veterinarians often face many psychological problems in clients; every veterinarian knows that people often use their animals as a lever for discussing their own problems. For this reason veterinarians do well to effect liaisons with mental health professionals. In addition, getting rid of a pet may signal a suicidal state of mind.) A plausible step, therefore, is for the veterinarian to inform the client, in a sensitive but honest way, that he believes that the client may be having some difficulty with grief, and that he or she would recommend that the client talk to an individual with expertise on grief.

If such a referral is not an option, the veterinarian should still share his or her feelings and understanding of the situation with the client. Were I the veterinarian, I would not attempt to pressure the client to keep the animal, but I would assay a different tack. I would point out that the dog seems capable of giving and receiving love and can therefore still be of value to a lonely person, although for the client the animal evokes painful memories. I would thus offer to attempt to place the animal in a home where a person has need of giving and receiving the degree of affection the animal is used to—perhaps an elderly person who has just lost a beloved pet. In this way, the dog can both be happy and make someone happy—a fitting memorial, I would add, to the client's wife.

If the client were adamant and simply insisted that the animal be euthanized, I would ask him to go elsewhere, pointing out that I was committed to avoid killing healthy animals, at least until I had explored every viable alternative option. I would further explain that this policy stemmed primarily from my definition of my role as an animal advocate, which in turn followed from my moral principles. I would finally point out (as we did in Case 6) that only by adherence to this policy could I mitigate the "moral stress" that would inevitably compromise my effectiveness in the profession.

Case

14

Supernumerary Teat Removal

Question

A valuable three-year-old Holstein cow freshened recently, and the right front quarter is larger than normal. This quarter has a small accessory teat at the base of a normal-sized one. You examine the cow and can strip a liter of milk out of the "extra" teat. The udder asymmetry is probably due to this abnormality (which is known as a *webbed teat*). You have a good relationship with the owner, but it has been a difficult financial year for him. You could inject the accessory gland with a sclerosing agent to reduce its secretion and surgically remove the small teat, but there is a risk of significant scarring. You have had some short-term success with surgery to join the two glands and remove the extra teat, but re-obstruction often occurs within six months. The owner is adamant that everything possible be done because the heifer is potentially very valuable if she classifies well.

Is it ethically correct to perform this surgery?

Response

The confluence of circumstances described in this case does yield a putative dilemma. Were this an ordinary milk cow whose economic value lay exclusively in milk production, there would be no difficulty. Treatment of the supernumerary teat and extra mammary gland, being necessary in order to forestall mastitis and other medical problems, would be dictated by economic and animal welfare considerations. In this case, however, the major economic interests of the owner lie in having the cow classify well, and in selling the progeny. The owner's interest and the cow's interest again militate in favor of performing the procedure since, as before, mastitis would be detrimental to both. But another dimension relevant to the owner's interest looms even larger, namely, that the presence of the teat will forestall the animal's being classified well and thus will diminish the animal's value. Since owner interest and animal interest coincide, it might prima facie appear to be a simple case.

The dilemma arises, however, when one considers the veterinarian's moral obligations, not to animal or owner, but to society. This becomes relevant because the teat abnormality is strongly suspected, but not known, to be a heritable defect. It has long been generally held, as a principle of ethics in veterinary circles, that it is not morally acceptable to correct a heritable defect in a way that cosmetically conceals that defect while leaving the undesirable gene to manifest itself in subsequent generations, to the detriment of future animals, owners, and society in general. Thus, equine veterinarians generally consider it unacceptable to correct surgically an undescended testicle so that the owner can then conceal the defect and breed progeny who carry the problem.

This case is more complex than the horse case, however, for the just-mentioned medical and functional considerations militate in favor of removing the teat, but, by doing so, the veterinarian could be implicitly colluding with the owner's desire to conceal the defect! The case is further complicated by the uncertainty surrounding the heritable nature of the trait. If the veterinarian treats the animal and the condition is indeed heritable, he is possibly involved in unwittingly colluding with concealment of the trait. On the other hand, if the veterinarian doesn't treat and the condition is heritable, he or she has avoided colluding with the possible concealment but has also failed to treat a patent medical problem likely to lead to disease.

However, what if the condition is not heritable? Obviously, if he or she treats, then everyone wins and no one loses—cow, owner, veterinarian, or society. On the other hand, if he or she fails to treat under these conditions, then everyone has lost, especially the owner, being now cheated of the value of the cow, which could possibly have classified well. Failure to engage the issue is not an answer, for it simply transfers the perplexity to the next veterinarian whose counsel will inevitably be sought.

Where there is no certainty, one must proceed on probabilities. According to the experts in veterinary medicine, dairy science, and genetics with whom I consulted on this case, the condition is "probably" heritable. If this is so, one is forced to balance the interests of the owner, qua milk producer, against the interests of society in forestalling transmission of the trait. Clearly the owner and animal are better off with a treated cow. On the other hand, there is reason to believe that the owner might be prepared to conceal the defect out of a desire to market the progeny. The issue for the veterinarian, then, becomes this: How does he or she treat the animal, while at the same time garnering reasonable assurance that the trait will not be concealed?

One veterinarian offered me a reasonable solution: The veterinarian should treat the animal but inform the owner of the veterinarian's obligation to prevent transmission of the defect. Toward this end the veterinarian also informs the owner that the veterinarian will notify the breed association of the correction of the defect. The breed association will then not classify the animal well if it considers the trait heritable. If it does not, that is outside the veterinarian's purview; the veterinary ethical obligation has been met.

Given this solution, it is manifest that the veterinarian should choose the most efficacious therapy relevant to preventing mastitis and assuring a healthy and productive animal.

I should like to thank Drs. Ken Odde, John Schlipf, Tony Knight, and Ellen Belknap for dialogue regarding this case.

Case

15

Breeder Seeking Euthanasia for Puppy with Overbite

Question

A breeder of rough collie dogs brings you a six-week-old healthy, well-grown puppy with a moderate overbite. She wants the dog destroyed because it is not show quality. She maintains that to let it go as a pet would be bad publicity for her kennel, and also that it may be a hereditary defect and she does not want to risk having someone use it for breeding purposes.

Is it ethically correct to euthanize the puppy?

Response

Because this case represents yet another instance of a veterinarian being asked to euthanize a healthy animal for nonmedical reasons, the reader should consult the preceding discussions on the subject for an account of some of the ethical considerations governing convenience euthanasia. I shall presuppose the results of these discussions here and thus assume that it is prima facie wrong to euthanize a healthy animal for owner convenience —all the more so if viable alternatives exist.

If such alternatives do exist, the veterinarian finds himself or herself in the familiar position of animal advocate, essentially arguing for the animal's life. The efficacy of such rational advocacy will of course depend in part on the veterinarian's rapport with the client, as well as on the client's receptivity to rational argument.

Were I the veterinarian, I would begin by responding first to the client's "arguments," then proceed to some more general principles underlying the issue at hand.

Although the veterinarian cannot confute the claim that the animal is not "show quality," he or she can point out that deviating from the standards involved in showing has little to do with either the animal's potential for living a happy, healthy life, or with its ability to bring love and joy to the persons with whom it might be placed. (On the contrary, the opposite is more likely to be the case, as show ring standards perpetuate many genetically based diseases and defects. Indeed, numerous genetic defects in dogs are in fact perpetuated by breed standards.) Thus, the fact that the animal is not of show quality is not a good reason for killing that animal.

The breeder's additional arguments are equally unsound. Even if one accepts her claim that she does not wish to see the animal breed, that concern can be easily allayed by spaying or neutering the puppy. Increasing evidence indicates that early spaying or neutering of the animal is not detrimental to the animal's health, happiness, and development —and that should be explained to the client.

As to her concern that the animal is a "bad advertisement for her kennel," that too is easily alleviated. You can simply request that she turn the animal over to you, and indicate that you will then place it without identifying the source. Indeed, if the breeder is still fearful that people will know that the animal is from her kennel, as she is the only breeder in town, you can call upon colleagues in other communities for assistance—a healthy collie puppy will be easy to place, whether or not it has papers, even if it has a moderate overbite. Thus all of her concerns are neutralized.

There remains the question of who pays for the spay or neuter. If the breeder is unwilling to do so, the veterinarian could recoup the cost from the person with whom the animal is placed.

So much for the specifics of the case. Were I the veterinarian, I would use this occasion to educate the breeder on certain moral and practical considerations that she could, in turn, carry to other breeders. First of all, I would suggest that if she and other breeders are worried about bad publicity, they should think about the kind of publicity that would accompany a newspaper story about breeders who destroy puppies not suitable for show. I would also discuss the unquestionable change occurring in the social ethic on animals, which becomes ever-increasingly concerned about the animal itself, as opposed to the animal existing merely as a tool for human use. Third, I would discuss the vulnerability of purebred breeders and fanciers to the demand for change—or legislation—emerging from this ethic. Finally, I would suggest to her that if her industry is to survive and thrive in the new ethical climate, it must proactively reassess some traditional practices. And I would point out that at the top of the list of practices it would be impossible to defend is the perpetuation of hurtful defects for the sake of aesthetics, and the killing of perfectly healthy animals because they do not meet these arbitrary standards. This, I believe, is an area in which veterinarians can exert a very positive force for change through education.

Case

16

Veterinary Anatomist Spaying Farm Cats

Question

A veterinary anatomist visits a friend's farm. The farmer is placing five young kittens and the queen in a bag full of stones. Cat overpopulation (presently eight to ten cats) is a problem on his farm, and he plans to throw these into the pond. All are unwanted strays that wandered onto the farm, and a local veterinarian has said that they may carry disease that can be transmitted to the sheep and goats (toxoplasmosis). The cost of vaccinating, deworming, and treating the cats for ear mites and fleas, along with spay and neutering charges, is prohibitive, as are euthanasia charges if each cat is injected by the veterinarian. The anatomist has not done surgery in ten years but offers to perform all the procedures on the farm for the cost of the materials, while admitting that there is an increased risk of problems. The farmer is willing to go along with the idea, as he doesn't really like killing cats and the total charges will equal only the price of one spay.

Is it ethical for this veterinarian to perform these procedures?

Response

Here is a veterinarian who has clearly embraced the moral principle I have discussed before, that it is prima facie wrong to kill healthy animals. This veterinarian is willing to do all in his or her power to prevent such killing from occurring in this case. Happily, the farmer agrees and is open to the veterinarian's offer—he, too, would like to find an alternative to euthanasia, let alone to drowning. There is thus no conflict between veterinarian and client—presumably the farmer is prepared to provide at least "farm cat care" to the cats in the future. Thus there is no need for the veterinarian to assume the animal advocate role and persuade the farmer of anything.

What, then, is the ethical issue in this case? It appears that the major problem is the question of the veterinarian's competence to perform the surgical procedure to which he or she has committed; the other procedures seem unproblematic. Unfortunately, the scenario does not tell us whether the veterinarian is a "born surgeon" or a marginal surgeon.

However, even if he or she falls into the former category, a decade with no practice clearly puts the animal at a greater risk than if the veterinarian had enjoyed regular surgical experience.

For the sake of discussion, let us assume that the veterinarian is an average surgeon whose skills are rusty due to his or her lack of practice; perhaps he or she is at the level of a fresh graduate. Were I the veterinarian, I would unhesitatingly enlist the assistance of a colleague, graduate student, intern, resident or practitioner whose expertise in surgery is more finely honed to scrub in with me. (I assume that the anatomist is probably based at a veterinary school.) Thus the procedure would amount to a bit of informal continuing education; this sort of collegial courtesy occurs on a daily basis among professionals.

If the animals die at the hands of the anatomist during the surgery, they are still better off than they would have otherwise been, for they will have experienced a painless death, no different from being euthanized. And no harm will have been done to the client, who was quite willing to see the animal killed. On the other hand, if the animals survive, they have a good chance for a decent life. If the choice is between these possibilities and drowning, there is no question that the relevant moral considerations militate in favor of the anatomist making the attempt. If he or she succeeds, not only will the animals benefit, but so will the anatomist, for he or she has again been put in touch with what most veterinarians and non-veterinarians see as the most dramatic capacity separating veterinarians from laypeople—the ability to perform surgery successfully to the benefit of a patient.

Case

17

Breeder Asking for Anesthetics So She Can Crop Ears

Question

A local schnauzer breeder with whom you have worked for the last five years wants to buy a bottle of Innovar-vet. When you ask the reason, she says that another breeder with whom you are not familiar has offered to teach her how to crop ears provided she supplies the anesthetic. Since the breeder will be operating on her own dogs, there is no problem with practicing veterinary medicine without a license. She says she has no complaints with the ear crops you have performed for her in the past; however, she needs to try to save money since her husband recently lost his job.

Do you sell her the Innovar-vet?

Response

A multiplicity of factors militate, in my view, against selling the drug to the client. Innovar-vet is an abusable drug for humans and, thus, is tightly controlled, at least in the United States. Although veterinarians can prescribe such a drug for a client to use, it should be prescribed for individual animals, not for stock. To prescribe blanketly a significant supply would be to place oneself in a difficult position, at the very least, vis-à-vis the Drug Enforcement Administration. This problem would be mitigated to some extent if one knew, for example, that the client was a competent, experienced surgical technician who had extensive experience cropping under veterinary supervision; by hypothesis such is not the case in this situation. Thus protecting oneself, and one's reputation, would loom large in my mind as a moral and prudential concern.

Second, and in the same vein, one must consider another possibility. Because the veterinarian cannot attest to the client's competence as a surgeon, it is very possible—perhaps likely—that she could subsequently get into trouble with anesthetic overdose, cardiac arrest, intractable bleeding, or some other problem, then blame the veterinarian for providing her with the wherewithal for doing so. Thus the veterinarian might be legally actionable; at the very least his or her reputation for responsibility and good sense could be tarnished. This discussion shows that moral obligations to oneself militate against providing the client with the drug. The risk to the practitioner is simply not outweighed by benefits to client or animals. Indeed, the question of one's obligations to the animals further militates against supplying the drug. The surgery is of no advantage to the animal—cropping simply caters to the whims of fanciers and the questionable "standards" of shows. Further, any surgical or anesthetic procedure involves risks and pain, and cropping is no exception. Such risks are minimized if the surgery is performed and monitored by a competent veterinarian, but it is surely maximized if performed by a novice taught by an amateur. This reason alone—the possibility, even likelihood, of increasing animal pain, suffering, and/or infection—would suffice, in my mind, as a reason not to sell the drug to the client.

Finally, and equally important, moral obligations to one's profession also vector against cavalier provision of the anesthetic. To encourage such practices is to sell veterinary medicine short, to treat surgery as simply rote carpentry. One can doubtless train people in a rote fashion to perform many surgical procedures—that does not mean that they are competent surgeons. Indeed, they are not—they do not understand a multiplicity of concepts, physiological processes, and pharmacological considerations that inform and provide the background for the mechanical cutting and sewing effected by a surgeon. One goes to school for at least four years to acquire such competence; it is neither right nor prudent to trivialize this dimension of veterinary education.

It is certainly true that many people, in fact, do their own cropping, and many other veterinary procedures as well, especially in agriculture. That does not mean, however, that this practice is desirable. Veterinary medicine currently constitutes an extraordinarily sophisticated body of technique and knowledge; it is not, scientifically, a poor cousin of human medicine. Just as physicians would surely not encourage amateur dabbling in surgery, veterinarians should also fiercely defend their hard-won expertise.

Case

18

Penicillin Residue in Milk

Question

A recent veterinary graduate in a mixed practice has had a long week. Late Friday afternoon he is called to examine a lame cow on a small dairy farm. The physical examination reveals uncomplicated foot rot. The veterinarian treats the cow with 20 ml of procaine penicillin G (300,000 IU/ml) given intramuscularly and rushes off to a case of milk fever. On Sunday evening he realizes that he never mentioned to the dairy farmer to withhold the milk. He calls the producer at home and finds that he has been putting the milk into the bulk tank. The tank's contents were picked up yesterday. The veterinarian then calls his employer and explains the situation. The employer says the chance of getting "caught" in such a situation is very small (around one in ten). However, reporting the incident could cost the farmer close to one thousand dollars in lost revenue and penalties and will also reflect poorly on the practice.

Should the veterinarian report this incident to the dairy involved?

Response

The fundamental issue here is, in essence, whether a person may violate the law if, first, it is in his or her interest to do so, and, second, he or she is unlikely to get caught. All of us are tempted to do so at one time or another; for example, when we are tempted to run a red light late at night. But, as the philosopher Immanuel Kant pointed out about ethical rules, we must consider what would occur if such a practice were to be universalized to all people in similar circumstances.

Kant's principle obviously applies here. If everyone broke the residue rule when he or she was likely to get away with it, the rule would lose any meaning, and so would breaking it. This might be rationally acceptable if one were dealing with an absurd rule that all of us would just as soon see disappear, for example, Prohibition. But it is not acceptable if we believe that the rule is basically just, and we are trying to get around it merely out of self-interest.

Clearly, the rule in this case is both sensible and just. First, it is designed to protect innocent people who might consume tainted milk and develop a hypersensitivity reaction, with a real possibility of sickness or even death. Second, it is designed to reassure an increasingly skeptical public of the safety of the food supply (food safety assurance is generally viewed as one of the three major issues facing agriculture as we enter the twenty-first century). Failure to so assure the public can damage the industry, and, indeed, put veterinarians' jobs and credibility in peril.

If I were the veterinarian, I would immediately notify the producer, admit my error, take responsibility, and tell the truth. I would then notify the processor. Although I may well incur a financial loss by doing so, I do not believe the credibility of my practice would be hurt. All of us make mistakes, and people tend to be quite forgiving when we are forthright about them. A reputation for honesty is invaluable to a practice. Getting caught trying to hide the mistake would be much worse than admitting the error, for both veterinarian and producer. Once lost, credibility is not easily regained, and processors might well stop buying from the farmer. Thus it is prudentially as well as morally wrong for the veterinarian to say nothing, and particularly to avoid telling the farmer.

The likelihood of being caught at such a cover-up has recently been greatly increased. In the United States, as of January 1, 1992, all tankerloads are screened for residues. The screening device used is the "charm test," which can pick up as small a residue as five parts per billion. Under such circumstances the load in this example would almost certainly come up tainted, and the residue would be traced back to the farmer, as all truckers take samples from each producer.

Case

19

Marketing Heartworm Regimen

Question

You are a member of a multiperson practice in a large metropolitan area in southern Ontario. Last year your practice tested 1,479 dogs for heartworm disease and found four dogs positive. This represented less than half of the dogs that had current files on the computer record-keeping system. The four dogs were over 25 kg in weight and had spent most of the summer out of doors. Three of these dogs were in the southern United States for two to three weeks during the mosquito season. The proportion of affected dogs and their signalment has been unchanged during the five years you have been in the practice. At your practice meeting this winter, a decision was made to send reminder cards to the owners of all dogs with active files, encouraging heartworm testing and the use of preventive medication. Among the seven dogs owned by the veterinarians in the practice, only one (a hunting dog) was tested last year, and none were given preventive medication. A large proportion of the dogs on file (approximately 60 percent) are house pets weighing less than 20 kg. The average cost per dog for heartworm testing and preventive medication in the practice last year was fifty-five dollars.

Is it ethical to make this blanket recommendation to the clients?

Response

The approach to heartworm practiced by this clinic is a common one. In many communities in the United States, including those where, as in this case, the dangers of heartworm are negligible, individual practices —and, indeed, veterinary associations—vigorously market heartworm testing and prophylaxis. In my own community, where the danger of heartworm is also extremely low, a large, vivid sign in front of one clinic warns of heartworm. Obviously, using the threat of heartworm as a marketing strategy is indeed effective. In the case of the clinic in question, the sum involved is $81,345, which represents fairly easy money.

In and of itself there is nothing wrong with easy money. The issue here, however, is whether clients who choose the heartworm regimen have given informed consent. Are they aware that only 1 dog out of 1,476 that had not traveled to a high-risk area had tested positive, which represents a risk of 0.067 percent showing a positive result? If this were known, it is doubtful that many people would choose to test.

To put this situation in perspective, consider a human analogue. Suppose one were to encounter an advertisement by a medical association that warned of the dangers of malaria and suggested a simple regimen of antimalarial medication. Let us further suggest that this ad appeared in Toronto or New York City. Medically knowledgeable people would laugh, for it is virtually impossible to contract this disease in these locations, except in a research facility. The suggestion of undertaking a preventive regimen, though not explicitly asserting the existence of a genuine risk, certainly implies the existence of such a risk. And "malaria," like "heartworm," is the sort of word that strikes fear into ignorant hearts (if anything, the images engendered by "heartworm" are even more vividly frightening than those evoked by "malaria").

If one were to undertake this antimalarial regimen and later find out—say, on an exposé appearing on the television program *60 Minutes*—that the risks of contracting the disease were infinitesimal, one would feel significantly betrayed by the medical community, even if the costs had been borne by insurance and the regimen posed no risks to one's health. How much more betrayed by their veterinarians would clients feel were they to find out the facts of the heartworm situation? Would this not do great harm to the credibility and professional image of the veterinarian in the eyes of the public?

It appears to me, then, that aggressively marketing the heartworm regimen in the manner described is both wrong and imprudent for veterinarians. This is not to suggest that one should not alert clients to the existence of heartworm and to the availability of the preventive regimen. Rather, one should present clients with all relevant facts and let them choose the course of action based on sound information. One can legitimately recommend testing and prophylactic medication if the dog will be visiting a high-risk area, but a strong recommendation does not appear justified in a general situation.

Case

20

Dairy Farmers Using Unauthorized Feed Additive Prescribed by a Veterinarian

Question

You are an associate in a multiperson mixed-animal practice in an area with a concentration of dairy farms. You hear through the local grapevine that a feed additive for beef cattle is gaining widespread popularity among dairy farms in the next county. It is being prescribed by the neighboring veterinary practice as a method to increase milk yield when fed on a continuing basis to lactating dairy cows. You phone the manufacturer of this product, who confirms your suspicion that the additive is in no way authorized for this use. Dairy farmers say it is a "wonder drug," there is no residue testing for the product, and that it is the only good thing that has happened during a period of decreasing profits.

Should you report this practice to the Bureau of Veterinary Drugs?

Response

If one looks beneath the surface and "x-rays" this case, one finds that its logical structure is virtually the same as Case 4 discussed earlier, wherein the veterinarian confronts the illegal but widespread use of hormones in veal calves. The primary issue identified in that instance was the issue of whistle-blowing. As we discussed, society is morally ambivalent about whistle-blowing. On the one hand, it is sometimes seen as "squealing," "ratting," or "tattling"; on the other hand, such behavior may be viewed as commendable if issues of public safety are involved. In this case, as in the earlier case, the use of a food additive in an unapproved way may well represent unknown dangers to the public, so the moral burden on the veterinarian to stop this behavior is significant.

One factor absent in the earlier case, however, is the involvement of a veterinarian. Whereas the veal case involved farmers using a drug on the recommendation of a feed salesperson, this case depends upon a veterinarian prescribing the drug in an unauthorized fashion. Thus issues of public safety and illegal drug use are interwoven with issues of intraprofessional conduct and ethical obligations to one's fellow professionals, which naturally tend to militate in a prima facie way against whistle-blowing, especially as the offending veterinarian is a "competitor" of yours.

Nonetheless, the ethical vectors of this case point in the same direction as those in the veal case. The primary concerns must be food safety and public confidence in the food supply. So the onus is on the veterinarian to stop this practice. There are also additional prudential and moral concerns involved. For one thing, the credibility of the veterinary profession as a guardian of the public trust is involved—if it became known that a veterinarian had essentially been involved in compromising food safety, the entire profession would be hurt, as well as the veterinary community's case for extralabel drug use, an issue currently in question in the United States. Finally, there are issues of self-interest: The veterinarian in a position to "whistle-blow" would surely be significantly harmed in public image by failure to report if the situation became known in any other way—say, by a press exposé. All of these factors far outweigh any moral force to remain silent for collegial reasons.

The question that remains concerns what form the whistle-blowing should take. I would, first of all, approach the offending veterinarian and demand that he or she desist from prescribing the additive; then I would ask the farmers to cease its use immediately and hold back potentially tainted milk. I would also enlist the support of the organized veterinary community to back me. If I could handle the situation effectively in this way, I would not enlist the government agency. If this approach was not effective, however, I would not hesitate to notify governmental authorities.

Case

21

Veterinarian's Responsibility When a Dog Is Suspected to Be Overly Aggressive

Question

A veterinarian is presented with an eight-month-old intact male rottweiler for rabies vaccination. During the prevaccination physical the dog is quiet until a stethoscope is placed over his chest. At this point the dog suddenly launches a vicious and seemingly unprovoked attack against the veterinarian. The owner pulls the dog away, but further examination requires a muzzle and two personnel to restrain the dog. The veterinarian suggests to the owner that this is a display of dominance aggression and that the unpredictable temperament of the dog has serious implications. The owner becomes upset at the suggestion and states categorically that the dog is not at all aggressive. He supports this statement with the observation that the dog is fine with his two children and that he probably just doesn't like women veterinarians. He refuses to discuss the matter further, and the veterinarian does not expect him to return to the clinic.

Do your responsibilities in this case extend beyond a simple warning?

Response

Veterinarians (and physicians) are not prophets. Even in matters of well-understood physical diseases, animals, like humans, defy predictability and often refute prognoses. In the area of behavior, human or animal, this is, a fortiori, the case. Few psychiatrists, psychologists, or other behavioral scientists will venture confident predictions on how even a closely studied patient will behave. And though ethologists may offer generalizations about species-specific types of behavior, few would generate confident predictions based on the facts of this case. Animals do behave differently in a veterinarian's office than at home. The dog may never have been in a clinic before and may have been reacting out of fear, not dominance. The dog may have had an injury, lesion, or sprain that the veterinarian unwittingly contacted. There are numerous possibilities.

In fact, aggressive behavior is not very well understood—witness so-called "idiopathic aggression," which many surmise is a result of a brain lesion or something resembling psychomotor epilepsy, but which, ultimately, no one fully understands. By the same token, I once had a dog that had been attack-trained and rented out to patrol construction sites, plants, and stores. When I acquired the dog, he was, judging by his teeth, well into maturity. His history indicated that he had been passed from owner to owner, sometimes as a form of payment for services, without ever establishing a true bond with any person or family. I was told that the dog was "vicious" and "unpredictable," and, in any case, incapable of bonding at this advanced age, all of which the passage of time revealed to be patent rubbish. Though he remained very aggressive toward strangers, the dog bonded quite well with my wife and me, even to the point where we could roughhouse with him. Even more remarkably, contravening "expert wisdom," he literally shared his food and house with a variety of other animals, including cats, kittens, and one mature male turkey, which, in fact, would curl up and sleep on the dog.

My point is that the veterinarian has made a reasonable remark based on her experience with the dog. The fact that it is reasonable, however, does not mean that it is correct, as the owner alleges that he has seen no evidence of similar behavior. Here numerous questions arise: Is the owner lying or telling the truth? Is the veterinarian's remark based, in part, on her having been shaken up, coupled with her view of rottweilers, the currently stylish "fear dog" in popular culture? Is the owner a novice or a seasoned and experienced dog person? Is the owner a macho type, for whom the dog is an extension of his own persona, or a reasonable neutral observer? Has the veterinarian seen the dog before? Has she talked to the wife or the children? Unfortunately, none of these questions are answered in the description of the case.

In my view the warning issued by the veterinarian is a reasonable and prudent response to the situation. Given the lack of information available to her, I do not see that she can do much more. If she is deeply concerned, she should test her intuitions against those of the other people in the practice and, if they concur, she should discuss the case with a practically oriented animal behaviorist. If she again finds support for her concern, she might consider writing a letter to the client, expressing her concerns and listing a series of other signs for which he should be vigilant.

Case

22

Painful Research Designed without Analgesia

Question

A veterinary surgeon is proposing to study the effects of two oxygen free radical scavengers on wound-healing in dogs. As part of the research each of two dogs will be subjected to two "wounds" involving both skin and underlying tissue debridement. Both wounds will be closed as per routine veterinary practice. Because the protocol submitted to the animal care committee does not specify any postoperative analgesia, the protocol is returned to the investigator with a request that postoperative analgesia be supplied to all the dogs and that information on the drug administered, route of administration, and the frequency and duration of the analgesia be provided.

The investigator's response to this request from the animal care committee is that "postoperative analgesics are not required, as they would not be used in veterinary practice following this type of procedure."

Is it acceptable to allow this research to proceed without the use of postoperative analgesia?

Response

This interesting case underscores a number of fundamental points relevant to veterinary ethics and the ethics of animal treatment. First, consider the surgeon's claim that there is no need to provide analgesia for the dogs, because such a regimen would not be provided in practice. The fact that many people behave in a certain way does not mean that their actions are correct, medically or morally. Indeed, over the last decade it has become clear that the scientific, human medical, and veterinary medical communities' traditional agnosticism about, or ignoring of, pain felt by animals is neither morally, scientifically, nor medically acceptable. I have, in fact, devoted an entire book to this issue (Rollin, 1989, 1998), as well as numerous articles in veterinary journals; furthermore, the report of the American Veterinary Medical Association (AVMA) Panel on Pain and

Suffering in Animals (Panel Report, 1987) has underscored the same point (Morton and Griffiths, 1985; Taylor, 1985).

Perhaps the most significant recent event relevant to animal pain was the encoding in U.S. federal law of the requirement to control pain, distress, and suffering in laboratory animals, which served notice of the changing social ethic regarding animal treatment. The late Dr. Hiram Kitchen, who chaired the AVMA pain panel, pointed out that with the passage of such a law comes a change in the standard of practice for veterinarians regarding all animals, and that control of pain and suffering must therefore assume a much larger role in veterinary medicine than it has traditionally played. Dr. Lloyd Davis (1983) pointed out that veterinarians often prescribe antibiotics without documenting infection, yet withhold analgesia because they are not absolutely sure there is pain. Yet it is now known that humans and animals heal better and faster if they routinely receive postsurgical analgesics.

So the investigator is quite wrong in this case. First, rather than a researcher referring to what is done in practice as a justification for withholding analgesia, how much more fitting that the research situation should be exemplary and provide a model for practice! Second, research will almost certainly be more reliable if a potentially confounding variable is removed, that is, the pain experienced by the animal. There is no question that wounded dogs do suffer significant pain. Third, and perhaps most important, it is by no means clear that humans have the right to hurt animals in research for human benefit. This is the subject of much debate, and powerful arguments have been mustered against such use. The pain that is being inflicted on the dog does not benefit the dog—it benefits humans, or science, or the researcher's career. At best, it benefits other dogs in the future. Even if the procedure were to benefit the dog, it seems clear that there is a moral obligation to control the animal's suffering if it is possible to do so. A fortiori, when pain and suffering are not accompanied by any benefit to the animal, we are all the more obliged to control these things when we undertake such experiments.

Finally, there is a burgeoning literature (Benson et al., 1989; National Research Council, 1992) on animal analgesia that can help veterinarians control pain in contexts too long ignored.

Case

23

Clients Who Insist on Continuing Treatment for Failing Cancer Dog

Question

You have been treating an eight-year-old cocker spaniel with lymphosarcoma for nine months with chemotherapy. Although the initial response to treatment was good, the dog has now relapsed and has failed to respond to subsequent therapeutic interventions. The dog is extremely thin and has eaten very little during the past three days. The owners want you to continue treatment. They are firmly convinced that the dog can be cured. They are outraged at your suggestion to cease therapy and euthanize the dog. They threaten to take the dog to another veterinarian for treatment. They insist they have the right to keep on trying to effect a cure in their pet.

Is it ethical to continue treatment under these conditions?

Response

It is in some measure paradoxical that because animal life has, in the Judeo-Christian tradition, never been deemed "sacred," veterinarians have been granted a powerful weapon in the armamentarium against pain and suffering whose use is officially denied to physicians. That weapon is euthanasia. In earlier cases we have discussed some of the moral problems that arise when the veterinarian is asked to perform euthanasia for client convenience, rather than for curtailment of otherwise intractable suffering. The case at hand, however, raises an opposite, but equally dreadful situation, where the clients' desire to preserve life at any cost has blinded them to the very suffering that only euthanasia can redeem. The animal is thus cheated of the final gift that loving owners can bestow: an easy end before the animal ceases to be a dog, for all intents and purposes, and becomes instead a locus of agony. So the veterinarian is called upon once again to serve as an animal advocate, this time in the face of a different sort of client selfishness—an unwillingness to let go.

If the veterinarian has done his or her spadework assiduously, vis-à-vis client communication, an issue like this should not arise or, mercifully, should be rare. In what may well be the largest animal oncology unit in the world, located at our veterinary school, clinicians inform me that such a situation arises, at most, once every two to three years. Discussion about when to let go should thus be an integral part of veterinarian-client conversations from the beginning of treatment for diseases like cancer. Just as one lays out therapeutic options, alternatives, and prognoses to clients, so one should anticipate with them the possibility of failure or decline. Clients should be made to understand that a veterinarian's concern for his or her patient extends just as much—indeed, more—to ameliorating suffering as it does to prolonging life. Further, they should be led to examine their own views and to articulate a grasp of the notion of quality of life, as applied to an animal.

It is essential that the veterinarian stress, in the course of such conversation, that he or she will not make the choice of an endpoint for the clients; to do so is to set himself or herself up as a future target for hostility and sublimated grief. ("You made us quit!" or "You killed our dog!") But it should be explained to clients that there are rational criteria accorded to suffering, such as cessation of pleasurable activities, inappetence, weight loss, weakness, and signs of pain and suffering. It should also be stressed that the best guide to stopping heroic efforts can come from the animal itself; many pet owners who have been through these experiences will eloquently articulate the point that "the animal told me when to give up" or "let me know that he or she wanted to quit."

Having said and done all this, the veterinarian can always encounter clients who are in a state of denial, or who believe in miracles, or who are, for whatever reason, unable to let go. In the overwhelming majority of these cases, I am told by my colleagues doing clinical work, there is probably some underlying reason for their attitude; the dog is a substitute for a deceased child, or is identified with a dead parent, or is all that is left of a ruined marriage. In such cases, I believe that the veterinarian should honestly, but diplomatically, point out to the clients that they have lost sight of the animal's interests, or of reality, then perhaps recommend counseling with a professional who specializes in grief, if one is available in the community, or with a psychologist or psychiatrist—or perhaps with a trusted client who has been through a similar experience and has realized that one must, for the sake of the animal, stop trying at a certain point. The ability to communicate this kind of painful, ego-threatening point will again depend on the sort of rapport one has established with the client, and on one's ability to use one's Aesculapian authority.

If all else fails, and the client has truly ruled out euthanasia, I would still not cut the tie to the client, for the sake of the animal. Severing that link could result in the animal's being taken to opportunists or quacks who do not have the interests of the animal at heart, or simply being left at home to die, with nothing to control suffering. Thus, I would insist on continuing to monitor the animal for indications of pain and suffering. If the latter could be managed on an outpatient basis, with clients bringing the animal in regularly, even twice a day, for pain medication, I would allow them to do so. If it could not be managed, I would request that the animal be hospitalized. In this way I could at least do my best to ensure that the animal's pain and suffering were mitigated, and that it did not die in unrelieved agony. In such a no-win situation the veterinarian's primary duty must be, as far as possible, to relieve pain and suffering. If the only way to accomplish this is to humor the client, I would do so for the sake of the animal. At a certain point, of course, the only effective control of pain will be euthanasia.

If none of this worked, I would invoke the threat of the anticruelty laws. Keeping a suffering, debilitated animal alive, with no hope of survival, is deviant and shocking, and closely enough related to such wanton negligence as depriving an animal of food and water to count as cruelty. Indeed, the U.S. laws for laboratory animals have established a much earlier endpoint for animals used in cancer research, and one could argue thereby that these have become the standard for euthanasia in practice.

I am grateful to Drs. Greg Ogilvie, Steve Withrow, Lynne Kesel, and Jim Wilson, and to Linda Rollin, Ph.D., for stimulating comments on this case.

Case

24

Tail Docking in Dairy Cattle

Question

One of your dairy producers has a problem with mastitis and high bulk somatic cell counts (SCCs). He has read in Hoard's Dairyman that veterinarians in the United States dock tails on dairy cows with elastrator bands to decrease teat contamination with environmental bacteria. Veterinarians in your neighboring practice also advocate this procedure. Your local dairy specialist assures you that there are no controlled trials to show that docking tails reduces SCCs. Tail docking is not without risk. Complications include decreased milk production following the procedure, and deaths due to infection and tetanus. The producer is convinced that tail docking will solve his mastitis problems. He will find a veterinarian who will do it if you will not. You do not want to lose this client.

Is it ethically correct to perform this procedure?

Response

One of the earliest precepts of medical ethics, articulated in Greece by the school of physician-philosophers known as Hippocrates, was "Do no harm." As relevant to veterinary medicine as it is to human medicine, this dictum is highly applicable to the situation described in this scenario.

Conversations with dairy specialists in animal science, dairy veterinarians, and a lactation physiologist have convinced me that the dairy specialist mentioned in this case was correct—there is absolutely no scientific basis for the claim that docking tails reduces SCCs or eliminates mastitis. As veterinarians know, problems with mastitis are largely a function of hygiene, arising when animals are regularly down in unclean stalls. The client's desire to remove the tails from the cows is an example of attempting to deal with what is essentially a management problem by mutilating the animal. Other examples of a similar mind-set are patent: "devocalization" of dogs, declawing of cats, and docking tails of confined piglets. In this situation, however, unlike the others, the procedure will not deal with the problem.

Not only is docking the tail, in fact, not curative, it can exacerbate the problem. The use of elastrators, contrary to the belief of some farmers, is quite painful. As case material indicates, use of an elastrator can also cause infection, death, and decreased milk production. In purely prudential risk-benefit terms, then, it is irrational to choose to dock the tails, and because there is no potential benefit from the procedure, the farmer is not rationally warranted in taking any risk whatsoever. The same point, of course, holds regarding surgical docking of the tail.

Indeed, there is reason to believe that docking the tails is likely to increase the very problem that the farmer is trying to eliminate, namely, high somatic cell counts. Kilgour (1978) and others have reported that stress elevates SCCs, and the subsequent pain and distress that docking causes the animal would certainly represent a stressor, as would any resultant infection. Furthermore, because stress results in immunosuppression, an animal experiencing the docking procedure would surely be more prone than ever to mastitis, since its immune system is being compromised.

If I were the veterinarian, I would make these points forcefully and persuasively to the client, and show him that the procedure would work against his interests. I would further suggest helping him modify his management to reduce infection. If he continued to insist on docking the tails, I would suggest the noninvasive alternative of clipping the switch; doing this should be functionally equivalent to docking the tail, if his theory of the source of mastitis is correct. If he persisted in demanding that the tails be docked, I would refuse, informing him that my ethics would not allow me to perform a painful procedure that doesn't work, and let him learn the hard way that he will not solve the problem in this manner. Presumably, when he has discovered this fact for himself, respect for my experience will be augmented, and he will return to my practice. Even if he does not, having a reputation for honesty and avoiding the "quick buck" will probably serve my practice better than acquiescing to questionable demands.

I thank Dr. Jerry Olson for dialogue on this case.

Case

25

Killing of Neonatal Buck Kids

Question

A large goat dairy in your area is an infrequent client. On a recent visit you see an employee kill a newborn goat with a single blow to the head. When you inquire about this practice, you are told that there is no market for buck kids, so they are routinely destroyed at birth with the exception of one or two having potential value for breeding. Further inquiries on your part reveal that there is no economically viable market for these goat kids in your area.

Is it ethically correct to condone this practice?

Response

The situation in question addresses an unresolved and perplexing dimension of social attitudes toward the treatment of animals, namely, does killing an animal in a humane manner pose a moral problem for our social ethic? (I am assuming here, based on the report of the American Veterinary Medical Association's panel on euthanasia [Panel Report, 1986] and on the recommendations of the British Humane Slaughter Association, that the kid is being killed humanely, and thus that pain and suffering are not an issue.)

Societal attitudes are not clear on this point. On the one hand, we accept the killing of pigs, cattle, sheep, chickens, of all ages, for food. On the other hand, we (officially) deplore the killing, painless or not, of healthy dogs and cats in pounds and shelters. On the terminal use of laboratory animals, even if no pain is involved, society's views are not clear; our intuitions vary with species, purpose, and so on. Similarly, we are undecided about hunting.

In the circumstance described in this case, many people who do not see the killing of food animals as morally problematic would nonetheless experience revulsion. Indeed, many people who think they do not find slaughter morally problematic change their views when they witness it for the first time. It is not clear whether the source of such revulsion is moral concern at taking a life; aesthetic revulsion or squeamishness; or, in this case, perhaps a sense of waste or a feeling of regret that the tiny, paradigmatically innocent creature has not had a chance to gambol, eat grass, or fulfill its *telos*.

"Is it ethically correct to condone this practice?" I am not sure what the question means. Does it mean, should we be killing any animals at all? For some people it more likely means, isn't there any way to give these animals some chance to live? I shall take it to mean the latter, because surely the average veterinarian involved in a food animal practice is typically not going to question the validity of raising animals to be killed for food.

Were I the veterinarian who was upset by the waste of the life of an innocent, beautiful creature before it ever really began, I would look to creating a win-win situation for the farmer and the animal. For example, in many suburban and semirural areas where people own acreages, "hobby farming" is growing. Thus, the single largest source of beef in the United States is hobby farming, that is, farming not functioning as a primary source of income. Many people raise animals not for money, but for lifestyle. Goats can be extremely lovable, friendly, albeit exasperating, animals, and they bond well with humans. They do not require much space, can be trained to pull a cart, and can keep down weeds—although it is true they can also butt, jump fences, and eat foliage. When mature, they can be used for meat; for example, a friend of mine sells his mature bucks to the Mexican-American community, where goat meat is a delicacy.

Thus, the veterinarian working with the farmer could create a network for placing the baby goats. If this plan worked out well, with good owners demand could spread and prices rise. In addition, the veterinarian could augment his or her practice, the farmer could realize a new source of income, and the animal could have a chance for a decent life. This alternative might or might not work, but at least the veterinarian could alleviate personal unease at the practice in question by giving the problem his or her "best shot."

I am grateful to Bill Slauson for dialogue.

Case

26

Veterinarian Discovers Violations in Religious Slaughter

Question

You are working for a small government-sponsored abattoir in a Muslim country and discover that the person responsible for slaughtering the animals is stunning them before cutting the throat. Although this practice is illegal, he does it because he believes ritual slaughter is inhumane. You agree with him, yet, as head veterinarian, you are responsible for ensuring that meat from the abattoir meets acceptance requirements. Although your manual sets out standards only for meat hygiene and disease prevention, you know that meat from animals not slaughtered in the traditional manner will be unacceptable to consumers.

Should you report your finding?

Response

The first point that must be settled in discussing this case is an empirical one. Is the ritual slaughter in question indeed inhumane, as both the veterinarian and the slaughterer believe? Work by Daly et al. (1988) on cattle showed that there was a significant difference in time for the loss of visual and somatosensory evoked response, and the loss of spontaneous cortical activity, between animals that were stunned and those that were killed by throat cutting in ritual slaughter. In animals stunned by captive bolt, the loss of evoked response was immediate and irreversible. Loss of spontaneous cortical activity occurred in under 10 seconds. In nonstunned cattle evoked potentials were lost between 20 and 126 seconds after cutting, with a mean of 77 seconds for somatosensory responses and a mean of 55 seconds for visual responses. Spontaneous cortical activity was lost between 19 and 113 seconds (mean 75 seconds) after cutting. The time difference was less in sheep, with sheep losing consciousness within 2 to 15 seconds (Grandin and Regenstein, 1994). The difference between species is probably a function of differing anatomy in cerebral blood supply.

All of this seems to indicate that what is plain to common sense is correct: Being stunned is preferable to not being stunned, assuming that consciousness during bleeding out is not pleasant (Religious slaughter, 1985). In New Zealand, Muslim slaughter is forbidden without stunning (Grandin and Regenstein, 1994). Significantly, some Muslim authorities permit either mild mechanical stunning or electrical stunning of the brain.

In the face of this information, it seems clear that the slaughterer and the veterinarian are displaying reasonable and morally sound concerns. The question, then, is whether the veterinarian's obligation to the animal trumps his obligation to his employer.

Because Islamic law is essentially the consensus ethic in most Muslim countries, the slaughterer is violating both the law and the social ethic for reasons stemming from his personal ethic—engaging, in a sense, in civil disobedience. Because the veterinarian shares the slaughterer's ethic, and because his job concerns meat hygiene and disease prevention, not the policing of adherence to religious standards, I do not see that he is morally obliged to go beyond his job description. (I assume here that the veterinarian is not Jewish.) Most university faculty members know students who smoke marijuana, yet very few feel a moral obligation to report them to the police, whether or not the faculty member agrees with laws against marijuana smoking. Though there is a prima facie moral obligation to report a crime, faculty members generally believe that reporting would cause greater harm than allowing the minor crime to go unreported. Similarly, in effect, by not reporting, the veterinarian is preventing a greater wrong.

In a positive vein, the veterinarian could approach religious authorities with information regarding the sort of stunning that has been accepted by Muslim religious authorities in New Zealand and Australia and attempt to convince them to incorporate such stunning into the plant. If he can accomplish this, he has resolved the dilemma in a win-win fashion.

I thank Dr. Temple Grandin and Judy Schindler for dialogue on the case.

Case

27

Using Information about Alternative Surgical Training in Hiring

Question

Two new graduates respond to your advertisement in the "Veterinarians Wanted" section of the journal. One has recently completed a new "no live animal use" option at veterinary school, whereas the other has completed a traditional curriculum. After interviewing both, you have no strong preference for one over the other.

Is it ethically correct to use the information on their different educational backgrounds to choose between the two candidates?

Response

A good deal of understandable discomfort exists among veterinarians regarding graduates of veterinary schools who have taken the sort of alternative programs dealing with surgical training here identified as a "no live animal use" option. This nomenclature naturally suggests that students who have been through such a program are ill prepared, because they have never touched a live animal. On the basis of my own experience with alternative programs in veterinary schools all over North America, I would argue that such a description of these programs is inaccurate and misleading, and paints a false picture both of students electing such options and of veterinary schools offering them.

During the late 1970s and early 1980s, many veterinary colleges reexamined the traditional invasive laboratory exercises required of veterinary students in the light of changing social-ethical concerns about animal use. The operative question was "Can the goals of these laboratories be achieved in other ways?" As a result, such labs as strychnine poisoning of animals, hemorrhagic shock demonstrations, and pharmacological manipulations of animals were videotaped or modeled on computers. Veterinary educators now generally agree that such alternatives respect growing sensitivity with no educational loss. Indeed, in most cases, the principles are better communicated now.

It was inevitable that such questioning of traditional teaching practices would extend to surgery as well, and this development was catalyzed by students who did not wish "to hurt or kill an animal in order to learn to heal," as many students have said to me. In all of the cases with which I am familiar, the alternative surgery teaching programs growing out of such concerns are not programs of "no live animal use," but, rather, programs that use live animals but minimize or eliminate hurting and killing. For example, at Colorado State University a major part of the search for alternatives has led to a very closely supervised spay-neuter rotation accomplished with adoptable humane society animals. The students are certainly doing live animal surgery, learning to deal with live tissue, hemostasis, anesthesia, analgesia, and recovery, yet are not inflicting needless pain and death on healthy animals. Students not wishing to do the traditional terminal surgeries will thus spend additional time with cadavers, on the spay-neuter rotation, and as surgical assistants on clinical cases. At other schools students may apprentice with approved practitioners.

The point is, as many surgeons have told me, there are many ways of teaching surgery, and the traditional labs that consumed large numbers of animals are not necessarily best or even viable, as cost and availability of live animals increase and decrease respectively. Today's "alternative programs" often become tomorrow's mainstream teaching programs. As one surgeon told an audience, students choosing the alternatives are often at the top of their class, are the sort of highly sensitive persons the veterinary profession should nurture in today's world, and very rarely emerge as the worst surgeons in the class.

Another veterinary surgical educator stressed that surgeons are not going to approve any program that compromises student education or the quality of the graduates they produce. In my view, demand for alternatives has generated healthy self-examination and reflection among faculty, which has resulted in better surgical education, with habituated and outmoded teaching approaches replaced by more innovative and effective ones.

A prospective employer concerned about a graduate who has chosen an alternative program should thus not assume that the student is inferior. The veterinarian should contact the school for full particulars on the alternatives program and, if he or she is satisfied that the program is reasonable, concentrate on the end product, not on the means thereto.

Case

28

Pig Farmer Asking for Euthanasia Solution

Question

On a routine visit to a three-hundred-sow, farrow-to-finish operation you observe two pigs that are very thin. One has severe, chronic septic arthritis, and the other has sustained permanent intestinal damage as a result of a severe enteritis suffered several weeks earlier. The owner states that he has about one such individual per month and would like you to leave him a bottle of euthanasia solution, which he can use to destroy such pigs humanely. He does not like to use a gun for fear of ricochet and because he prefers not to have a gun on the farm with his three small children. He does not believe that using blunt trauma to the head of such poor doers is truly humane and knows of no other workable alternative for humane destruction.

Is it ethically correct to dispense euthanasia solution to this producer?

Response

From what I can determine, it would not be legal, at least in the United States, for the veterinarian to do what the client has asked. With the disappearance of T-61, all euthanasia solutions with which I am familiar are essentially pentobarbital, which, like any barbiturate, is an abusable and thus a controlled substance. Although what is legal and illegal is not always isomorphic with what is moral and immoral, the illegality of dispensing the solution is very reasonable in this case. Not only could the drug be attractive to addictive personalities, but I know that, for certain individuals, the availability of euthanasia solutions can lead to thoughts of, and flirtations with, suicide. Further, if the client is concerned with firearms around children, he should surely be equally concerned about euthanasia solution. Given that there are reasonable humane alternatives to his request, there is absolutely no reason to involve oneself in the risks—moral, legal, and in terms of liability associated with dispensing euthanasia solution.

What can the producer do? Let us assume that the pigs in question are finishers no larger than 250 pounds. If this is the case, they can be killed humanely with a captive bolt pistol utilizing the heaviest load available. This same regimen would also work for sows. A good-quality captive bolt pistol, with all the ammunition one could ever use, would cost about two hundred dollars—actually less than an ordinary high-quality handgun. This would be a reasonable outlay for the farmer and would assuage his concern about firearms. He would, of course, need to be trained.

By the same token, firearms are a reasonable, though unaesthetic, method of euthanasia approved by the AVMA Euthanasia Panel. Certainly, a medium- to large-caliber pistol will do everything the captive bolt will do, plus. For example, you cannot euthanize a boar with a captive bolt but could do so with a large-caliber pistol. If one is knowledgeable, or properly trained, death by gunshot is instantaneous. It is still a method of choice for many large-animal practitioners. The issue of safety is relatively easy to resolve. One should ideally shoot the animal on dirt rather than on concrete so that the bullet will not ricochet. Preferably, one should have a backstop (for example, a dirt mound) in the direction one is firing. The concern about children can be assuaged by keeping the gun unloaded, employing a trigger lock, and locking the gun in a cupboard or store box, with the bullets stored elsewhere. In any case, it is a good idea to train children in firearms safety.

If the client is uncomfortable with all of these options, he can easily arrange with the veterinarian for euthanasia. The client should be reminded that pentobarbital, being caustic, can be inhumane if improperly injected and is better administered by a veterinarian.

Case

29

Feeding Kittens to Snakes

Question

You are in a three-person small-animal practice in a city. A man comes in and tells you he owns two boa constrictors, which consume one rat per month. He purchases these rats at a pet store for four dollars. He feels guilty that these rats, which are intended for pets, are being fed to his snakes. He has found out that you euthanize two to four kittens every month. He thinks that there is no point in both the kittens and the rats dying, since the kittens are going to die anyway. He is willing to pay four dollars for every kitten. This money can be put into a fund for helping to feed stray animals until they are adopted or euthanized.

Should you sell him the kittens?

Response

This case seems quite straightforward. The answer is an emphatic "Of course not!" for two reasons. In the first place, and of paramount importance, the veterinarian is pledged to provide euthanasia, that is, a "good death," for the kittens. Being subjected to an indefinite period of terror, crushed, asphyxiated, possibly consumed alive, does not count as a good death. Thus one would be violating one's moral obligations to the kittens by agreeing to the arrangement.

Furthermore, a boa does not require live prey. In any large city containing research facilities, one can generally find a source of laboratory mice or rats who have been euthanized using CO_2 (so there is no residue for the snake to consume) and feed it to the animal, thereby circumventing the whole "dilemma." The veterinarian should explain all this to the snake owner.

The second reason for shunning the suggested arrangement is a prudential one. Unless one were seeking to commit professional suicide, no veterinarian would want to be known as a purveyor of live kittens for feeding snakes. Public reaction would be inestimably negative and would effectively destroy one's credibility within the community. In addition, one would be subject to peer action for violating AVMA euthanasia guidelines, which indeed enjoy a quasi-legal status in the United States. For these reasons, prudence and ethics combine to provide a clear-cut answer to this case.

Case

30

Veterinarian Seeking Maternity Leave

Question

You are the owner of a two-person mixed-animal practice in a small rural community. You have employed a woman veterinarian for the last two years, and you are very pleased with her performance. On Monday morning she announces that she is pregnant and expecting a child next fall. She would like to take a four-month maternity leave and then return to work part-time.

Do you

1. *Give her three-months notice?*
2. *Begin looking for another veterinarian to work full-time during the pregnancy leave, and then part-time following the return of your employee?*
3. *Return to a one-person practice?*

Response

When I first became involved with veterinary medicine in the mid-1970s, such a case would have been a rarity, there being very few women in veterinary practice. Today, however, the situation has changed considerably. At one U.S. veterinary school, over 90 percent of the freshmen class is female, and most veterinary-school classes now contain a majority of women. Over 25 percent of practicing veterinarians are now female, with that number increasing consistently.

There are legitimate pulls in opposing directions here for the employer. On the one hand, he or she is very pleased with the employee. On the other, the practice is too large for one person. It would be foolish for the owner to take on the work of two; that is a sure path to high stress, low job satisfaction, and poor health. This leaves only options 1 and 2 as viable.

Option 1 is unpleasant. The owner has presumably built a good rapport with the veterinarian and works well with her, a relationship worth keeping. Furthermore, she has done nothing blameworthy or questionable by becoming pregnant. She is clearly attempting to balance career and family in a realistic and reasonable way in her desire to take a brief leave and return to work part-time. As more and more females enter veterinary medicine, this scenario will become increasingly prevalent—part, as it were, of the veterinary landscape. Thus any employer is likely to face such a situation unless he or she chooses not to hire women, a strategy that is neither fair nor prudent, since society in general is moving to accommodate women who wish to have both career and family, and since the best candidates may well be female. So employers must begin to adjust to such scenarios.

Perhaps the fairest move is for the employer to place the burden of finding a qualified substitute upon the woman wishing to take the leave, conceivably another woman looking for a part-time position. It may well make sense (in many occupations, not only in veterinary medicine) for two people to share a position, when both wish a family and a career. If finding such a person is part of the conditions for the veterinarian's taking the leave and keeping the job, and if she knows she must work with her substitute in the future, she is very likely to find someone who is compatible with the practice. If such a Solomonic solution can be accomplished, everyone wins.

On the other hand, if the woman seeking the leave is unwilling to participate in seeking potential replacements, her commitment to the practice is probably limited, and the owner is thus justified in feeling fewer compunctions about letting her go.

I am grateful to Drs. Linda Rollin and Tim Blackwell for discussion of this case.

Case

31

Surgical Procedures Performed by a Technician

Question

A veterinary colleague uses his veterinary technician to perform dog and cat castrations in-clinic and to castrate and dehorn calves in the country. Although the veterinarian is always present during the in-clinic surgeries, the technician generally performs the on-farm procedures without supervision.

Is it ethically correct for a non-veterinarian to be allowed to perform these types of procedures?

Response

One might think that this question would have been dealt with by the laws governing veterinary medicine and, indeed, in the United States—and this is true to some extent. State laws do speak to what may and may not be done by technicians—both certified Animal Health Technicians (AHTs) and noncertified technicians. However, these laws vary widely from state to state. Some states allow non-veterinarians to perform these procedures, but only in the presence of a veterinarian, whereas others allow the veterinarian to be absent but make him or her "responsible" for the technician's performance. Some states distinguish between what can be done by an AHT and what can be done by a non-AHT. Others distinguish between procedures involving anesthesia and those not involving anesthesia—and so on. This variegated legal situation mirrors society's mixed ethical intuitions on the subject.

On the one hand, it could be (and has been) argued that a non-veterinarian—indeed, even a layperson—could be trained in a rote fashion to be extremely adept at certain surgical and medical procedures and, indeed, after a good deal of practice, be better at such procedures than a veterinarian who does them infrequently. This claim is buttressed by our commonsense knowledge that nurses are usually better at drawing blood and giving injections than are physicians; or that laboratory animal technicians are often far superior to senior researchers in gavaging animals, or performing cervical dislocation.

On the other hand, it is surely the case that the ability to perform one or even a few procedures well does not make one a veterinarian! As Aristotle points out, there is a major difference between one who has mastered some activity as an art, and one who has mastered it as a science. The person for whom it is a science "knows the reasons why"; the person for whom it is merely an art does not. The veterinarian, then, as a function of his or her education, knows what to do if unusual problems or circumstances occur during a procedure; the technician does not, or at least cannot be expected to. When a client contracts to have a procedure done, he or she in part and implicitly contracts for the veterinarian's ability to handle the unforeseen problems that can emerge.

One can argue that the veterinarian is on sound ethical ground in the case of the in-clinic surgeries, provided he or she has ascertained that the technician has mastered the procedures. Most important, the veterinarian is present to supervise if the technician errs in anesthesia or surgery, or if an unforeseeable emergency arises. This is, of course, how veterinarians themselves are typically trained—they perform procedures under close supervision.

When the veterinarian is not present, however, the situation can change in ethically relevant ways. Unfortunately, the case does not give us details of the on-farm procedures, but we can consider various possibilities. Dehorning is a relatively minor procedure if paste or electricity is used on the horn buds of a very young animal. Most important, nothing of an emergency nature is even remotely likely to occur. Thus the technician can proceed unsupervised. However, if an older calf is being dehorned surgically, and saws or spoons are required, much can go wrong. If the latter is the case, it would be unethical for the veterinarian not to be present to supervise and manage problems.

With regard to castration, one can make a similar point. If elastrators are used, and the veterinarian has confirmed the technician's competence, he or she can be dispatched without supervision. On the other hand, if the castration is surgical, even "easy" surgical in a very young animal, it would be wrong to permit the unsupervised technician to perform it. Although it is true that cowboys and farmers regularly castrate young (and even old) animals, that is not the point here. In the case in question, the farmer has obviously hired you, a veterinarian, for a reason—he surely knows that many non-veterinarians do these things. Perhaps he believes that veterinarians perform the procedure with less trauma. But, for whatever reason, he wants a veterinarian and is paying for it. Because there are untoward eventualities that might arise, it would be wrong merely to send the technician (Wilson et al., 1988).

Case

32

Veterinary Liaison with Pet Store Chain Providing Poor Animal Care

Question

You are on a locum in a multiperson, small-animal practice in a large metropolitan area. The practice provides a discount on services to a large pet store chain in return for client referrals. One afternoon you are presented with four recently weaned puppies. All are dehydrated, hypothermic, and hypoglycemic. Two have bilateral ocular discharges and diarrhea. Another has a deep corneal ulcer, and a fourth has an abscessed suture line from an umbilical hernia repair. The pet store manager reports all puppies were healthy that morning. Two of the puppies die, and two respond to treatment and are discharged with instructions regarding follow-up care at the pet store. Three days later one of the puppies is returned with a temperature of 34°C and is euthanized. The hospital staff report that this pet store chain is notorious for poor-quality pets and pet care. When you voice your concerns to the owner and the other veterinarians employed in the practice, you are discouraged from pursuing the matter because the pet store represents a significant source of revenue for the clinic.

Is it ethically correct to follow the wishes of your employer?

Response

There are a number of interconnected issues raised by this case. In the first place, one may ask if the sort of arrangement between the pet store chain and the clinic in question is intrinsically morally problematic. I do not believe that it is, as long as the clinic provides high-quality care to the pet stores, and as long as the referrals by the pet store are honest, indicating to the potential clients that the veterinarians in fact provide animal care to the chain in part in return for the referral, and honestly describing the sort of work the veterinarians have done. If these conditions are met, everyone wins. In essence, the veterinarians are taking part of their fee from the pet store in publicity, rather than in cash. The client is free to choose whether or not to employ the clinic's services, the animals get good care, the pet stores get a break on fees. Although one might argue that disclosure of the arrangement to clients blunts the value of the referral, I do not think this is necessarily the case, as long as the pet store can buttress the referral with a description of the clinic's track record.

So, for purposes of our discussion, we shall assume that the type of arrangement described can be ethically acceptable if these conditions are met. However, in the particular case described, the basic elements of an ethically acceptable arrangement are not met. A significant part of good medicine is prevention, and removing or changing conditions that lead to disease. Clearly, the clinic has not met its obligations in this area, or alternatively, the pet store has ignored the recommendations of the veterinarians—we know this both from what the hospital staff report and from the fact that the veterinarians in the practice do not wish to "rock the boat." But if this is the case, the ethical acceptability of the arrangement is significantly blunted, as the veterinarians should not tolerate low standards of care by the pet store and repeated incidents of disease arising from such poor care.

Given that the veterinarian on the locum has unearthed a significant flaw in the medical and ethical acceptability of the contract, and given that preventable animal suffering and disease are created and perpetuated by the clinic's inaction, it is neither ethically nor medically correct for him or her to drop the matter—to do so would in fact violate the Veterinarian's Oath. Nor, in fact, is it *prudentially* wise for the clinic to proceed as it has been. In today's climate of concern for animal welfare, the poor animal care provided by the pet stores is very likely to become a subject of press and public attention, and, if so, the risk to the clinic's reputation surely outweighs the pecuniary benefit of keeping silent.

The veterinarian on the locum should make these points forcefully to the members of the practice, indicating that he or she feels morally and medically obliged to pursue the matter of improving conditions at the pet stores and will do so whether or not the clinic cooperates, but that the clinic would do well to lead such a thrust for improvement. The clinic can in turn use the concern of the veterinarian on the locum as a lever to effect change in animal care in the pet store. If the practice still persists in turning a blind eye to the problem in the face of these legitimate points, the veterinarian on the locum is morally justified in going outside the practice, perhaps directly to the pet chain management or to the local veterinary association as first steps to seek a way to ameliorate an intolerable situation.

I am grateful to Dr. Steve Roberts for dialogue on this case.

Case

33

Freeze-Firing Racehorses

Question

You have been employed in a standardbred racetrack practice in Nova Scotia for one year. It is routine practice there to freeze-fire tendons and ligaments of horses in training. Your employer demonstrated the simple technique of freezing the skin in small round spots over the affected tendons with the comment, "I don't know if this does any good, but the trainers all seem to believe in it." This technique was not taught to you in veterinary school, nor was it practiced in your first job. It appears to be harmless enough, and the method is in regular use by practitioners in the area. Many of the trotters and pacers at the track sport the white-dot scars on their legs. A thorough search of the textbooks and appropriate journals for any description has been fruitless. Discussions with colleagues at the last American Association of Equine Practitioners meeting revealed only one who was aware of the technique, and he believed it was of no therapeutic value at all. This procedure is so entrenched in local racing circles that for any one veterinarian or practice not to provide this form of treatment would have little or no effect in your area. It would, however, result in a financial loss to the practice.

Is it ethical for you to continue to freeze-fire horses with the knowledge you now possess?

Response

The case at hand has some conceptual affinity with the one discussed in Case 24, dealing with the question of tail docking for mastitis. As in that case, the veterinarian is being asked to perform a procedure that is scientifically baseless but nonetheless believed by the client to have a salubrious effect. Although freeze-firing is presumably not as traumatic an insult as tail docking, it must surely cause a certain degree of pain and suffering, and for essentially no reason. If there is no benefit in the procedure, reason dictates that even minimal suffering by the animal is not warranted.

Equally important, in my view, such cases point to the core of being a medical professional. One's role as a professional is to bring state-of-the-art, scientifically based, informed diagnostic and therapeutic modalities to one's practice. If one's clients believe that bacterial diseases are caused by demons and evil spirits, you are surely not obligated to perform exorcisms or to discontinue use of antibiotics, though you may wish to explain what you are doing in a language your clients can understand. By the same token, in this case you are not obliged to perpetuate folk treatments that are clearly ineffective.

Indeed, it seems to me that one has a positive obligation to educate clients away from such treatments. If trainers continue to believe that freeze-firing is an effective way to deal with tendon and ligament injury, they will undoubtedly continue to follow training regimens that eventuate in such injury. On the other hand, if they understand that such firing is a bent reed, they may exercise more care in training, thus producing less injury. From the point of view of preventive medicine, then, resisting such an ineffective method can lead to a reduction in injuries.

Finally, I am reminded of a story told to me by a dean of a major veterinary school in an agricultural state. Upon assuming the deanship, he polled the users of his school's veterinary services regarding their satisfaction and dissatisfaction with the school's services. Although the respondents gave the school high marks in herd health, they criticized the veterinarians for accepting all innovations in confinement agriculture without raising concerns about animal welfare: "We depend on you veterinarians to tell us when we are pushing the animals too hard. Too often you tell us everything is fine, and we get blindsided by the general public." As I pointed out in an American Association of Equine Practitioners (AAEP) lecture a few years ago, the equine industry is very vulnerable to a number of criticisms on welfare grounds. Veterinarians do not serve their clients, themselves, or the animals well if they fail to call the industry's attention to these problems, for eventually enemies of the industry will publicize them, and then it is too late. Training methods that lead to injury—and useless practices like firing, which "treat" them—are paradigmatic examples of activities that veterinarians should be eliminating, not perpetuating (Rollin, 1992).

Case

34

Performing Cat Castration on the Farm

Question

You are called to a mixed farming operation to castrate and dehorn ten calves, castrate and vaccinate fifty pigs, and castrate a two-year-old colt. After you have completed these surgeries, the farmer asks if you will castrate a stray tomcat, which has been hanging around the farm for the last month. The last tomcat that the farmer castrated himself died. Your provincial veterinary association requires that cats be castrated in an approved surgical facility. The cost of in-clinic cat castration is equal to your charge for castrating fifty pigs and seems excessive to the farmer. In addition to the cost, he will be forced to make two trips to town. The farmer doesn't understand the difference between the calves, pigs, colt, and this stray tomcat. "If you don't want to do it here, Doc, I guess I'll give it a try," he replies.

Is it ethical to allow him to attempt this surgery?

Response

Any rule—moral, religious, or professional—binds us presumptively but can be overridden by weightier moral pressures. In the Talmud the rabbis argue that saving a life can trump even the Sabbath prohibitions, which are among the most profound rules in Judaism. And common law tells us that one may break the law to prevent a greater crime. A moment's reflection shows us that rules cannot be applied algorithmically—few things are more frightening than the thought of a computerized policeman. Those situations wherein we have faced mindless application of rules—be it in the military or in elementary school—vividly remind us of the vital role of common sense in mediating between the universality of rules and the particularity of real situations.

The point behind the veterinary association rule that cat castration occur in a surgical suite is a good one, designed to provide an ideal of state-of-the-art, scientific medicine that should govern one's behavior in a clinic. Obviously, such rules do not apply to emergency conditions—a sophisticated surgeon will perform a tracheotomy with a ballpoint pen or amputate a limb with a penknife if it is necessary to save a life.

The situation described is, in certain salient respects, analogous to an emergency. The cat does not belong to the farmer, and his desire to castrate it is reasonable and laudable given the number of stray cats that can starve to death in rural areas. At the same time, one can hardly expect him to expend the time and money to provide an in-clinic castration. But letting him undertake the castration is very likely to lead to pain, suffering, injury, and death for the animal. At the very least, the procedure will involve surgical pain, since the farmer will not use anesthesia and may do something as barbaric as the venerable "boot method" routinely practiced in the American West.

You, as a veterinarian, have a significant moral obligation to alleviate animal pain and suffering, and a fortiori to prevent it when possible. In this case your obligations to animal, client, and society converge to militate in favor of your performing the castration at the farm. Indeed, you are not violating the spirit of the veterinary association rule either, since its primary import is presumably to raise and maintain the level of performance at veterinary hospitals. Given that a cat castration is a procedure that is very likely to be successfully performed, to the benefit of animal and client, under the conditions described, one would be remiss *not* to perform it.

Case

35

Irresponsible Veterinarian-Breeder

Question

A veterinary colleague asks your help in diagnosing the cause of a reproductive problem that is occurring in his dog-breeding operation. He explains that he has upward of one hundred breeding bitches, representing fifteen breeds, from which he produces puppies for a number of pet stores. Further inquiry reveals that inbreeding is a common practice in his kennel. The consequences of this practice are difficult to determine, because the majority of puppies leave his farm at six weeks of age. From his description it appears that the level of cleanliness, nutrition, and medical attention is adequate. However, you doubt whether operations such as this can produce quality dogs, because no follow-up can be made to ensure that appropriate genetic selection is practiced. You are also concerned with the lack of human contact, which you believe is essential to produce a good pet.

Should you refuse this colleague's request for help and inform him that you are opposed to his type of breeding operation?

Response

In an article published in the *Journal of the American Veterinary Medical Association*, I argued that the veterinarian is in a unique position to help society make progress on what is sloppily called the "pet overpopulation problem"—the mass euthanasia of healthy dogs and cats. In reality this is a misnomer; the problem is with humans, not with companion animals, and involves much more than "too many animals." Among the issues that must be dealt with are people's lack of understanding of their animals, leading to an inability to deal with them; euthanasia for behavioral problems, a major cause of companion animal death; acquisition of animals for purely aesthetic or impulse reasons; perpetuation of genetic defects by breed standards and irresponsible breeding; unwitting abuse of animals growing out of ignorance of their needs and natures; euthanasia or surrender of animals for trivial reasons. I have also argued that high-tech refinements in contraception, such as pet food containing birth control drugs or advances in immunocastration, will not provide a magic bullet, since they address at best a narrow segment of the tissue of problems. Only education and increased awareness can create the requisite attitude changes and levels of knowledge for society to engage the issues properly. As a highly respected medical professional, possessed of significant Aesculapian authority, the veterinarian is in a unique position to advance this public education and change social thought on companion animal issues as dramatically as has occurred in the last two decades regarding environmental issues.

In this case we have a veterinarian unfortunately instantiating a paradigm case of companion animal irresponsibility. He is, in essence, running a puppy mill. With one hundred bitches representing fifteen breeds and inbreeding practiced, he is almost certainly perpetuating genetic diseases and problems that will cause later suffering for animals and owners. In other words, he is not practicing preventive medicine. He is, furthermore, making no effort to socialize the animals to humans during what is generally considered to be a crucial stage of life, thereby increasing the likelihood of future behavior problems. He has absolutely no control over the subsequent treatment of the puppies, nor any voice regarding the sorts of homes they will eventually belong to. Nor does he have any influence in assuring that the purchasers understand the physical and psychological needs, behavior, and problems associated with owning a dog. In short the veterinarian-breeder represents a classic example of the source of the "pet problem," rather than serving as part of the solution.

It is understandably tempting for you, as the veterinarian he has approached, to reject his request for a consultation. But this will accomplish little as far as changing his behavior is concerned; indeed, it is likely to make him defensive and intransigent. It would be better, in my view, to educate the breeder to the problems and consequences he is causing. It may well be that he does not care, but it is likelier that he has not thought the issue through in moral terms. If he respects you enough to seek your counsel, he probably respects you enough to attend to your concerns. In addition to the moral dimension, it would be judicious to point out that he is putting veterinary medicine in a bad light; at a time when many veterinarians are and should be seeking a solution to these pet issues, he is aggravating the problem and is lending ammunition to those who portray veterinarians as insensitive to animal welfare issues. Such peer pressure may well shock him out of his dogmatic slumber (Rollin, 1991).

Case

36

Annual Rabies Vaccination

Question

A client has come into a clinic in Alberta with his older dog and a vaccination reminder card. Your employer has sent this reminder stating that all dogs should be vaccinated for rabies every year. The client asks you, the employee, if yearly rabies vaccination is necessary for his older dog. (Rabies vaccination is not required by law in Alberta. For the import or export of dogs between the United States and Canada, rabies vaccinations are considered to be adequate for three years.)

Is it ethical to encourage this practice?

Response

Current scientific opinion supports the view that rabies vaccination is efficacious for three years. Indeed, the FDA requires of vaccine manufacturers that they demonstrate three-year efficacy in their products. Regulatory and legal considerations, however, vary considerably from locale to locale, with some jurisdictions requiring annual boosters and others, such as Alberta, requiring no vaccination at all.

Although it is possible that a given animal may not meet the general rule of three-year vaccine efficacy because of individual differences—for example, when a dog suffers from an immunosuppressive disease militating against the development of a full immunological response—such a situation is extremely rare statistically. If a veterinarian had reason to believe that such a condition obtained in a given case, he or she might be justified in recommending annual vaccinations. Such relatively rare circumstances do not, however, justify an across-the-board recommendation of annual immunizations.

This caveat about annual immunizations is strengthened by some preliminary results in cats reported in *Cancer Research* (Hendrick et al., 1992). A group of researchers at the University of Pennsylvania working with the Laboratory of Pathology noted that, beginning in 1987, there was a marked annual increase in the number of cases of subcutaneous inflammatory injection site reactions in cats, a phenomenon that had previously been rare. This increase coincided with the passage in 1987 of a state law mandating rabies injections of cats. Further, between 1987 and 1991, the lab saw a 61 percent increase in the number of feline fibrosarcomas presented for biopsy. The article presents epidemiological, histological, and ultrastructural evidence that suggests that the increase in fibrosarcomas is related to the increase in vaccination. The authors conjecture that the development of the neoplasms may be related to aluminum-based adjuvants used for injection.

If it is the case that rabies vaccination can cause cellular insult resulting in, as the authors say, "derangement of . . . fibrous connective tissue repair response," in turn leading to neoplasia, it is plausible to guess that similar problems can arise in the dog. In the face of this additional concern, it would seem wrong to suggest superfluous vaccination regimens.

In sum, it does not seem to be good medicine to suggest annual vaccination for rabies, both because there is reason to believe that a triennial regimen is adequate and because of the suspicions evoked by the report we discussed. I would thus not encourage the animal vaccination, and explain my reasons to my employer.

I am grateful to Dr. Greg Ogilvie for dialogue on this case.

Case

37

Government Policy Regarding Export of Breeding Swine

Question

Breeding swine from Canada intended for export are required to originate from herds not "affected" by a recently identified disease. This disease seldom causes clinical signs, although it is endemic in Canada. Most herds have never experienced clinical signs, nor have they ever been tested for the disease. A herd that had never experienced clinical signs of the disease tested one pig for private sale. This pig tested positive. Government authorities are now preventing this herd from exporting swine to other countries, because seroconversion in this one pig is interpreted to mean that the herd is "affected."

Is it ethically correct for government authorities to prevent the export of breeding stock from this herd that is not showing clinical signs of the disease, while allowing the export of breeding stock without a requirement for serological testing from other herds not showing clinical signs of the disease?

Response

The governmental policy described in this case appears to me to be neither fair nor equitable, as it does not affect all relevantly similar parties in the same way. In essence it does not touch a breeder who does not happen to test his herd voluntarily, whereas it punishes a breeder who happens to have done so. At the same time, it fails to protect recipients of exported animals from receiving infected animals.

No governmental policy should discourage people from doing the right thing. Yet this is precisely the effect that the current policy will have on breeders. If testing is not required of all breeders, and if a breeder who does test runs the risk of being prohibited from exporting his animals, clearly rational self-interest will militate against a breeder ever testing. Thus knowledge of the extent and duration of infection among herds will be truncated, and important information potentially relevant to preventing and controlling the disease will be lost. Foreign markets will be unprotected from the disease, and at least some countries will very likely eventually begin to demand that any animals exported from Canada be tested. Since breeders risk having their entire export business aborted if they do test, they will not agree to do so. Eventually, large amounts of potential export business will be lost, and foreign buyers will grow increasingly leery of Canadian swine.

What would a fair and rational government policy be in such a situation? One possible policy is to demand tests only of those breeders whose herds do display clinical signs. This, however, would not assure that asymptomatic animals that were exported would not later turn symptomatic or infect other animals in a symptomatic way in the importing country. Were this to occur to any significant degree, other countries would very likely curtail importation of Canadian breeding swine and look elsewhere.

A more plausible, though unpopular, strategy would be to demand tests of all producers who export swine, whether or not their herds display symptoms. The results of those tests—namely, that the exporters' herds are uninfected, infected and asymptomatic, or uninfected and symptomatic—should be provided to the importer, who would be free to decide whether or not to import the animals. In this way the government policy would be nonarbitrary and would provide for—not work against—the acquisition of knowledge relevant to managing the disease. At the same time, it would prevent the swine industry from getting a bad reputation abroad, which could well persist even after the disease in question is under control.

A third possibility is, of course, for the government to stay wholly out of the issue, so one would essentially create a situation of caveat emptor equally affecting all buyers and sellers.

The key point is that any of these three policies affect all relevant parties equitably. They do not, like the current policy, penalize anyone happenstantially while allowing someone else in essentially the same position to emerge untouched. Although one can debate the relative merits of these three policies, they at least meet some fundamental necessary conditions for any morally acceptable government policy, namely, fairness and nonarbitrariness.

I am grateful to Dr. Tim Blackwell for dialogue on this case.

Case

38

Improperly Labeled Prescriptions Swallowed by Child

Question

A woman you have never seen before rushes into your office distressed that her child has just eaten "some of these pills." She hands you a vial containing three different types of tablets and capsules. The vial is labeled only with the previous veterinary clinic's name and the instructions, "Take one of each pill twice daily as directed." You immediately direct the woman to the appropriate emergency care.

Is it your responsibility to tell the woman that the vial was improperly labeled? Should you contact the provincial veterinary association? Should you contact the veterinary clinic involved?

Response

An excellent discussion of the sort of situation described in this case may be found in James Wilson's standard reference book, *Law and Ethics of the Veterinary Profession* (Wilson et al., 1988). Wilson points out (p. 233) that despite the fact that 95 percent of veterinary drugs dispensed for small animals are subsequently kept around the home where they may be ingested by children, a large number of veterinarians do not place all relevant information on the drugs they prescribe. In addition, many veterinarians do not dispense pharmaceuticals in child-resistant containers. Although use of the latter is not required by law, it is encouraged by both the AVMA Council on Therapeutic and Biologic Agents and the Consumer Products Safety Commission. Proper labeling, however, is required by state or provincial law (p. 233). It is further noteworthy that drugs are in fact responsible for the majority of serious accidental poisonings that occur annually.

Obviously, if accidental poisoning occurs, it is vital for physicians to be in a position to identify the drug ingested as well as its quantity and its potency. In the face of this, Wilson argues that veterinarians are morally and prudentially bound to supply relevant information on the containers of dispensed drugs, and that failure to do so would render them morally and legally liable if tragedy occurs. Such information, says Wilson, following the California law, should include name of prescriber, name and address of dispenser, name of patient, name of drug, date dispensed, volume and strength of drug, expiration date, and clear directions for product use. Wilson's summary statement is a model of moral clarity:

> The simple policy of never dispensing any medication without at least the majority of the above information on the label seems morally right even if it might not be legally required in all states. When veterinarians see incomplete labels from other veterinary hospitals, they should encourage clients not to accept drugs with label omissions in the future. If the life of only one child or one animal is saved by this minimal professional effort, the modest cost and inconvenience are worth the effort. (p. 234)

The situation in question in this case thus represents a paradigmatic example of violating the points Wilson makes, with the addition of an extra component—mixing three drugs in one container. How, then, should the veterinarian respond? In my view the veterinarian should warn the client never to accept such poorly labeled prescriptions. By implication, one would of course be telling the client that the prescribing veterinarian had done something wrong, but that ought really not be a major concern in such an instance. I would further phone the prescribing veterinarian immediately and explain the consequences of his or her sloppiness and the points so forcefully made by Wilson. Only a truly reckless or irresponsible individual would fail to learn from such a call. Indeed, he or she should be grateful for your efforts.

Whether or not I notified the veterinarian association would depend both on the prescribing veterinarian's response and on the outcome of the ingestion. If the child is fine and the veterinarian chastened, I would take the matter no further. On the other hand, if the veterinarian is unrepentant or unwilling to change his or her behavior, or if the child suffers lasting damage or death, I would feel compelled to notify the association. Not to do so would appear to me to violate the special trust I have received from society.

I am grateful to Stu Forney of CSU Veterinary Teaching Hospital for dialogue on this case, and to the other veterinary pharmacists who responded to his queries by electronic mail.

Case

39

Referral Practice "Stealing" Clients

Question

As a general practitioner, you routinely refer specialty work, such as orthopedic surgery, to a relatively close, larger practice that employs a qualified individual to perform these surgeries. This practice has always represented itself to you as a referral practice for your benefit, but it is also engaged in general medicine and surgery.

For the third time this year you have received complaints from clients whom you had referred to this specialty clinic for orthopedic care. They say that the receptionist at the referral practice aggressively pursued them to have some type of routine medical procedure performed—once heartworm test, twice annual vaccinations. In these cases the individuals declined, advising the receptionist that they preferred to have these services performed by their regular practitioner.

Is it ethical for this referral practice to try to pick up this extra work?

Response

The relationship between a referral and a general practice is, at root, a symbiotic one. The referral practice benefits from cases first seen by general practitioners, cases calling for expertise and skill beyond what is expected in a general practitioner; the referring veterinarian benefits from having a ready source of expertise for such cases. As in all symbioses, both parties must take great care to preserve mutual benefit. Failure to do so by either party essentially destroys the basis of the agreement.

In this case, the behavior of the referral practice (or at least that of the receptionist therein) is clearly inimical to the continuation of the symbiosis. No general practitioner will send clients to a practice that attempts to steal them. Not only will such behavior sour the extant agreement, it will very likely make it impossible for the referral practice to enter into such relationships with any other veterinarian once its behavior is known, and thus it will lose its referred clientele. Such behavior is therefore not only back-stabbing, and thus unethical, but also highly imprudent from a self-interested perspective.

Were I the general practitioner, I would want to ascertain whether the receptionist or the owners of the practice were responsible for what took place—it is quite possible that the receptionist is an "eager beaver" and that the behavior in question is not even known to the veterinarians. Pursuant to this goal, I would confront the veterinarians who own the practice. If they are guiltless, they will quickly stop the receptionist from trying to steal clients. If the policy originated with them, and they show no remorse, I would make sure that every veterinarian in the area was aware of such underhanded tactics.

Case

40

Confidentiality and a Breeder Perpetuating a Line of Dogs with Seizures

Question

You are presented with a two-year-old springer spaniel that has a history of an increasing incidence of seizures. You have treated another springer spaniel from the same breeder for occasional seizures. The breeder is a client of yours and, in fact, has one bitch that has seizures. You have not mentioned to either of these clients the problems with the other dogs, due to client confidentiality. However, you do know that the two clients who purchased their dogs from the breeder have contacted the breeder regarding this issue. The breeder never mentioned to either purchaser that this problem existed in her line of dogs. When you confront the breeder with your suspicion that her breeding practices are contributing to the problem, she tells you that she breeds an excellent line of dogs and that this seizure problem is sporadic, affecting fewer than one in thirty dogs. She believes that most breeders have some problems inherent in their breeding programs that they do not publicize. She believes that she is producing a superior springer spaniel 97 percent of the time and claims that that is good enough for her.

You refer the latest client to a neurologist for further diagnostic work. In your letter you mention the background of seizures from the breeding operation. You inform the neurologist that the breeder wants this information to remain confidential.

Are either you or the neurologist ethically bound to honor the breeder's request for confidentiality?

Response

This case is similar to the situation discussed earlier (Case 5) regarding a client whose cattle was being treated for BVD and who sold some of his cows to another one of the veterinarian's clients without revealing that the animals were viral shedders. Here, as there, the ethical tension arises from the veterinarian's prima facie obligation to preserve confidentiality as opposed to the harm done to innocents if he or she keeps silent.

In this case the breeder is behaving in a patently immoral way. In the first place, she is not attempting to rectify the genetic defect, which could, of course—and very likely will—spread genetically as the gene(s) are perpetuated and disseminated in subsequent generations. This in turn leads to ever-increasing amounts of animal suffering occasioned by the seizures. Furthermore, owners of the animals will also be harmed—emotionally, as they are compelled to watch the animals suffer, and financially, as they attempt to treat the disease.

Thus, as a veterinarian, you are placed in a difficult position of moral conflict between your obligation to the breeder on the one hand, and to the other client, society, and the animals on the other. Indeed, responsible breeders of springer spaniels could also be harmed, since the breed will possibly develop a reputation for seizures, which could diminish its popularity. The operative question is whether the combined harms occasioned by keeping confidentiality outweigh the harm caused by its violation.

Though it is difficult to see immediately a middle way through this conflict, there is a strategy worth assaying. If I were the veterinarian, I would contact the breeder, and tell her the issue had reached the point where you could no longer turn a blind eye to it. (Not only do you feel that way as a responsible professional, but presumably the neurologist does as well.) Maintaining the status quo, you should tell her, is not only likely to proliferate harm to innocents, it could also damage your own reputation when the truth emerges. For this reason you urge her to seek genetic counseling to eliminate the problem (indeed, part of the answer may be to stop breeding the one bitch with symptoms). Until it is eliminated, inform all subsequent purchasers that their dogs may be seizure-prone and advise previous purchasers not to breed their animals. Continuing to ignore the problem exposes the breeder to being sued, especially in an age when laws are increasingly being passed to protect buyers against defective animals. If she accepts your advice, the problem is resolved, for she has now in essence made the problem public. If she refuses to do so, you cannot in good conscience continue to cover up for her behavior. Thus you would feel obliged to tell the next client with a seizuring animal that the problem is, in all likelihood, a genetic one, *something you would be likely to surmise on the basis of your experience with these dogs, even if you hadn't known the breeder.*

Thus, we have come down on the side of public disclosure but have done so in a way that allows both you and the breeder the option of taking the high road. This choice also allows you to circumvent having to reveal privileged information or break confidentiality. Not to act in some such way is tantamount to the veterinarian's colluding in harming innocents.

Case

41

Should Veterinarians Be Required to Report Animal Abuse?

Question

Medical doctors are required to report cases of child abuse.

Should veterinarians be required to report cases of animal abuse?

Response

Concern about cruelty to animals is as old as recorded human thought. It can be found in the Old Testament, in classical philosophy, and in various strains of Eastern thought. Beginning in the early nineteenth century in Britain, concerns about cruelty to animals began to be codified in anticruelty laws, and one can find virtually no civilized society that does not include such legislation in its legal system.

Sources of social and philosophical concern about cruelty to animals have been twofold: In the first place, there is a direct concern for the suffering of the animals themselves as conscious beings. This is specifically expressed in the ancient Rabbinic tradition in Judaism as the concept of "Tsaar Baalai Chayim," literally the "suffering of living things." Second, and of great historical importance, is the notion that those who are cruel to animals are likely to "graduate" to harming people, and thus such behavior must be disallowed. This was the position of St. Thomas Aquinas and is in fact official Roman Catholic theological doctrine. (Aquinas believed that animals, lacking immortal souls, were in and of themselves not of moral concern, but that cruel behavior tended to spread.) One can also find elements of this argument historically in judicial decisions interpreting the anticruelty laws in the United States.

Contemporary social ethics seems to embody both of these traditional concerns. First, society is in the process of developing an expanded ethic for the treatment of animals that addresses even animal suffering that is not the result of cruelty, such as that arising out of research, testing, and industrialized agriculture. In such a milieu, there is a fortiori greater concern with the sort of wanton actions addressed by the cruelty laws. Second, contemporary research has confirmed the intuition connecting animal abuse with human abuse (Kellert and Felthous, 1985). It is now known that most of our recent prominent serial killers had histories of cruelty to animals. Of particular interest is the close connection that has been established between the abuse of animals and the abuse of children.

Interestingly enough, for much of our history—well into the nineteenth century, and in some ways even today—children enjoyed a moral status somewhat similar to animals: Both were, in essence, property. It is ironic that, in the United States, laws against cruelty to animals were promulgated *prior* to laws forbidding cruelty to children; indeed, the first case of child abuse was prosecuted using the animal cruelty laws! (The American Humane Association to this day has both an animal protection division and a child protection division, which bespeak this close historical connection.)

Conceptually, it is not hard to speculate about the connection between animal abuse and child abuse. Both children and animals are totally dependent, vulnerable, helpless, and innocent. The sort of coward, bully, and/or psychopath drawn to hurt one gratuitously would surely be equally drawn to harm the other, both groups being such easy victims. Indeed, an article in *JAVMA* has explicitly spelled out the connection between the two forms of abuse, with special reference to veterinarians (Arkow, 1994).

In the face of our discussion, the conclusion is evident: Yes, veterinarians should be obliged to report suspected animal abuse for two excellent reasons. First, they need to be at the forefront of response to the new social concern about animals. I have argued for fifteen years that veterinarians are the natural, rational advocates for animals in society, and furthermore, that society expects them to fill this role. If they do not act against animal cruelty, which even the traditional social ethic for animals condemned and codified in law, how can they possibly be credible in responding to new and growing social ethical concerns about all other kinds of animal use, from agriculture to zoos? Second, as health care professionals with an obligation to public health and welfare, they must act to ferret out those individuals likely to move from animal abuse to human abuse, particularly to child abuse. And, finally, they owe it to themselves. Veterinarians see a great deal of animal abuse that is not so much the result of cruelty as it is a product of ignorance, greed, or stupidity. Often they have little power to prevent the problems that demoralize their professional life—for example, the constant requests for euthanizing healthy animals. In cases of overt cruelty, at least, they can be empowered to address the situation.

At the Colorado State University Veterinary Teaching Hospital, we have long had a policy requiring every clinician who suspects cruelty to report the case to the hospital director, who then takes responsibility for reporting the case to the authorities.

Finally, such reporting should be legally mandated so that there is no dilemma for the veterinarian—he or she should be obliged by the social consensus ethic to report.

I am grateful to Dr. Tim Blackwell for discussion and valuable suggestions.

Case

42

Two Cases of Found Dogs

Question

A. A regular client brings in an adult dog for an examination and annual booster shots. When you examine the dog, you notice that it has one of your spay/neuter tattoos in its ear. The owner tells you that he found the dog wandering near a shopping mall two months earlier. He checked the mall for notices regarding lost dogs and decided to keep the dog when none was seen. No other inquiries were made.

You check your files and find that you vaccinated the dog as a puppy and neutered and tattooed it six months ago. The original owner did not inform you that the dog was missing. The present owner is adamant that he is going to keep the dog, and you are quite sure that he will provide it with a good home.

Do you inform the original owner that you know where his dog is? If not, do you send the original owner an annual vaccination reminder?

B. One day the staff of your practice receives a phone call from people who have recently moved to your area. They explain that they have lost their dog, which they describe as a mature female tricolor sheltie with short hair on its belly and a scar. A few days later new clients arrive at your clinic with a dog for vaccination. The dog is a mature female tricolor sheltie. It has shorter hair on its abdomen, although no scar can be seen. You question the new clients about where and when they acquired their sheltie and explain that one with a description fitting their dog's appearance had been lost several days ago. The clients respond by saying that their dog was found as a stray, but it is theirs now and they are keeping it. As they are leaving the clinic, one of your staff calls out the dog's original name, and the dog responds by turning its head. You are suspicious that this is the missing dog but cannot prove it. The next day the people who lost their dog phone to tell you their dog is still missing and ask if anyone has heard anything.

Given that the new clients have come to your clinic with their pet expecting the full respect and confidentiality you give all your clients, what should you do?

Response

In both of these cases the veterinarian is faced with conflicting obligations. How you act has ramifications for the original owner, the person in possession of the animal, and your own reputation and feelings. Only by weighing all of these considerations can you morally make a decision.

Consider Case A: The veterinarian certainly has a prima facie obligation to protect the confidentiality of the new owner. On the other hand, failure to inform the original owner involves a betrayal of trust as well. As a client, he would certainly be entitled to expect you to notify him if you had located his dog, especially as you have identified the animal with certainty. Though the dog will have a good home with the new client, two months of bonding does not normally compare to the bonding that has very likely been established with the original owner since the animal was a puppy. A dog is not a car, and it surely has a preference for being with the people who raised it. By the same token, the original owner is likelier to suffer a greater sense of loss than the new owner if the dog is not returned to him. In terms of your reputation, you are pretty much in a "damned if you do, damned if you don't" situation. If you do notify the original owner, you will probably lose the new owner as a client, and he will probably attempt to sully your reputation for betraying a confidence. On the other hand, if it becomes known that you did not notify the original owner, your reputation will also suffer, as many, if not most, people would favor the return of the animal to its original owner. In terms of my own feelings in such a situation, if I were the veterinarian, I too would feel worse about being party to disrupting a long-standing bond than a short-term one.

One might argue that the failure of the original owner to notify you that the dog was missing bespeaks a lukewarm commitment to the animal. I do not believe this to be the case, necessarily, as it may never have occurred to him to check with the veterinarian—most people do not think in those terms. If he truly doesn't care about the animal, he may well let it stay with the new owner. So, in balance, I would argue that the situation militates in favor of notifying the original owner. As a courtesy, I would tell the new owner what I was going to do and attempt to explain my reasoning. What transpires after that is between the two clients.

Case B differs from Case A in two relevant ways. First, you have no definite evidence, comparable to the tattoo, that the dog brought in by the new clients is in fact the lost dog. Second, the people who have lost the dog are not your clients. Otherwise, the same considerations previously discussed obtain.

I would probably handle this case by calling the new clients and telling them the truth—that people have phoned you twice seeking a lost animal meeting the general description of the one they brought in. I would then urge them to contact those people and arrange a meeting with them to look at the dog. I would explain to the clients what the loss of an animal long established in a family can mean to both the animal and the owner, and also explain that the animal may well not be the lost animal, since you did not find a scar. If, however, they did not choose to make the call, I would not do so myself. First of all, I have no assurance that the dog is in fact the missing animal (indeed, in the absence of the scar, I have some evidence that it is not; furthermore, the fact that the dog apparently responded to its name being called out means very little—dogs often respond to such a stimulus, especially a sensitive and responsive sheltie). My prima facie obligation to respect client confidentiality is not outweighed by other considerations, especially given the fact that the people looking for the lost animal are not themselves clients.

I am grateful to Dr. M. L. Kesel for dialogue on this case.

Case

43

Should a Biting Dog Be Adopted Out?

Question

A veterinary technology program obtains stray dogs and cats for teaching purposes. At the end of the school year the animals are adopted by students, staff, or local residents. This year a purebred Siberian husky in the program bit students on two separate occasions. In both instances the attacks were unprovoked, and the bite wounds were not serious. Obedience training, increased exercise, and behavioral modification techniques recommended by a local animal behavior authority were ineffective in altering the dog's behavior. The dog was to be euthanized when a student found a couple living on a farm who were looking for a watchdog. The couple have no children and are fairly isolated.

Should the dog be given to them for adoption or should it be destroyed?

Response

In the case described there are too many unknowns to make a reasonable judgment. For example: Were the attacks on the students genuinely unprovoked, or did the students perhaps unwittingly release aggression by something they did, for example, by palpating something painful or unknowingly taking a threatening posture? What is the source of the dog's aggression—fear? dominance? Are the people who are considering taking the dog knowledgeable about dog behavior, or naive? Is the dog in fact a good potential watchdog? (Siberian huskies generally are not.) What do they mean by a watchdog? Will the dog be confined? Will it live indoors or outdoors? So we must make certain assumptions in order to facilitate discussion.

Let us assume that the dog's aggression is incomprehensible, not predictable, and not organically based (that is, there is no discernable lesion). In other words, we are dealing with an animal who will bite apparently at random. Let us further assume that the dog is a reasonable watchdog, else the couple would not consider adopting it. Since the farm is isolated, the major question is whether they are prepared to deal with this sort of animal, and how they plan to do so. If their answers suggest that they are familiar with such animals—for example, by having owned them before—one's concerns are mitigated. By the same token, if they plan to keep the animal confined in a yard, in the house, or on a chain, they have reasonably planned for protecting the innocent. Since the animal is healthy, such a life is better than no life. Because the people know enough to understand the risks they are taking, and are prepared to do so, they should be allowed to choose.

The only question remaining is one of liability. The school providing the animal needs some assurance that it will not later be sued if the dog bites someone else. I would ask the couple to sign such an affirmation, detailing their cognizance of the risks and dangers involved. I do not know whether such a document would ultimately protect the institution from lawsuit, but one cannot make decisions based largely on the fear of being sued.

I am grateful to Dr. M. L. Kesel for dialogue on this case.

Case

44

Euthanizing Sick Animals without Their Owner's Permission

Question

You are called to a small organic hobby farm where the owner complains that his sheep are lame and not doing well. When you arrive, the owner is absent, but his fourteen-year-old son is present. Two older ewes have severe secondary infections extending up the leg. When forced to rise, these two ewes will stand for only seconds before they collapse. They are emaciated and dehydrated. You believe they should be destroyed immediately on humane grounds, but the owner will not be back until after midnight.

Is it ethically correct to euthanize these two ewes without the owner's permission?

Response

This case contains a number of conflicting and vexatious elements that we have encountered before in earlier cases, and that make veterinary ethics so interesting and challenging. There is, first of all, a conflict here between the veterinarian's obligation to the animals and his or her obligation to the owner. From a humane and indeed a medical perspective, one should unquestionably euthanize the animals. On the other hand, one is also obliged to let the owner participate in making decisions on treatment modalities, including euthanasia. Indeed, one's moral obligation to euthanize is at loggerheads with the legal status of animals as property, whereby the owner must ultimately make such a decision. (I have earlier discussed cases wherein moral issues are raised both by owner unwillingness to euthanize a suffering animal and by owner desire to euthanize a healthy animal.)

What, then, is the veterinarian to do? I presume, from the case description, that the death of the animal is inevitable, and that no viable treatment exists. Thus the only question is whether or not the animals are allowed to suffer. Federal law in the United States, and national law in Britain, both mandate that, if these sheep were research animals, they be euthanized immediately, ideally with researcher (owner) permission, but without it if necessary. Because national law expresses the social ethical consensus, it appears that our current ethic for animal treatment demands euthanasia for intractable suffering. Thus a standard for veterinary practice is implicitly set, which could be appealed to by the veterinarian if the owner were to protest the euthanasia of the animals or even attempt to sue.

If one weighs the alternatives, one also sees that the animals suffer a great deal if the veterinarian awaits the owner's return, whereas the owner suffers little harm if the veterinarian does not, as the animals' deaths were inevitable. So, were I the veterinarian, I would perform the euthanasia, perhaps after confirming and documenting my course of action with a colleague as the only medically viable alternative.

The denouement of the situation will really depend upon how the veterinarian relates to and communicates with the owner, both in previous interactions and upon the client's return home. If one has established a good rapport with the client, and if he respects the veterinarian's Aesculapian authority and goodwill, the veterinarian will probably encounter no problems, especially if he or she makes it a point to contact the owner that night and explain what happened in detail. But if your communication is not solid and effective, you can indeed suffer negative consequences, ranging from loss of a client to being sued and defamed in the community. This is indeed a textbook case for educating veterinary students who may have perhaps been drawn to veterinary medicine rather than human medicine because they "do not wish to deal with people," for it is manifest that successful resolution of this situation depends on how the veterinarian deals with people, not with animals.

Case

45

Partner's Misdiagnosis

Question

You are employed in a two-person practice in a rural setting. You examine a dog with a persistent cough, which your colleague has seen on two previous occasions. He has prescribed two different cough medications, but the dog has not responded to either treatment. On physical examination you identify a severe heart murmur and pulmonary congestion. You suspect this has been the source of the cough all along. You prescribe a diuretic and digoxin. The owner asks if this is a stronger cough medicine.

Do you openly discuss the diagnosis with the client or sidestep the issue?

Response

This case raises the question of whether a veterinarian should openly criticize the diagnoses made, or treatments ordered, by a colleague. Although veterinarians often confront this issue with reference to peers in other practices, in this case it is the judgment of your own partner that is at issue.

On the one hand, there is a prima facie obligation incumbent on all human beings to tell the truth, since, as Thomas Reid pointed out, veracity is a presupposition of discourse, and discourse is of course a presupposition of all social interaction. On the other hand, this prima facie obligation can be reasonably overridden under special circumstances. We do not, for example, consider it wrong to lie to a murderer about the whereabouts of his intended victim, or in other instances wherein telling the truth would produce great harm.

Do such pressing considerations exist here that absolve the veterinarian of the presumptive obligation to tell the truth? I think not. Certainly the temptation to sidestep exists—by ducking the question, you could possibly prevent conflict between the client and your partner; forestall the possible loss of a client; forestall negative publicity in the community; or avoid an acrimonious showdown between yourself and your partner. On the other hand, you would be patently misleading the client and failing to provide the answer he is paying you for. In any case, you run the risk of his asking the pharmacist or someone else the same question, thereby eventually raising in the client's mind the specter of a "cover-up," which can cause even more harm to you and your practice. In addition, the client needs to understand the severity of the disease and be faithful to the medication regimen, which regimen you must also monitor.

The way to resolve this apparent dilemma lies in your ability to communicate. In my view you can tell the truth, but do so in such a way as to avoid ascribing blame to your colleague. I would respond to the query as follows: "No, this is not a stronger cough medicine. We know that cough medicines have not helped, and I am now considering the possibility of the heart being involved. If there is a heart problem, these drugs will help by . . ." and so on.

If the client asks why your colleague did not suspect heart problems on the basis of the same evidence you have, you can explain that many dogs have heart murmurs without resultant coughs. With the failure of the cough medicine, it is reasonable to try something else.

There is no element of dissembling in this forthright explanation to the client. Whereas you may *suspect* that the heart has been the problem all along, you cannot *know* that this is the case; the initial cough could, after all, have been caused by completely other things. Indeed, one of the bases for your current diagnosis is the knowledge that the two cough medicines didn't work!

I would certainly discuss the case with my colleague and examine the animal's record. If my partner did not perform a physical examination, or did not connect the results of that examination with the cough, it is incumbent on me to educate him. Once again, communication is paramount, so that I can accomplish this goal without triggering a strong and counterproductive defensive posture.

Case

46

Heavy Metal Toxicosis and Slaughter for Food

Question

Should animals that have been treated for, recovered from, or are suspected of having heavy metal ingestion/toxicosis be slaughtered for human consumption?

Response

This issue represents a clear-cut example of the conflict that can arise between a veterinarian's obligation to a client and a veterinarian's obligation to society. On the one hand, society has articulated clear concerns about food safety and the "wholesomeness" of the food supply; indeed, most agriculturalists see social concern about food safety as one of the three major issues confronting agriculture as we move into the twenty-first century. On the other hand, the veterinarian is obliged by the very nature of professional obligation to help the client make a living and to minimize client losses.

The form of the conflict is clear. Heavy metal deposits in the food supply are a major environmental health concern, since heavy metals accumulate in both human and animal tissues. When a human consumes an animal that has suffered heavy metal toxicosis, the person can also ingest the heavy metal with which the animal was afflicted, thereby increasing the amount stored in his or her own tissues. The extent to which this represents a serious health threat is variable, and dependent in part upon the person's previous ingestion of heavy metal (or heavy-metal-contaminated food), and in part upon what portion of the animal is consumed. Lead, for example, tends to accumulate in the liver, kidney, and bone, with relatively minute amounts deposited in muscle. Thus, a child fed great amounts of organ meat who may have also ingested additional lead from a room painted with lead-based paint is at far greater risk than an adult not previously exposed to lead.

In the face of the cumulative risk of ingestion, U.S. society, at least, through the vehicle of the Food and Drug Administration, has set extremely low tolerance levels for heavy metals. USDA meat inspection, in turn, follows these guidelines and would condemn any carcass containing any trace of heavy metals above minimum tolerance levels. Thus, there is a clear message from the social ethic to veterinarians not to ship such animals to slaughter.

On the other hand, the veterinarian realizes that not shipping the animals can impose an enormous financial burden on clients, as the client is likely not to be insured. If a large number of animals have been exposed to the toxin, the loss can be catastrophic. Furthermore, the veterinarian knows that only the organ meat is likely to contain any significant accumulation of toxins, so why should the client lose the entire carcass? In addition, little random or routine testing for heavy metals is performed; meat inspection does not target heavy metals in the relentless way it seeks residues of antimicrobials. So it is very unlikely that the residue will be detected, unless there is so much in the liver or kidneys that it can be seen on gross inspection, in which case it will be condemned. Thus, some veterinarians would choose to ship the animals.

In the end, in my view, adherence to the social ethic must trump obligation to the client. For a profession to remain autonomous, its professional ethic must accord with the larger social ethic. Failure to do so can result in the imposition of intolerable regulation and the loss of such vital privileges as extralabel drug use.

The way to mitigate the severity of the point we have just made is clear. It would seem reasonable that meat inspection rules could be changed to allow condemnation of liver and kidneys, without necessarily condemning the entire carcass. If heavy metal deposition in muscle is indeed minute, and thus human consumption of that muscle essentially risk-free, perhaps the regulations could be changed. It would fall to the veterinary profession as a whole to try to make the case for such regulatory change. But until that happens, individual veterinarians are obliged to respect the social ethic.

I am grateful to Drs. A.P. Knight, Lynne Kesel, Frank Garry, Mo Salman, Tim Blackwell, and to Dr. Zemca of the USDA for patient and helpful dialogue on this case.

Case

47

Conflict of Interest

Question

Is it ethical for veterinarians to practice veterinary medicine while employed directly by a feed company, a drug manufacturer, or the government?

Response

As stated, the question is radically ambiguous, and can mean three very different things. Because each possible interpretation is significant, we will briefly consider them all.

In the first place, the question may mean, Is it *ever* possible for a veterinarian to be engaged in a morally acceptable activity while serving a corporate or bureaucratic master? Presumably such a job may be seen as radically different from merely serving animal owners directly, for the larger entity has some vested interests that constrain the way one practices. The feed company, for example, wants to sell feed, not merely improve the health and well-being of animals.

If the question is interpreted this way, the answer is clearly yes. Although it is true that the person working for the feed company may experience conflict as a result of being so employed—for example, if he or she finds that a feed ration touted by the company is unhealthy—so too does the veterinarian who directly serves animal owners. The pet owner may want a healthy animal euthanized, the farmer may wish a fetotomy, or may be using an illegal growth promotant, and so on; these are the problems that make veterinary ethics so interesting, and that are indeed the stuff of these cases. The issue here is not whom one works for; it is, rather, how one deals with the inevitable ethical pulls that arise in the course of one's job. If dealing with tensions and vested interests makes a job inherently unethical, then there are probably no ethical jobs.

A second possible interpretation of the question is a less sweeping version of the first: Is it morally acceptable for a veterinarian working for a feed company, drug company, the government, or some other large corporation to follow the company line even in the face of flawed company policy—such as an absurd regulation, or a harmful feed formulation? This interpretation of the question is a good deal more plausible than the first. We all know the fate of whistle-blowers—as Ibsen's *An Enemy of the People* demonstrates, it is often not a happy one. Failing to follow the company line even in universities, the alleged bastions of free thought, can have disastrous consequences.

This does not prove, however, that one cannot be an ethical practitioner in such situations. The fact is, many people do behave morally despite such pressures. Such behavior may take courage, but moral behavior does not come cheaply. Furthermore, there are often ways of rectifying morally unacceptable situations that do not entail committing professional suicide or even losing one's job.

A third interpretation of the question is of far less global consequence: If you are employed full-time by a feed company, or some other such entity, can you ethically practice on the side? For example, if a large animal ambulatory practice is essentially a weekend hobby for you, your main source of income emanating from your job with the company, can you afford the fully outfitted truck, or whatever else may be essential to state-of-the-art practice? Can you pursue the continuing education requisite to being a good practitioner?

Again, I see no reason that this is impossible or even unlikely. The feed company salary may be sufficiently generous to let you buy better equipment than would a poor practice, for example. The company may encourage you to keep up-to-date through continuing education, and so on.

The point is that in all versions of the question, there is no a priori reason to deny the possibility or even likelihood of ethical practice. What in fact occurs will depend more on the character of the practitioner than on the nature of the job.

Case

48

Rabies Vaccine for Livestock

Question

Should rabies vaccine for livestock be sold as an over-the-counter item?

Response

The issue here is quite complex. On the one hand, controlling rabies is an exigent public health concern, and one wishes to do everything possible to expedite such control. In rural areas where rabies is prevalent, farm animals are a potential source of the disease spreading to the human population, yet there is rarely if ever a legal requirement for vaccinating these animals. Thus it would make good epidemiological sense to vaccinate the farm animal population. Because veterinarians typically mark up the price of vaccine significantly, because a farmer may have a great many animals, and because having a veterinarian visit a farm to inoculate animals is extremely costly, few farmers pursue this route. Thus, it might be argued, selling the vaccine over the counter relatively inexpensively would significantly accelerate inoculation, thereby serving to prevent dissemination of the disease.

On the other hand, it can be argued that if laypeople perform the vaccination, there are likely to be some missteps. Although non-veterinarians, especially farmers, can probably give an injection, they are likely to be far more cavalier about proper storage of the vaccine and could well compromise its efficacy by exposing it to extremes of temperature, by failing to respect expiration dates, and so on. In addition, in the event that the vaccination fails and someone contracts the disease from a farmer's animal, there is no authoritative attestation that the farmer in fact administered the vaccine properly or at all. Such an attestation is useful both for public health purposes and for defending the farmer on issues of liability. Furthermore, veterinarians might argue that selling the vaccine over the counter for livestock purposes might encourage dog and cat owners to perform their own vaccinations, resulting in both a loss of revenue to veterinarians and in a less formidable barrier against the spread of rabies in urban areas. Furthermore, some veterinarians would claim that if pets are not brought in for vaccination, they will correlatively receive fewer health checks, and thus good medicine will suffer.

In my view it seems most plausible for veterinarians to retain control of rabies vaccine, but to be prepared in high-risk epidemic areas and on high-risk farms to dispatch technicians or to be prepared to do the vaccination themselves without marking up the vaccine significantly. In this way veterinarians meet their public health obligation, assure that vaccination is properly done, and attest to its having been done, yet essentially retain control over the vaccine. A good start would be to vaccinate the animals whenever one is called to a farm for other reasons. Such a policy would very likely be compensated by public goodwill toward veterinarians as a result of positive publicity from the media about the veterinary professions' "pitching in during a crisis."

I am grateful to Dr. Tim Blackwell for detailed discussion and explication of the issue, and to Drs. Lynne Kesel and A.P. Knight for helpful suggestions.

Case

49

Female Veterinarian Receiving Unwelcome Attention

Question

A recently graduated female veterinarian is employed by a progressive mixed-animal practice. During the first few months of work one of the senior partners appears overly anxious to assist in training the new employee. He often leans over her when teaching her to perform some procedure and has offered to accompany her on late-night emergency calls. Last night he suddenly appeared at 11:30 P.M., when she was admitting an emergency "hit-by-car." When she mentions her concerns to her co-workers, they tell her to lighten up—the senior partner is "harmless" and just trying to be helpful. The new employee is afraid that if she mentions her concerns to her employer, she may spoil what is otherwise an ideal job.

Should she:

1. *Make up an excuse to leave the practice without mentioning her real concerns?*
2. *Put up with the status quo and wait to see if the situation worsens?*
3. *Tell the senior partner she is feeling harassed and hope he doesn't overreact?*

Response

When I first became involved with veterinary medicine in the mid-1970s, the relatively small number of women in the field had limited options in such a situation. Society as a whole was quite cavalier about rape, let alone harassment, and women experiencing this sort of unwelcome attention were often advised to "grin and bear it." For example, I recall one veterinary student telling me that if she and other women did not accept such behavior on the part of a certain clinical faculty member, he would ignore them during their rotations on his service, and their training would be compromised.

Much has changed during the ensuing decades—the notion of sexual harassment has significantly entered social consciousness and social ethics and is being codified and refined in the legal system. The key insight is a very commonsensical one: People should be allowed to do their jobs without having to fend off unwelcome advances, touches, and machinations aimed at finding the person alone or in a vulnerable situation. It is bad enough when such pressure comes from a co-worker who does not stand in a relationship of power to the object of the unwanted attention; at least in such cases one can respond with anger and tell the offender off. When the harasser stands in a position of power over the victim, as occurs in Michael Crichton's *Disclosure* and in this case, the situation is far more difficult to manage.

To ignore the situation is untenable, since it will certainly continue, if not escalate, all the while eroding the employee's job satisfaction. Thus option 2 is likely to lead to some variation on option 1—it is just a matter of prolonging the agony. On the other hand, apart from the harassment, we are told that the job is ideal. Thus rationality dictates that one should attempt to end the harassment without losing the job.

What of option 3? This does not appear very promising, as the possible negative outcomes outweigh the positive ones. A person capable of such behavior is very unlikely to respond to what is in essence a plea to stop; if he were sensitive to these issues, he would not engage in such behavior to begin with. Furthermore, such situations are often as much or more about power and domination as they are about sex. If this is the case, the harasser may actually be positively reinforced by the complaint. And if, perchance, he is unconscious of what he is doing, the likely response will be one of angry denial: "I'm trying to help you find your way in a new job, to mentor you, and you make filthy accusations."

Were I the female veterinarian, I would meet with the other senior partners privately and discuss the situation. We are told that the practice is "progressive," and thus there is some reason to believe that at least someone in power is possessed of some level of awareness. I would explain that though I loved the job, the unwelcome advances were poisoning the well for me. The partners are doubtless aware that an employee leaving the practice for reasons of sexual harassment could do great harm to the practice's image, both in the general community and in the veterinary community. A lawsuit would constitute even more of a nightmare. Since the partners stand on an equal power footing with the harasser, it is possible that they can at least get him to desist in his behavior, if not change his underlying attitude.

This option is at least worth a try—though it may not succeed, I don't think that the employee is worse off in virtue of the attempt. If nothing changes, she should probably quietly resign. Why quietly? Consider the alternatives. She could confront the harasser and tell him off. But that is unlikely to have any impact other than to make him a vindictive enemy and, if he has in fact been behaving objectionably as a domination ploy, might well bring him satisfaction! She could tell the veterinary community, but they are more likely to believe an established colleague than a young graduate. ("Oh, hell, Joe would never do anything like that—must be another oversensitive woman.") Finally, she could sue. But on what grounds? Objectively, she doesn't have much to bring forth. Further, a lawsuit is highly erosive of one's energy and in any case would very likely mark her as a troublemaker and compromise her career.

One person I discussed this case with suggested that, even if her career is compromised, the young veterinarian should take a stand "for the sake of other women to come." For my part, I never feel comfortable soliciting others to become martyrs—that is a role one must choose for oneself with great care.

I am grateful to Roselyn Cutler for dialogue on this case.

Case

50

Female Veterinarian Offended by Colleagues' Humor

Question

A three-male mixed-animal practice in rural Saskatchewan has recently hired a new female graduate. Every morning, as the work schedule is put together over coffee, one of the partners tells a few jokes he heard on his rounds the day before. Some of these jokes are quite mild, though others could be construed as being demeaning to women or minority groups. Some of the jokes make fun of men. Everyone seems to enjoy the humor, and it has obviously been part of the workplace for several years. The new graduate is treated as a respected professional by everyone in the practice. She has no complaints, other than the odd joke that she considers to be in poor taste.

Should she risk the excellent camaraderie established to date by mentioning her concerns to this veterinarian?

Response

In Case 49 I discussed the issue of sexual harassment of the sort that society ignored—or expected working women to grin and bear—for much of our history. As I indicated, over the past two decades the social ethic has grown increasingly sensitive to both overt and subtle sexual harassment, and this sensitivity is reflected in laws, regulations, popular fiction and film, art and literature. This is, of course, all to the good. Professional life is difficult enough without being colored by the sort of fear, anxiety, and discomfort created by unwanted sexual attention.

The downside of this laudable social change is a tendency that seems to characterize the ideology underlying all social revolutions in our society. We change relentlessly from feast to famine, yin to yang, without passing through anything in between—a peculiar skill possessed, it seems, only by human beings and quanta. As we once tended to see sexual harassment nowhere, we now find it everywhere.

To the untutored, ideologically zealous, and conceptually unsophisticated, anything that makes them uncomfortable is perceived as harassment. And administrators and managers, motivated by the Eleventh Commandment (Protect thy rear end) rush to ferret out the hapless offenders. The intelligent person who has once borne the brunt of such righteous indignation will rarely make the same mistake again. Perhaps he or she has told a joke that offended someone (very few good jokes don't offend someone), or complimented a co-worker of the opposite sex on a new outfit or hairstyle, or admitted being attracted to some cultural icon. Rest assured, his or her future conversational gambits will be restricted to the weather.

This is a great pity, for as Mill forcefully pointed out in his classic *On Liberty,* freedom of speech is the bedrock of a free and democratic society. Yet there are those (many in universities) who would curtail free conversation to blunt the allegedly greater mortal sin of "hurting someone's feelings."

To be sure, one can certainly harass with language. But all that offends is not harassment. Some distinctions borrowed from the twentieth-century Oxford philosopher, J. L. Austin, will help make this point forcefully. In a classic little book entitled *How to Do Things With Words*, Austin distinguishes three separate senses of what we can loosely call "meaning." The first sense is the simple content of an utterance. For example, the sentence "The cat is on the mat" asserts of a particular animal that it is situated on a piece of fabric. The second dimension of meaning is the use to which the speaker is putting the sentence. For example, if your nonhousebroken cat has positioned itself on my priceless ancient-Egyptian mat from one of the Pharaoh's tombs, my purpose in uttering the sentence in a hysterical voice is to have you remove the cat posthaste. The third aspect of meaning distinguished by Austin is its effect on the hearer. Ideally, the effect should match the purpose, and in this case you would rush to remove the cat. But you may not act at all and instead be grievously offended. (Austin calls these three dimensions respectively the locutionary, illocutionary, and perlocutionary aspect of speech acts.)

Using these distinctions, we can analyze this case. When a person makes a remark, they may indeed intend to offend. Typically, when one tells a joke, one generally, but not always, intends to amuse. Intention here, as in all areas of life, is judged by context—if I tell a violently anti-Catholic joke to the Pope, I probably intend to offend. If I, a Catholic, tell it to other Catholic pals of mine, I probably do not.

Excessive ideological sensitivity to any issue causes a person to look only at the first and third dimension of speech, and to ignore the second. In the situation described, it is clear that the joking is a manifestation of comfort and familiarity among the partners, and is good for morale and esprit de corps. Whereas perhaps in the recent graduate's milieu, one does not tell such jokes, she is here, as it were, a visitor to another culture. Just as one would (or should) consider it unacceptable, when visiting another culture, to declare, "Yuk, how can you eat that crap?" the new veterinarian should respect the presumably long-established, well-functioning culture of that practice. Indeed, the fact that she is now considered to be part of the daily circle of stories is probably as genuine a compliment and statement of acceptance as she could hope to get. The culture of rural North America is not the culture of urban North America; this is the stuff of common sense and literature since Aesop. If she is not comfortable with her colleagues, she is unlikely to be comfortable with many of their clients, and should consider a practice more in harmony with her mores. She will not, and probably should not, change these practitioners' long-established interaction— she will only create an uncomfortable and ultimately untenable awkward silence in her presence. "When in Rome . . ." is the operative dictum here.

Case

51

Client Refuses Euthanasia for Sick Cat

Question

An eight-year-old neutered male domestic shorthaired cat is admitted to your clinic with a complaint of lethargy and anorexia. The cat was last examined two months previously with a urinary tract infection and severe cellulitis at the site of a ventral abdominal urethrostomy. The urethrostomy was performed several years ago at another clinic. Euthanasia was recommended during your first examination, but the owner insisted on treatment. The cat improved after receiving fluids and systemic and topical antibiotics, but its condition suddenly deteriorated two days ago.

Physical examination reveals severe dehydration, bradycardia, hypothermia, and an infected and flyblown urethrostomy opening. Euthanasia is again recommended. The owner refuses and leaves the clinic, apparently intending to seek a second opinion.

Should you have:

1. *Attempted treatment again as requested by the owner?*
2. *Euthanized the cat on humane grounds against the owner's wishes?*
3. *Notified all nearby clinics of the situation and the likelihood that the owner will be seeking treatment elsewhere?*

Response

I am not quite clear about the point of this case, since some key information is lacking. The operative question is whether the recommendation for euthanasia is justified and reasonable. On the basis of the information provided, it is not clear that the animal is untreatable—for example, is the cat in a state of extreme renal failure? So in order to discuss the case in a viable way, I must examine some alternative assumptions.

Let us first assume that the animal *may* be treatable, but that such treatment is outside the expertise of the practitioner in question. If that is so, the desirable course of action for the veterinarian is to refer the case to a specialist. Failure to do so is wrong, since the euthanasia recommendation is based on imperfect knowledge. On this assumption, then, the case is straightforward.

The alternative assumption is that the euthanasia recommendation is totally justified by the facts of the situation, and we are dealing with a case analogous to the situation we discussed earlier (Case 23), wherein the clients insisted on prolonging the treatment of a suffering animal afflicted with terminal cancer, and the veterinarian advocated euthanasia. The current situation is similar, except that, in the previous case, the client merely threatened to go to another veterinarian, whereas in this case he has terminated his relationship completely. The veterinarian thus no longer has the opportunity to negotiate with the client and deploy his or her Aesculapian authority for the benefit of the animal.

What ought one do in this scenario? Option 2, euthanizing the cat on humane grounds against the owner's wishes, is patently illegal and morally unjustified unless all possible avenues have been explored, which they have not. A more reasonable approach is to attempt a dialogue with the client leading to palliative treatment, including pain control, which might relieve the animal's suffering. As mentioned in the earlier case, effective control of the animal's suffering may be tantamount to euthanasia. Thus option 2 collapses into a version of option 1, with the veterinarian focusing attention, above all, on relieving pain and suffering.

Option 3, of course, assumes that the owner is irrevocably gone from your clinic. Notifying "all nearby clinics" does not seem reasonable. Aside from the fact that this may well be a herculean task, what are you notifying them of? That the client is irrationally committed to refusing treatment? That is something the other veterinarians will determine quickly enough on their own, in which case, why notify them? Indeed, attempting such notification may be perceived by other veterinarians as bespeaking a resounding lack of confidence on your part in either their medical ability or their morality. In the absence of contrary evidence, one needs to assume that other veterinarians are as medically astute and morally concerned as you are. If they are not, your notification will accomplish nothing.

I am grateful to Drs. Tim Blackwell, Mike Lappin, and Lynne Kesel for dialogue.

Case

52

Should Veterinarians Prescribe Drugs to Increase Productivity?

Question

Should veterinarians prescribe medications that are neither therapeutic nor prophylactic in order to increase productivity in livestock?

Response

Historically, drugs prescribed to increase productivity have included antibiotics, hormones, and—if one counts equines in the class of livestock and success at the racetrack as an instance of productivity—analgesics, diuretics, and anti-inflammatories, which mask pain or other symptoms of an underlying condition rather than treat it.

There are three reasons that militate in favor of the view that it is wrong to prescribe such medicaments. The first reason pertains to the welfare of the treated animal. The clearest instance wherein such a regimen can cause significant harm to an animal arises in horse racing. The drugs just mentioned suppress pain or other manifestations of a medical problem without in any way treating the problem. Thus a horse runs with an injury and is placed at risk of further injury for the sake of being able to compete. Since the overwhelmingly compelling moral dictum for any medical practice, human or animal, is *primum non nocere* (above all, do no harm), prescribing such a regimen is patently wrong.

A similar example might arise were a veterinarian to prescribe a drug that serves to mask the feeling of satiety in a food animal, so that the animal continues to eat long after it would normally stop. (Cholestocystokinin has been used in such a way with swine.) Suppose the increased weight gain benefits the producer but harms the animal in ways not affecting productivity, for example, by engendering leg and foot problems from excess gain. (Animals genetically engineered to produce excess growth hormone have evidenced this phenomenon.) Again, this practice is wrong.

A third example can be found in the use of BST or BGH, which, according to some authorities, increases mastitis. Assuming this is the case and BST is a prescription drug, once again the primary moral medical directive is violated by prescribing it.

A second way in which using drugs merely for increased productivity can be seen as wrong arises if the drug doesn't harm the animal but might harm people who consume the animal or its products. DES provides a classic example of such a problem, as does clenbuterol, recently found in some show animals. A less esoteric example is provided by the widespread traditional use of antibiotics in food animals, despite patent biological reasons to believe that such use, in essence, amounts to selection for antibiotic-resistant microorganisms that could be dangerous human or animal pathogens. This phenomenon has in fact been confirmed. In at least one case, the Centers for Disease Control traced human death directly back to antibiotic use in a dairy.

The third way in which using a drug to increase productivity can be seen as morally wrong is if the substance is part of a causal chain leading to environmental despoliation, in the way in which pesticides and herbicides contaminate the aquifer. Although I personally know of no such situation occurring, it is not difficult to imagine a possible scenario. Suppose some such drug is excreted in significant amounts by a food animal and leaches into the soil or streams. Let us further suppose that, in the manner of DDT, it has pernicious consequences for wild animals, plants, or the ecosystemic balance. Once again, such a use is clearly wrong.

In the absence of such conditions, there is nothing inherently wrong with chemically enhancing productivity. Nonetheless, since untoward consequences are often detected much later, it is better to be circumspect rather than cavalier in such use. As I have often remarked, we must recall that there are other values besides efficiency and productivity that need to be respected.

Case

53

Previous Practitioner Leaves Sponge in Dog's Peritoneum

Question

You perform a laparotomy on a vomiting dog and find a gauze sponge walled off by omentum in the peritoneal cavity. The dog recovers uneventfully, and the vomiting problem resolves. The dog's only previous surgical history was an ovariohysterectomy performed at another clinic.

Do you tell the owners what you found? Or do you avoid mentioning the gauze for fear that it could create problems between you, the owners, the other veterinary clinic, and the provincial association?

Response

The basic issue here is one that is familiar to most veterinarians and was indeed a major focus of traditional veterinary ethics: Does one inform a client of another veterinarian's error? Given that any profession must form a cohesive unit, with members of the profession united in mutual respect and common cause in order to be effective in securing its place, authority, and autonomy in society, most professions condemn any behavior that would jeopardize such cohesion, and that could lead to what Hobbes called "a war of each against all." On the other hand, members of a profession must effectively self-regulate and not appear to be protecting each other under all circumstances, regardless of incompetence, else society in general will usurp that regulation, leading inevitably to less professional autonomy and effectiveness.

In a previous case I discussed an ambiguous situation wherein a veterinarian assumes another's case, changes the diagnosis and treatment, but lacks a sufficient basis for affirming that the previous practitioner acted incorrectly. The present case differs significantly. Here the previous veterinarian has been unambiguously careless and has patently erred, to the detriment of the animal. What are the current veterinarian's obligations in such a situation?

Consider some alternative possibilities. Suppose the client does not ask what you have found. It might be tempting not to say anything; after all, there is no prima facie obligation to tell a client more than he or she asks for. Such an easy way out, however, would be a mistake. In the first place, there is no guarantee that you will not get a phone call from the client in a few days, asking, "By the way, Doc, what was wrong with Fido anyway?" If you tell him what happened at that point, you will appear to have been initially covering up. Second, you do not want a discrepancy between what you have said (or not said) and what you have put in your medical records—that alternative leaves you in a very vulnerable position.

If the client does ask what you have found, you are certainly a fortiori morally and prudentially obliged to tell him. Thus the issue becomes, in my view, not *what* you tell, but *how* you tell it. Were I the veterinarian, I would explain to the client that virtually every veterinarian, at some point in his or her career, makes a mistake like this, just as all people doing carpentry bang their thumbs. Further, I would tell the client that I will talk to the other veterinarian and would, indeed, follow through on this. Presumably the original veterinarian will then wish to call the client, apologize, or otherwise make amends.

This approach is of course predicated on the assumption that leaving the sponge was a fluke on the part of the other veterinarian, rather than a regular occurrence or part of a pattern of oversight and error. If you know that the latter is the case, one needs to bring the situation to the attention of the local association in order to protect clients, animals, and the profession.

Case

54

Illicit Importation of Boar Semen

Question

You are called to examine a problem of diarrhea in some recently weaned piglets on a breeding stock farm. While you are taking the history, the producer mentions that these pigs and several other litters on the farm were sired by a friend's boar in Europe. Each year this producer returns home for a holiday and on his return carries several doses of fresh boar semen back to Canada in his carry-on luggage. He uses the semen only to inseminate sows on his own farm.

How should you respond to this information?

Response

In both Canada and the United States, laws regulate the importation of various animals and animal products, including semen. These laws exist to protect the domestic herd from infection with serious foreign diseases. Boar semen, as in the case in question, can carry brucellosis (a human zoonosis), African swine fever, pseudorabies, hog cholera, foot and mouth disease, leptospirosis, and chlamydia, diseases that can spread rapidly and cause significant animal suffering as well as major economic loss, as, for some of these diseases, infected animals must be destroyed.

Thus the farmer in question is breaking the law. Though the veterinarian certainly has a presumptive duty to maintain client confidentiality, he or she also has significant obligations militating in favor of not ignoring the situation. In the first place, as I have indicated many times before, the veterinarian has a general duty to society to promote and maintain the health of humans and animals. Clearly, the farmer's practice flies in the face of sound practice in this area. Second, the veterinarian has a duty to animals, and the possibility of disease transmission via the illicitly imported semen certainly has major potential for damaging animal welfare. (African swine fever or foot and mouth disease, for example, can create major animal suffering.) Third, the veterinarian has duties to other clients, whose herds may suffer from the outbreak of disease originating in the illicitly imported semen, and to peer veterinarians, whose herd health programs may be jeopardized by the actions of the client importing the semen. The moral weight thus seems clearly to press in the direction of not ignoring the client's practice.

Were I the veterinarian, I would respond to the situation by talking to the client and explaining the potential dangers entailed by his activities, as well as indicate to him my own moral responsibilities in the case. Perhaps that alone might suffice to get him to desist from illicit importation. More likely, however, he will protest that he has been engaged in this practice for years, with no adverse effects—his animals have never gotten sick, neither have the animals that are the sources of the semen. If he takes that tack, I would respond with an analogy: We have all been tempted to run a red light at a lonely intersection late at night. However, we generally refrain from doing so when we realize that we would not wish to see such behavior universalized. That is, we would not wish to see everyone exercising their own judgment about when it was permissible to run a light (especially teenage drivers). The risk is too great if everyone simply uses his or her own judgment.

Similarly with importation of the semen. Although the risk created by any given producer illicitly importing semen may be minimal, the risks engendered by *every* producer doing so when he felt like it are cataclysmic. Thus the client's behavior subverts the system designed to protect all producers. I would also point out that he is not prohibited from importing boar semen, simply that he is required to go through the regulatory steps designed to prevent disaster.

I am grateful to Drs. Tim Blackwell, Michael Hill, and John Maulsby for discussion of this case.

Case

55

Misreading of Radiograph

Question

A racing Thoroughbred is presented to you because of a left forelimb lameness that developed during a race. The horse is mildly lame at the trot. Perineural and intra-articular nerve blocks, up to and including the fetlock joint, do not improve the lameness. Radiographs of the splint bones, carpus, and elbow fail to identify a reason for the lameness. You advise the owner to rest the horse for one week and then return it to training. If the lameness does not improve, you request that the horse be brought back for a reevaluation. Three weeks later the horse breaks its left front cannon bone and falls during a race. The jockey is hospitalized with multiple injuries. You review the radiographs with a colleague. On the second viewing, and with the advantage of hindsight, there appears to be a hairline fracture of the left cannon bone.

Do you:

1. *Keep quiet and hope that no one comes looking for the radiographs?*
2. *Call the owner and your insurance company, admit your mistake, and wait for the calls from the lawyers and provincial licensing body?*
3. *"Accidentally" misplace the incriminating evidence?*

Response

Whereas this case certainly raises a serious and common ethical question—namely, does one cover up one's mistakes or forthrightly admit them?—it also raises a more subtle conceptual issue related to the epistemology of diagnosis.

In a fascinating paper delivered at the CVMA meetings in Victoria in 1995 (Papageorges, 1995), Dr. Marc Papageorges, a radiologist, points out that "both interobserver and intraobserver error rate in identifying subtle radiographic abnormalities is between 20% and 30%." In attempting to account for this, Dr. Papageorges points out that his discussion "may give the impression that radiology is less reliable than other fields of medicine, but a similar error rate has been found when the ability of clinicians to detect and describe lesions such as heart murmurs was studied." Such errors arise not only at the level of *detecting* lesion, but also at the level of "description and estimation of (the lesion's) clinical significance."

In his account of the origins of such errors, Dr. Papageorges makes a point familiar to philosophers since Kant: We see (or otherwise perceive) not only with our eyes (or other sense organs), but with our theories, expectations, predilections, moods, background knowledge, and experience. Where a woodsman sees a deer track, an urban person sees only grass. Indeed, where a radiologist sees an organ, a layperson sees only light and shadow. Common sense recognizes the variability of perception in the homily that "a pessimist sees the glass as half-empty, the optimist as half-full." Indeed, the ability of ideology in science to blind members of the scientific community systematically to the presence of felt pain in animals, or to the existence of ethical judgments in science (particularly in animal use), forms the subject of a hefty book I have written: *The Unheeded Cry: Animal Consciousness, Animal Pain, and Science* (Rollin, 1998).

Having pointed this out, let me return to the case at hand. Unfortunately, we are lacking some prima facie relevant information in this scenario. Specifically, it would be valuable to know if the fracture turned out to be a common, predictable fracture or an esoteric one—a horse, as it were, or a zebra. A condylar fracture is one of the three major fractures in horses and thus would seem to be less likely to be missed; a stress fracture on the proximal palmar cortex, on the other hand, is very easily missed. This would appear relevant in that one is more likely to blame the veterinarian for missing the expected rather than the unexpected.

In either case, however, I believe that the veterinarian's response ought to be the same—namely, to face up to the mistake in a forthright fashion and notify the owner and the insurance company. The other options are both morally dishonorable and prudentially unwise. If, for example, one "keeps quiet and hopes that no one comes looking for the radiographs," one will be sorely disappointed—the horse owner, his lawyer, and his insurance company will certainly come looking, and the veterinarian's failure to come forth looks both cowardly and incriminating. "Accidentally" misplacing the evidence is the same, only worse.

If the fracture was a rare, esoteric one, the veterinarian has nothing to fear—chances are most people would have missed it. On the other hand, even if the fracture was a common one, the veterinarian does not deserve to be pilloried. In the first place, we have been told only that in the veterinarian's reexamination of the radiograph—even armed with the wisdom of hindsight and with the expectation of finding a fracture—"there appears to be a hairline fracture of the left cannon bone." The locution "appears to be" suggests that even when one is specifically looking for a fracture, this fracture is far from unequivocally patent.

Human beings make mistakes. "To err is human," the homily goes. As Dr. Papageorges's paper notes, mistakes are inherent in the perceptual process. A judgment of veterinary incompetence should thus not be based on a single incident of this sort. Although there are egregious, inexcusable medical foul-ups, such as performing surgery while drunk or missing classic, unequivocal symptoms, the present case seems to fall well within the range of understandable human error. Only if there is a pattern of error that goes beyond the isolated mistakes that all humans make should aspersions be cast on a person's competence to practice.

Were I the veterinarian, for my own peace of mind, I would take the radiograph to a number of colleagues with comparable experience and tell them only the same information I had when first reading the radiograph. In this case, at least, the veterinarian is likely to find that others err in the same way.

I am grateful to Drs. Tim Blackwell, Lynne Kesel, Ted Stashak, and Jim Voss for dialogue on this case.

Case

56

Cattery Serving as Source of FIP

Question

A client presents you with a mature cat suffering from feline infectious peritonitis (FIP). The only other cases of FIP in the community have come from a local cattery. The history reveals that this cat has been in contact with a cat from this cattery. Although you have recommended to this cattery on several occasions the need to control or eradicate this disease, the owners have declined to follow your advice.

You call your veterinary association regarding what actions you may take regarding this irresponsible breeder. You are advised not to mention your concerns to anyone, including your veterinary colleagues within the community, because of the possibility of a libel suit. You are further advised not to treat the cattery's animals.

Is it ethically correct to turn a blind eye to this source of infectious disease that threatens the health of cats in your practice area?

Response

FIP is a devastating, incurable, and tragic disease. I personally watched helplessly as my small son's kitten, afflicted with FIP, deteriorated before his eyes while he begged me for help. "You have so many friends in the veterinary school, Daddy, can't anybody do something?"

Here we have a situation where a veterinarian *is* in a position to do something—indeed, can pursue the only available course for limiting the spread of the disease, which is to eradicate the disease at its source. Furthermore, in this case all the usual pulls creating ethical tensions for veterinarians converge in pointing out the practitioner's duty.

As we have mentioned in previous columns, veterinarians have obligations to clients, animals, peers, society, and themselves. Although there is often significant conflict among these obligations, such is not the case here. The obligation to clients is clear: One must do all one can to avoid disease in people's animals. As the case indicates, you have already had clients lose animals (and money) to the source of the disease. The same point applies to one's obligation to animals: It is certainly against their interests to ignore the reservoir of FIP. Again, one's obligations to one's fellow veterinarians is, clearly, to help them protect their clients and patients. Similarly, public health obligations incurred by veterinarians in virtue of their station militate in favor of closing the door on sources of infection. Only the obligations to oneself may give the veterinarian pause. After all, why risk a libel suit? Why make oneself a target? Why not look the other way?

The answer, of course, is that often one does run a risk by doing the right thing. As citizens, we deplore those urban dwellers who do not respond to mugging victims' cries for help, and we do not excuse the response, "I didn't want to get involved because I might have to lose time testifying," or "It might interrupt my dinner," or even "I might risk recriminations from the mugger." Similarly, it is ignoble to be paralyzed by fear of lawsuits, unfortunately epidemic in our society. Part of one's obligation to oneself, after all, is to be able to look oneself in the mirror.

Were I the veterinarian, I would approach the cattery firmly and decisively, marshaling the relevant evidence and demanding that they address the problem. If they refused to do so, I would point out to them that they are in a highly vulnerable position. After all, the situation is very newsworthy, and adverse publicity would be likely to put them out of business. Again, they are extremely susceptible to lawsuits from the many people who have lost animals. And, in fact, such lawsuits would be far more plausible than a lawsuit against the veterinarian in this case for libel.

I would also confront the veterinary association with the same logic. The stance they have taken is professionally irresponsible and pusillanimous. It is their job to join with the veterinarian to stop such irresponsible behavior, and to help forestall any lawsuit that might ensue from doing the right thing, not to counsel the veterinarian away from his or her clear duty in such a case.

Case

57

Injured, Unowned Animal

Question

A man comes into your clinic on a Friday afternoon with a golden retriever that he hit with his car. No one in the area where the dog was hit recognized it or knew who the owner might be. One person directed the driver to your clinic. The dog is unconscious and in shock. There is an open fracture of the femur and crepitation in the pelvic area. The driver is upset but unwilling to accept financial responsibility for the dog's treatment. The dog has a collar, but no identification, and is not a regular patient of yours.

Should you:

1. *Euthanize the dog?*
2. *Treat it for shock and put it in a cage for the weekend to see if anyone calls?*
3. *Repair the femur and the pelvis and give the dog the same pre- and postoperative care you would for a regular patient?*
4. *Call the provincial veterinary association to check on your legal responsibilities?*
5. *See if the driver will take the dog to the humane society or a twenty-four-hour emergency clinic?*

Response

Every veterinary practitioner has been exposed to this sort of situation, wherein one is presented with an injured animal with no one to bear financial responsibility for treatment. The five choices presented in the case also represent a reasonable account of the possible modalities facing the private practitioner.

Option 2, as far as I am concerned, is categorically ruled out by one's moral obligation to the animal as well as by sound medical practice. The animal may be bleeding internally, would certainly be in severe pain if it recovered consciousness, and is likely to injure itself further. By the same token, the severity of the situation militates against option 5, which is, in any case, passing the buck, unless one knows for sure that another veterinarian or the humane society has special funding earmarked for such situations. Even if the latter were the case, I would not be comfortable sending the animal away with such severe injuries, nor would I want to risk the negative publicity that doing so might occasion.

As for calling the veterinary association, I might have a staff person do so if I had definitely made the decision to euthanize the dog and was concerned that the owner might later bring legal action against me. But I would first make a medical decision—is there a good chance that the animal could be saved? Only if I had proceeded far enough in diagnosis to assure that the animal was not salvageable would I choose euthanasia. And if this were the case, I would proceed with the euthanasia regardless of what the association told me.

As far as I am concerned, the only option I would feel comfortable with is some variation of 3. Given that most veterinarians adhere to what I have called in other columns the pediatrician model of veterinary practice (as opposed to the garage mechanic model), the course of action is predetermined—to go ahead and treat the animal as I would any other.

The obvious problem with such a course of action is that it seems to conflict with a veterinarian's obligation to himself or herself. After all, one cannot expend time, energy, and materials practicing for nothing. Indeed, it is undoubtedly concern about this dimension that drives practitioners to choose one of the other options.

One of my practitioner friends once gave me a wonderful response to this concern. He informed me that he and his partner always treat the animal in a state-of-the-art way in such a case. "First of all," he said, "the practice is invaluable in keeping our surgical and medical skills sharp. We consider it continuing education. Second, we have worked out a marvelous agreement with the local newspaper. Whenever we treat such an animal, we take before and after photos. In addition, the newspaper runs a story after the animal has recovered, indicating the nature of the injuries, the nature of our treatment, and running a photo of the dog. If the owner comes forward, he probably will pay the bill. If not, the newspaper asks for volunteers willing to adopt the dog. There is never a shortage of volunteers."

My friend went on to point out that he could not buy more effective advertising for his practice for any amount of money. Local television and radio stations could be enlisted to provide similar coverage. In this way the veterinarian can both do good and do well.

In some communities humane societies or other groups concerned about animal welfare maintain a fund to pay veterinarians who care for unowned animals. Undertaking the establishment of such a fund in a community is another opportunity for veterinarians to create a win-win situation for themselves and for animals while increasing the positive visibility of veterinary medicine in the community.

I am grateful to Dr. Lynne Kesel for dialogue.

Case

58

Writing Prescriptions for Branded Drugs in Return for Financial Incentive

Question

Recently, research has identified that a specific in-feed medication improves performance and is cost effective. This research involved an off-label use of the medication. As a result, the feed manufacturer requires a prescription to mix the feed. The brand-name manufacturer of the medicine (who also sponsored the research) offers veterinarians a financial incentive to write the prescription using their trade name. A generic equivalent to the brand-name product is available at a significantly reduced cost over the branded product.

Is it ethically correct to write the prescription for the branded medicine and accept the incentive?

Response

The first question relevant to this case is whether the generic product is truly equivalent to the brand-name product. Assuming that it is, one cannot justify a financial incentive arrangement with the brand-name manufacturer. The ethical principle underlying this claim is that, in such a situation, a veterinarian has primary obligation to his or her client. When a client hires a veterinarian, inherent in this professional relationship is the presumption that the veterinarian is deploying his or her expertise to the benefit of the client. Obviously, as we have seen in other cases, the presumption can be overridden by other moral obligations the veterinarian has, for example, obligations to public health or to the animal. But such situations must involve powerful ethical reasons: if the client is endangering public or general animal health, perhaps, or cavalierly disregarding basic social morality, or ignoring animal suffering.

In this case no higher moral principle overriding one's obligation to one's clients is served. Certainly veterinarians have obligations to themselves, but in this case the veterinarian is meeting those obligations by virtue of being paid by his or her clients. So the financial benefit gained by prescribing the brand name would come at the client's expense—in effect, the client would be paying twice.

Furthermore, even disregarding ethical considerations, the veterinarian would be prudentially unwise to take the money from the drug manufacturer. If it became known that the veterinarian was accepting "payola" in order to impose an additional financial burden on clients, his or her reputation would be seriously—perhaps irrevocably—damaged. Any client who learned of this would distrust the veterinarian and would certainly spread word in the community. As veterinarians and other professionals know well, nothing is more precious than one's good name.

Even if the generic were not as good as the brand name, or if I, as the veterinarian, believed it to be not as good, I would not accept the money. If I did, I would be placing myself in a position wherein clients and the community could impugn my motives for using the brand name, by accusing me of failing to prescribe, for self-serving reasons, an "accepted generic equivalent." Again, my reputation could suffer irrevocable damage. One's image as a professional possessed of integrity is not worth risking for significant gain, let alone for peanuts.

Case

59

Negligence of an Emergency Clinician in Treating Trauma

Question

You are an associate veterinarian working in a day clinic from which an affiliated emergency clinic operates on evenings and weekends. Monday morning a vehicular trauma case is transferred to your care from the emergency clinic. The dog is depressed and in pain. It is lying in its own feces and urine. Intravenous fluids and antibiotics are being administered. No analgesics have been given. Your diagnostic work-up reveals a strangulated inguinal hernia (not noted on the emergency clinician's record) and a tibial fracture (amputation recommend by the emergency clinician). Surgical correction of the strangulated hernia, including an intestinal anastomosis, is performed. When you mention your findings to the emergency clinician, he states there was no hernia present over the weekend nor did the dog show signs of pain. The owners are not dissatisfied with the emergency treatment. The close affiliation between your clinic and the emergency clinic makes it difficult to criticize the service provided, even though you feel a proper work-up was not performed.

How should you respond?

Response

This is clearly a case of negligence at best, or incompetence at worst. The animal in question was patently in shock, and seriously injured. For the emergency clinician to say that the animal showed no signs of pain at the same time as he has diagnosed the animal as having a tibial fracture sufficiently severe to elicit from him a recommendation for amputation is incredible. Even if the animal showed no overt signs of pain upon being brought to the clinic, any reasonable medical person would realize that the animal is either too depressed to show the signs, or the injury had only just been sustained and the pain was temporarily held in check by endogenous opiate release—or else the veterinarian simply ignored what was manifest. In any event, the dog is showing pain now. Had the veterinarian been responsible, he would have seen to pain management between the time he received the animal and the time you saw it.

If this evidence does not suffice to prove negligence or incompetence, failure to note the strangled inguinal hernia does. It is extraordinarily unlikely that the hernia somehow occurred through something the traumatized animal did to itself while at the emergency clinic. This in turn means that the emergency veterinarian did not do a thorough examination or else ignored what he found and is prevaricating in a weak effort to protect himself.

In the same vein, the fact that the dog is transferred to you lying in its own excrement bespeaks either negligence or a bad attitude on the part of the emergency veterinarian. When this latter point is considered together with the other problems already discussed, it is manifest that one cannot simply ignore the problem.

One might argue that if the animal's owners are satisfied, why create trouble? The answer is obvious: If the clients are indeed satisfied, it is almost certainly because they are medically naive. This does not of course change the fact that egregious misdeeds or omissions are attributable to the emergency veterinarian. It only means that he was lucky to encounter such naive or trusting clients.

In the situation described, we do not know your relationship with or background knowledge of the emergency veterinarian—how long you have known him, how well you know him, whether he has behaved similarly in the past, and so on. Such knowledge can have significant bearing on how you approach him. But approach him you must. If his past medical track record has been exemplary, perhaps his behavior in this case is a fluke—maybe he is ill, under stress, undergoing personal problems. If this is the case, he might need time off while coping with the difficulty. On the other hand, he may have a long history of such behavior, perhaps associated with substance abuse.

In either case you cannot morally or pragmatically ignore the situation. Although you may have a good relationship with the emergency clinic, your primary moral and professional duty is certainly to your clients and to the animal patients. Furthermore, preserving your own good name and the clinic's good reputation necessitates that you not allow such sloppy or heedless medicine to go unchallenged. Were I the veterinarian, I would therefore confront the emergency clinician with the significant evidence of his mismanagement of this case and ask for an explanation. My subsequent behavior would depend on the plausibility of his response. But whatever course I took, be it talking to his boss, my boss, the veterinary association, or whatever, it would be aimed at assuring that such a situation would not recur.

Case

60

Poor Air Quality in Swine Barn

Question

You provide routine herd health services to a five-hundred-sow farrow-to-finish swine farm. Over the last several years the air quality in the buildings has deteriorated markedly. Several employees (all smokers) complain to you that despite wearing paper masks, they are coughing and wheezing excessively. Pig health and performance are above average and have not been affected by the deteriorating air quality. The absentee owner says that current profit margins prohibit investing in a new ventilation system, especially when performance is satisfactory. He reminds you that if these employees are so worried about their health, they should quit smoking. He recommends that you concentrate on the health of the pigs if you want to keep his account.

Should you take his advice?

Response

It has been recognized since antiquity that farmers and farm workers are at risk for respiratory problems resulting from their exposure to agriculturally related air pollutants. This insight has been increasingly refined in the twentieth century. In 1932 Campbell first described "farmer's lung," a form of pneumonia arising from mold forming in wet hay, and subsequent researchers have identified a variety of other respiratory diseases specific to an agricultural context (Warren, 1989, p. 47).

Beginning in the early 1980s, researchers have become aware that those who work in confinement swine barns risk "a number of pulmonary manifestations, including pulmonary edema, asthma, bronchitis, bronchiolitis, airways obstructions, and organic dust toxic syndrome." Pollutants giving rise to these problems include toxic dust containing animal fecal material, animal dander, feed material, mineral dust, insect parts, pollen, fungi, bacteria, and bacterial endotoxins (Merchant and Donham, 1989, p. 58). Toxic gases may also be present. The resulting diseases cause significant amounts of lost work time for farm workers. Research has also shown that smokers and former smokers are at significantly greater risk than those farm workers who have never smoked (Donham and Gustafson, 1982, p. 140). One can thus conclude that the advent of confinement swine rearing has engendered major risks of respiratory problems for those who work in such facilities. This group includes veterinarians managing the health of these animals (Donham and Gustafson, 1982, p. 139). Not surprisingly, these risks are increased in a manner inversely proportional to degree of ventilation in the swine barn (Donham and Gustafson, 1982, p. 138).

This background information provides us with a context for evaluating the case in question. Clearly, the workers in this case have already been adversely affected, and the data rather surprisingly indicates that cessation of smoking at the stage the veterinarian finds them will make little difference (Donham and Gustafson, 1982, p. 140).

The veterinarian is thus faced with significant conflicting moral pulls, stemming from his diverse obligations in this case. Once again, obligations to clients, animals, peers and the profession, society, and self are all operative here to varying degrees, and some involve conflicts even within the category in question. In the first place the veterinarian has obligations to the client, the person who pays the bills and contracts for his services. The client has clearly indicated that he wishes to make no changes in the air-handling system, since productivity is not affected. On the other hand, the client may be losing money he has not considered, due to worker time lost to sickness. Further, the air quality may well be affecting the animals in subtle ways, for example, by stressing them through subclinical infection, which can impede production and reproduction.

Second, the veterinarian has obligations to animals. Whether or not bad air affects production, it certainly creates a poor quality of life for the animals, already living (compared to extensively reared swine) a questionable existence.

Third, the veterinarian has public health obligations to society, here represented by the innocent workers. As veterinary medicine has become increasingly sophisticated scientifically, its involvement in public health has grown exponentially. That obligation looms large in this case.

Fourth, the veterinarian has obligations to peers and the profession. As we indicated earlier, veterinarians too are put at risk in confinement swine operations. Further, the credibility of the profession is eroded when veterinarians turn a blind eye to pathogenic agricultural systems. When the public inevitably comes to know about the respiratory problems in swine barns, it will not be seemly for veterinary medicine to have kept silent.

Finally, the veterinarian has obligations to himself. On the one hand, he must be able to look himself in the mirror, something that will grow increasingly difficult if he does not attempt to alleviate the plight of the workers and animals. Further, he himself is at risk breathing the air in the swine barn. However, aggressively challenging the owner can possibly result in the veterinarian being replaced by a less morally sensitive colleague.

In the end, the moral balance sheet seems to militate in favor of the veterinarian not letting the matter drop. Were I the veterinarian, I would forcefully suggest modifying the ventilation system and, in the meantime, demand that the owner immediately provide the workers with proper respirators. In making my argument, I would educate the owner on potential losses incurred via worker illness and the inevitable erosion of efficiency. I would also point out his moral obligations to animals and employees and the negative public relations dimensions of failing to take them seriously. I would also remind him of his potential for liability vis-à-vis the workers. Finally, I would attempt to put him in touch with other operators who had dealt with the problem in a reasonable fashion.

If none of this proved effective, I would terminate my relationship with that owner. It is not good for me, as an individual or as a veterinarian, to work in a pathogenic facility, or to be associated with one. Although I would not go out of my way to publicize my reasons for quitting, neither would I hide those reasons if asked. And I would certainly explain the risks to the workers in the swine barn.

I am grateful to Dr. Lorann Stallones for invaluable dialogue and references.

Case

61

Supplementing Income with Prescription Drugs

Question

You have recently joined a four-person mixed-animal practice. The office manager and the senior partner want to discuss your charges on farm calls. You are consistently billing two to three hundred dollars less per day than the other associates. Review of your records reveals you are seeing as many, or more, cases each day as your colleagues. The hourly rate is a set fee. The difference in billing is due to treatment charges. You are using labeled dosages of over-the-counter drugs for conditions traditionally treated in this practice by the off-label use of prescription drugs. There have been no complaints regarding the efficacy of your treatments. The partners believe that the clients will not tolerate a higher hourly rate, so the practice must generate income based on drug sales. You are strongly encouraged to follow the clinic's practice.

What is your response?

Response

When I first read this case, its resolution appeared totally straightforward to me. My initial response was that the practice is "double dipping" unfairly, charging not only for practitioners' time, but also for more expensive drugs than necessary. If an over-the-counter drug does the job, I reasoned, what else but greed explains the dispensing of prescriptions?

A moment's reflection mitigated my initial reaction. If the practice were indeed cynically overcharging, surely it would be losing clients to other practices, and its reputation in the community would have suffered. Thus, I concluded, there must be more to this situation than meets the eye. In order to understand what was going on, I telephoned a prominent veterinarian in Canada and asked him if I had misread the situation.

Our conversation was revelatory. He told me that, in various locales, veterinarians are convinced that their clientele will tolerate only a certain hourly charge. That charge in turn will simply not pay the overhead on the practice and return a reasonable (*not ex-*

cessive) profit. Thus, the veterinarians are driven to drug sales as a significant source of their income. In the case in question, the veterinarian who prescribes over-the-counter drugs is in effect not pulling his or her weight in the practice.

My communicant went on to draw an analogy between the situation for veterinarians and that for other service industries. Physicians may charge considerable amounts for a vaccine or a knee brace, much more than the product would cost over the counter. People who repair automobiles or other machinery similarly charge top dollar for parts. They could, of course, charge less for the parts, but only if they were to raise their hourly rates, rates that consumers already find excessive.

In the wake of our discussion, my initial reaction was blunted considerably. However, the situation still leaves me somewhat uneasy, even though the client is not being overcharged. Rather, the charges are being made for drugs instead of for professional time. It is difficult to articulate exactly the source of my unease, but I will try.

I once heard a lecture by a veterinary practice manager (a non-veterinarian) in which he stressed that "veterinarians make as much money as they think they deserve." He was talking to an equine practitioner audience, and his examples were drawn from the equine area, but they could be modified to fit all areas of veterinary medicine. He spoke of how equine veterinarians will feel sorry for even a rich client when the stock market has taken a downturn, and not bill what they should. He spoke of veterinarians' failure to bill for bandages and similar items, and of their failure to charge for telephone conversation time. Pediatricians and attorneys charge for phone time, he pointed out—why not veterinarians? Why should veterinarians give away their hard-won expertise?

It is in this same vein that I am disturbed by the veterinarians' circuitous way of earning a fair living in this case. It bespeaks too low a self-concept, assuming that clients won't ever pay the hourly rate necessary for the veterinarian to turn a profit. It would seem to me better to educate the client to pay for value received than to bury the extra charge in drugs. For, in the long run, a practice could come along that charges less for prescription drugs, either because of large volume or because it is part of a superstore chain, and undercut your prescription prices. If that occurs, you are left with having to make ends meet without the aid of drug charges. So I believe that it is better not to obfuscate and to be paid for expertise and quality of service—this is ground that cannot be cut from under you the way drug prices can.

I am grateful to Linda Rollin, Ph.D., Lynne Kesel, D.V.M., and my Canadian practitioner colleague who prefers to remain anonymous.

Case

62

Client's Request to Euthanize His Dog after His Death

Question

The wife of a regular client arrives at your clinic requesting euthanasia for a healthy, well-behaved three-year-old sheltie. The dog belonged to her recently deceased husband. He requested that upon his death, the dog should be euthanized and cremated, so that their ashes could be spread together in the mountains. His wife is not fond of dogs and does not want this one.

Should you comply with this request?

Response

In a number of previous cases I have discussed the issue of euthanizing healthy animals for owner convenience. In these discussions, I have argued that carrying out such euthanasia is not only morally questionable vis-à-vis the animal, but is extremely erosive to a veterinarian's morale and psychological well-being. Indeed, my own experience in dealing with veterinarians for over twenty years has convinced me that the recurrent demand for convenience euthanasia is probably the most demoralizing and psychologically damaging feature of companion animal practice. Thus, I tend to believe that both the veterinarian's obligation to the animal and the veterinarian's obligation to himself or herself tend to trump one's obligation to the client requesting convenience euthanasia. (How this general maxim plays out will of course vary from case to case.)

In this case there is an additional wrinkle. I, the veterinarian, have not been directly asked by the client to euthanize the animal in the event of his death. Instead, I am being asked by his wife, who has promised her husband to euthanize the animal. Had I been asked by the husband, I would have refused to do so and would have attempted to make a case for the animal's life. Usually, sane people wish to see the animal destroyed after their own death only because they genuinely believe the animal cannot possibly be happy without them. As the late Dr. Leo Bustad, a pioneer in discussing the nuances of the human-animal bond, has pointed out, this is rarely the case. The belief that the animal "can't be happy without me" is usually wishful thinking. Normal, resilient animals adjust after the death of an owner, even as normal, resilient children adjust to the death of a parent. There are, of course, pathological cases of an animal who can't adjust, but these would be statistically insignificant. It is also hard to believe that, in this case, the dog has not bonded with the wife while in the home.

Dr. Bustad argued that the much-touted legend of Grayfriars' Bobby, the story of the Scottish dog that pined away at his owner's grave, and other similar sentimental stories rife in popular culture, have deflected attention away from the prosaic, but morally relevant, point that 99 percent of dogs can continue to enjoy life with another owner and therefore should at least be given a chance. I myself have adopted three dogs over the years, all of whom were relinquished by owners after five to seven years, and all of whom lived out their lives happily with us. Were this not the case, no one could ever adopt adult animals!

Thus, I, as a veterinarian, would never have committed to the client to kill the dog, and did not, in fact, do so in this case, though the client's wife may have done so. Therefore, I am under no direct obligation to euthanize and would not do so. I would further explain to the wife why I did not believe it was the right thing to do.

Presumably, at this point, the wife will do one of two things. She may attempt to find a veterinarian who will carry out her husband's wishes, or she may ask me whether she ought to do so—if she is justified in disregarding her husband's last wish, however irrational. If I were asked the latter question, I would say something like the following: "I do not believe that you would wrong your husband by failing to kill the dog. Had he talked to me, I would have done everything I could to dissuade him. Suppose he had asked you to burn a valuable Rembrandt painting he owned or to scatter his money to the four winds, you surely wouldn't feel bound to do so! The point is that the request was *irrational* and *morally* unjustifiable. You did the right thing by humoring him and agreeing to his request, but you also do the right thing by not following through with the killing. In any case, it is difficult for me to see how we can harm the dead. Indeed, even if it is sensible to believe that we can, we do far more harm to your husband (or to his reputation) if people find out that he insisted on having this young, healthy dog killed than if we fail to honor that request. If you wish to honor the rational core of his request, on the anniversary of his death take the dog somewhere where your husband and the animal shared good times together."

I would hope that approach to the wife would allow her to pass between the horns of the dilemma—that is, kill the dog or break her promise—unfairly foisted upon her by her husband through his request. (I say unfairly because whatever she does is likely to create some guilt.) But regardless of whether she accepts my argument or not, I would not kill the animal.

Case

63

Confidentiality and an Employee's History of Drug Abuse

Question

You discover that narcotics are missing from your clinic. Based on entries in the narcotics log book and an eventual confession by the technician, you determine that the abuse has been occurring for one week. The matter is reported to the authorities, who agree to allow you to deal with the matter internally. The technician has been under a large amount of personal stress recently, is repentant, and agrees to seek professional help. Prior to this incident the technician had been a valuable member of your staff. You keep the technician on staff but eliminate access to the narcotic cupboard.

A few months later the technician moves to another city. You discover, thereafter, that the professional counseling was discontinued after just two weeks. A week later you receive a call from another veterinarian who is contemplating hiring this individual. The new job entails full access to narcotics.

Should you inform this veterinarian of the technician's past history with narcotics abuse?

Response

Most prospective employers value personal references far more than more objective measures, for example, transcripts of one's academic record, when evaluating a candidate. My veterinary students, accustomed to working for grades, are invariably nonplussed when a prospective employer is not interested in even looking at their academic record. As one veterinarian told me, "Grades don't tell me a damn thing about what kind of person or clinician a candidate is."

Unfortunately, analogous to what academics call "grade point creep"—inflation of grades—society has also witnessed an inflation of personal evaluations and recommendations. While recently serving on a search committee, I screened 120 applications. If one simply read letters of reference, one would come away with the impression that everyone in the applicant pool was a remarkable cross between Einstein, Gandhi, and Jesus. So hyperbolic was the prose in these letters that our search committee found itself looking for any hint of negativity as grounds for disqualifying a candidate. For example, one comment suggesting that a candidate was sometimes perceived as "very assertive" elicited in us the fear of hiring an academic Genghis Khan.

There are many reasons for "reference inflation." These include fear of litigation should the person requesting the recommendation learn that you may have said anything negative. Equally important is the current social trend forbidding saying anything that might "hurt someone's feelings" or, God forbid, affect their "self-esteem." While feelings are protected, employers and society suffer because the clear distinctions between greater and lesser degrees of competence and reliability have been blurred and obscured.

Abuse of illegal drugs is one of the major problems in society today, judging by the amount of rhetoric devoted to the issue, as well as by the amounts of money expended (largely futilely) to curtail drug traffic. In the case in question, furthermore, we are told that the technician has been using "hard drugs"—narcotics. We also know that the technician has already abused the trust involved in working around narcotics. We know that the technician was not seriously committed to rehabilitation; abandoning the program as soon as enrolling in it has accomplished the goal of shielding him from greater penalties. To put it plainly, the technician has been caught, given a second chance, and has quickly violated the conditions of that chance. Now you are being asked by a colleague to evaluate this technician. Upon analysis, I find the question of the morally proper course of action relatively nonproblematic.

What are the sources of moral obligation relevant to this case? In the first place, one has a duty to society. Society has spoken against drug abuse, especially in the workplace, and most especially where drug impairment can cause harm (a railroad engineer as opposed to a clothing sales associate). The impaired veterinary technician can certainly cause significant harm. Thus, as a member of a profession serving society and whose autonomy depends on social dispensation, you cannot ignore the technician's history. Furthermore, we are all obliged to restore credibility to personal references, without which society cannot function effectively.

Second, one has a duty to peers, colleagues, and the profession. Your fellow veterinarian is entitled to an honest appraisal and to knowledge of relevant information that might affect his practice. In this case drug abuse by an employee can cause him and his practice incalculable harm. Similarly, the profession needs to be safeguarded against those who can damage its reputation in society.

One's duty to clients and to animals also clearly militates in favor of telling the truth. A technician impaired by drugs, as mentioned earlier, can cause significant amounts of harm to animals and thereby to owners.

The only considerations that might appear to militate against telling the truth are your obligations to the technician and to yourself. In the case of the technician, your behavior has already been supererogatory when you gave him a second chance and convinced the authorities to let you handle the infraction. The technician has gone on to violate your trust by discontinuing the counseling. Thus informing the veterinarian of the facts is hardly backstabbing. Indeed, it is no favor to the technician to continue to cover for him; such behavior will simply encourage further infractions. Insofar as not covering for him may lead him to take responsibility for his drug use, you will have actually done him a favor.

Regarding obligations to oneself, failure to inform the hiring veterinarian of the technician's history can come back on you, especially if the technician again violates trust and his previous history is unearthed. Your credibility would be undercut in such a situation, not only with veterinarians, but with the agency that trusted you to deal with the situation.

If one does inform the hiring veterinarian of the relevant history, one faces an additional decision: Should you inform the technician that you have done so and tell him the reasons why? The answer to this question will vary, depending on a variety of factors peculiar to the situation—the personality of the technician, how close your relationship is with him, whether you believe it might shock him into taking the matter more seriously, and so on. But whether or not you inform him, I strongly believe that you are obliged to reveal the history to your colleague.

Case

64

Convenience Euthanasia of a Dog without Proper Permission

Question

A five-year-old healthy Maltese is presented to your clinic for euthanasia. The dog is well behaved and the client gives no reason for the euthanasia. The consent form is signed and the dog euthanized. The following day the client's wife phones inquiring about the dog. The Maltese was her dog, and her husband had it destroyed as part of an ongoing fight with her.

Is it appropriate to contact all family members before agreeing to perform a euthanasia?

Is the veterinarian liable for the death of this woman's dog?

Response

I have already addressed the issue of euthanizing healthy animals in a variety of dimensions. I have argued that such euthanasia is a major source of stress and job dissatisfaction for practitioners, and that the way to mitigate such tension is to do everything possible as an animal advocate. These discussions bear on this case since, by hypothesis, the veterinarian did not engage the client in any dialogue as to the reasons for euthanasia. Since we are told that the animal is well behaved, and we know that behavior problems are a major cause for euthanasia of companion animals, it would certainly have behooved the veterinarian to probe the client about his reasons for euthanasia, since in many cases, including behavioral difficulties, there exist alternatives to killing. Merely to euthanize healthy animals on request is virtually a guarantee of significant job dissatisfaction at some point in the future. Furthermore, had the veterinarian taken his advocacy role seriously, in this case at least, the problems with the wife might not have arisen, as he may well have uncovered the fact that the husband was driven by spite.

Adopting a conscientious policy on convenience euthanasia does not absolutely assure that the veterinarian would have unearthed the husband's base motives. If the husband was a skilled liar, he could surely weave a highly plausible set of reasons for euthanasia, for example, affirming that a child in the family was allergic. But if the veterinarian probes and challenges this reason, for example, by requesting permission to try to place the animal, the truth might emerge, or at least the husband might be caught without an adequate answer. Thus, one's animal advocacy stance can certainly help diminish the probability of such unfortunate incidents—obviously to a far greater extent than would a policy of euthanizing on request—but probably cannot eliminate them all.

So let us assume that the veterinarian has left no stone unturned in questioning the husband and has still been duped. By "duped" I mean that the husband has told a story that leaves even a strong animal advocate convinced that there is no alternative to euthanasia—for example, the dog is dangerous and vicious (hard to believe with a Maltese); the dog has been pronounced incorrigible by numerous behavior experts; the dog has been placed in various homes and attacked everyone; the dog attacks babies on sight; no one else will adopt it; and so on. (The difficulty one has in constructing such a case bespeaks the rarity of situations wherein euthanizing a healthy animal is truly morally justified.)

If the euthanasia is in fact justifiable, it is hard to blame the veterinarian for listening to the husband and performing the euthanasia. As I have said before, veracity is a presupposition of discourse. If I have no reason to doubt the truth of a person's story, and the story is plausible, I assume that what that person says is true. In fact, people like this husband, and con men, rely precisely on this unspoken rule of civilized interaction. Having been burned in a given case as this veterinarian was, one might try to be more careful in the future. But what does this mean? Does one call every member of a family to assure that they have agreed to, say, a surgery? (A similar case could occur wherein one spouse gives consent for surgery, and afterward the wife claims it is her dog and *she* didn't consent.) As any paranoid knows, one can be endlessly suspicious.

In the end, people like the husband are very rare, just as swindlers are rare. Certainly one who has been bitten might be more wary in the future but, on the other hand, should not become excessively preoccupied with being bitten. Becoming excessively distrustful of all clients in the wake of an incident like this does not serve one's own peace of mind well, certainly does not serve the public well, and is likely to alienate most clients. Cases like this are thankfully rare; a policy of eschewing convenience euthanasia should further narrow the possibility of recurrence. For the rest, it is better to risk another incident than to treat clients (or others) with a constant attitude of distrust and suspicion.

Case

65

Veterinarian Who Ignores Roundworms in Puppies

Question

You have recently joined a rural mixed-animal practice in southern Manitoba. In this practice puppies are vaccinated and dewormed when they are first presented for examination. Booster vaccinations and a follow-up fecal examination are performed two to four weeks following the initial visit. You are concerned that this is not providing adequate control of roundworms and are particularly worried about puppies in homes with young children. You suggest to your employer that deworming new puppies every two to three weeks until three months of age would greatly diminish the risk of visceral larval migrans in children who have close contact with these young dogs. The employer assures you that this line of reasoning, although scientifically valid, would discourage people from owning pets and could be viewed by others as a money grab. He assures you that he has never had a problem with his regular deworming policy and does not want clients to be confused or feel threatened with fears of eye disease in their children.

How should you respond?

Response

The case described seems to me to be more a question of communication and persuasion than one of ethics. One of the primary obligations of a veterinarian is promoting public health, and the ocular disease potential in children growing out of zoonotic transfer from puppies is significant. According to Dr. John Cheney, Colorado State University parasitologist, the Centers for Disease Control reports some two thousand cases per year in the United States.

The key point is that this incidence is significant, especially since it is so easily preventable, simply by following the regimen indicated by the veterinarian who has recently joined the practice. Dr. Cheney points out that the fecal examination described would not rule out the presence of infestation, and that the eggs are so hardy they can survive five years in the ambient environment and have been known to survive even in formalin! Thus one's obligation to public health (that is, to the children) militates definitively in favor of the regimen suggested by the employee.

Correlatively, there is no ethical pressure against following the regimen. That the veterinarian has "never had a problem" bespeaks good luck rather than state-of-the-art medicine. His other points, that he does not wish to confuse or alarm clients or discourage people from owning pets, or that he does not want to appear mercenary, do not provide a morally adequate justification for failing to recommend the regimen, and in fact bespeaks a questionable view of client intelligence. It is his job to explain to clients in a manner they can understand that though infestation is a risk associated with puppies, that risk is totally manageable in an inexpensive way with the regimen suggested. As Dr. Cheney points out, this veterinarian surely does not cavil at recommending rabies vaccinations, despite the fact that the danger of contracting rabies is far lower! Thus there is no reason to believe that explaining the risk and the mode of dispelling it will discourage pet ownership any more than does rabies vaccination. (In my entire life I have never encountered a person who refuses to acquire a pet because of fear of controllable zoonoses.) If the veterinarian does a good job explaining the situation to clients, there is little risk of their being "threatened or confused."

What of his fear of appearing to be mercenary? Again, I think this concern is largely spurious. Few people would regard suggesting an inexpensive regimen that would protect their children's eyes as money gouging. In fact, I believe that expressing concern about protecting clients' children from zoonotic risks could only enhance one's image.

Not only does the veterinarian's obligation to public health support this recommended regimen, so does the veterinarian's obligation to himself. In the first place, I would have trouble living with myself if I had not done everything possible to forestall zoonotic risk to children. Although this does not seem to trouble the veterinarian in this case, it surely would if his luck ran out and a child did get eye disease from a puppy not properly treated by him. Indeed, if such a mishap occurred, his reputation would be seriously damaged and he could surely be sued for malpractice, as he has failed to recommend a regimen that is, by his own admission, validated as state-of-the-art scientific.

I am grateful to Dr. John Cheney for his lucid and penetrating comments.

Case

66

Stray Tattooed Beagle

Question

Your veterinary clinic advocates and performs tattooing on clients' animals. You recommend this procedure as a permanent form of identification. New clients arrive with a stray beagle, which is already tattooed. The tattoo was not done at your clinic. Apparently, the dog had wandered around the clients' neighborhood for a week before they decided to adopt it. You advise the clients that the tattoo indicates previous ownership. They respond by saying that they had called the local Society for the Prevention of Cruelty to Animals (SPCA), and there had been no reports of lost beagles. The clients do not want to take the dog to the SPCA, where it will be eligible for adoption if unclaimed after five days. Your local veterinary association states that your responsibility ends with notifying a new owner of the tattoo and its significance; you are not to actively pursue locating the original owner. You have been tattooing pets in good faith, assuring clients that it is a real safeguard against loss or theft. You now feel you have been misleading your clients.

What is your next course of action?

Response

I do not think that the veterinarian in this case should give up seeking permanent identification for pet animals, or even necessarily give up tattooing. The underlying assumption he has made in recommending tattooing is, after all, sound. It is unquestionably highly desirable to have all animals permanently identifiable, for numerous reasons, primarily to prevent loss and theft. This assumption is not at all undermined by what has occurred in this case.

What the case does do is underscore a point that the veterinarian has perhaps not sufficiently emphasized in his thinking, namely, that creating the permanent identifier, in this case the tattoo, is only half the battle. The second, equally important, component of such a system is an essentially unerring way of easily correlating the unalterable identifier with the relevant information about the animal's owners.

One can presume that, in the case in question, veterinarians who tattoo the animals maintain their own file correlating tattoos with owner identification information.

Someone who finds the animal, therefore, has no readily available algorithm for using the tattoo to find the owner. Are they presumed to know enough to phone every veterinary practice? Is that burden to fall on the SPCA, which has clearly failed to shoulder it in this case? Is the nature of the system common knowledge?

The strength of a system of identification varies in direct proportion to the extent that it is common knowledge. If a person receiving a blow to the head remembers nothing but his name, it will be relatively easy for authorities (or even good Samaritans) to track down his identity, address, and profession. On the other hand, if he remembers only his secret fraternity nickname, the task of tracking his identity is made immeasurably more difficult.

This is, of course, why fingerprinting and branding are such successful forms of identification in humans and cattle, respectively. If one finds a branded stray cow, it is a simple matter to establish ownership, since brand books are readily available, easily accessible, and carefully controlled. Regrettably, tattooing, as this case illustrates, is far more haphazard.

Tattooing and microchip injection are currently the most viable forms of permanent identification for companion animals. Yet both can be useless without a central well-known data bank to which those finding an animal are inexorably led. Because various manufacturers make different and incompatible microchip systems, implanting an animal is no guarantee of the inexorable tracing of ownership. The same holds with tattooing.

Instead of despairing, the veterinarian should work to establish a central registry of tattooed animals, at least covering his own geographical area, utilizing some viable and unique identifiers—the social security number of the owner, for example, would be ideal in the United States. All veterinarians, animal control people, and humane societies should be in a position to access that data bank by computer. Had such a system been in place, the SPCA and the veterinarian could immediately and simply have located the owner as soon as the person who found the beagle contacted them. Such a system would provide additional benefits, as well, including enabling municipalities to track down irresponsible pet owners who allow their dogs to run loose and do not bother to claim them if they are lost or impounded by animal control.

Case

67

Prescribing and Selling Pharmaceuticals

Question

Is it a conflict of interest for a veterinarian to prescribe and sell pharmaceutical products?

Response

As stated, the question is ambiguous and can mean two distinct things. First, it can be interpreted to mean "Can there ever be a conflict of interest occasioned by a veterinary practitioner prescribing and selling pharmaceuticals?" Second, it can be taken in a much stronger way, to mean "*Must* there *always* be a conflict of interest occasioned by a veterinary practitioner prescribing and selling pharmaceuticals?"

The answer to the first question is certainly affirmative. There are surely situations wherein a conflict of interest could arise. For example, a veterinarian could have a financial interest in a particular pharmaceutical—say, a vaccine he has developed that competes with other vaccines on the market. Were he routinely and exclusively to prescribe and/or sell that particular vaccine without explaining to the client his proprietary interest, that there are other vaccines on the market, and why he thinks his is best, he would certainly be generating such a conflict. Similarly, if he prescribes or dispenses an antibiotic by trade name solely because he gets a higher profit on it than he would get from the identical generic, and in so doing fails to inform the client that one can buy the generic easily and cheaply at a large, competitive pharmacy, he is again in a conflict of interest situation, the conflict, of course, arising from his role as medical professional versus his role as profit-making merchant. In short, a conflict of interest can certainly arise between the veterinarian's obligation to do the best for the client (a professional obligation) and his desire to maximize his income, if he fails to notify the client of different and cheaper alternatives to the regimen that benefits the veterinarian economically.

When one turns to the second question, however, one can readily see that it is not necessarily the case that a conflict of interest *must* arise just because a veterinarian prescribes and/or sells drugs. If the veterinarian is honest, straightforward, and open with the client, conflict of interest can be avoided. For example, suppose you are prescribing the aforementioned antibiotic, generic or not. It is very unlikely that you can compete with a high-volume pharmacy. On the other hand, it is perfectly fair that you be compensated for the convenience afforded to the client by not having to go to the store, or for the money you have locked into your inventory. In a small, rural community, with no pharmacy nearby, both the convenience for the client and the requisite inventory can be considerable.

As always, the proper course of action is a mean between extremes, in Aristotle's felicitous phrase. One ought not expect a veterinarian to provide the service of supplying drugs for no recompense. On the other hand, outrageously marking up those drugs for trusting clients is not only morally questionable, it is highly imprudent. For once you have earned a reputation for gouging clients in one area, it is difficult to mitigate that reputation. Even among medical peers your recommendations will be suspect if you are perceived as markedly enhancing your own income at the expense of your clients.

Though I have heard it argued that some veterinarians keep their fees down by overcharging on medicine, I do not accept that argument. It is better to practice, and to charge top dollar for, first-rate medicine that provides excellent service to clients than to attempt to compete by quietly charging too much for pharmaceuticals. If you do the former, the worst that clients can say is "he is really good, and he charges for it." Surveys have shown that cost is not a main factor for most clients, if the service is superb. On the other hand, overcharging on drugs is petty and is very likely to lead to people wondering whether you overcharge on everything, even if you don't. (Cf. Case 61.)

Case

68

Suspected Poisoning

Question

A six-year-old Shetland sheepdog has suffered three episodes of vomiting, diarrhea, and circulatory collapse. The dog recovered each time following treatment with IV fluids and cage rest. Radiographs taken after the most recent episode revealed a possible intestinal foreign body. You recommend to the nineteen-year-old woman who owns the dog that an exploratory laparotomy, after the dog has regained its strength, may help to better define the problem. The evening prior to the scheduled surgery, the client's mother phones. She requests that you collect the appropriate samples for a toxicologic investigation while you are performing the exploratory laparotomy. She suspects that her daughter's boyfriend is poisoning the dog. She wants to be billed separately for the testing and does not want her daughter to know of this arrangement. The same suspicion has also been troubling you.

How should you proceed?

Response

This case is best analyzed by looking first at the moral obligations borne by the veterinarian in this situation. Obviously, the veterinarian is primarily obligated to the animal and to the client, in this case the young woman. There is no tension between those obligations, as the client wants the dog healed and the episodes stopped, and the same result is, of course, in the animal's best interest. The client has hired you to effect diagnosis and treatment, and doing so is your primary concern.

Obviously, you have no direct obligation to the client's mother. She is serving as a source of possibly relevant information, in exactly the same way as if she called to tell you that she saw the dog rooting around in an area containing toxic waste or poisonous plants. So, initially, she is simply a source of a diagnostic clue. Since you have already suspected the possibility of poisoning, and presumably would pursue that possibility were the laparotomy to reveal nothing causative of the signs and symptoms, this additional information mainly serves to underscore the need for you to explore that diagnostic avenue, that is, to send samples for toxicological determination. Given that you would have done so without the mother's call, it is not appropriate to bill her for the tests. The situation is also much simpler if you have no formal paid relationship with the mother, for accepting money from her could lead to a conflict of interest.

Thus I would thank the mother, indicate that you are already prepared to explore the possibility of poisoning, tell her that you will report the results to her daughter, your client, and ring off. I would then call the daughter and inform her of the toxicological diagnostic pathway you intend to pursue should the laparotomy prove inconclusive, without mentioning the mother's phone call.

If the toxicology laboratory reports no suspicion of poisoning and is definitive in its conclusion, the matter is closed. If, however, the laboratory does find evidence of poisoning, I would inform the daughter and ask her who might be in a position to poison the animal. Unless the mother had given me unequivocal evidence buttressing her suspicion of the boyfriend—for example, if she claims to have seen the boyfriend feeding the dog rat poison—I would not involve the mother again. If she had given me such a strong claim, I would call her back and suggest that she communicate the fact to her daughter, since she is the person who witnessed the poisoning.

I might also suggest to the daughter various routes she could take to identify the poisoner—for example, the use of a hidden camera unknown to anyone but her, or limiting the people who can access the animal. If, for instance, she keeps the dog in the house except when she accompanies it, and no symptoms appear, the poisoner is likely to be a neighbor or an outsider. If, however, the animal does get sick again, she can legitimately conclude that the poisoning is accomplished by someone in the house. In the event that she does succeed in identifying the poisoner, I would urge her to pursue the matter, as such behavior can be indicative of a psychopathic personality.

Case

69

Euthanasia of Research Animal without Researcher's Permission

Question

You are the staff veterinarian at a research facility in a university medical school. An animal health technician presents you with a rat that has a badly infected hind limb following surgery. The research project involved has received full approval from the university Animal Care Committee. You know, both from the research protocol and from previous experience with the project, that long-term survival of the rat is critical to the success of the research. The principal investigator has always been very cooperative; however, he is out of the country for two weeks and cannot be contacted. His research associates suggest that you take no action until the principal investigator returns. Provision for treatment is not included in the experimental protocol, and a minimum number of rats have been assigned to the trial, so the loss of one rat could affect the significance of the results. You believe that this rat should receive immediate treatment or be euthanized.

What action should you take?

Response

This dilemma should never have arisen. Had the committee been doing its job properly, it would never have approved a protocol that did not specify both end points and treatment modalities covering plausible eventualities. And infection is certainly a foreseeable consequence of any surgical protocol. Thus, at the very least, this committee should learn from the situation and revise what it demands from investigators. Similarly, they should never have allowed the investigator to use so few animals that any unforeseen circumstance could vitiate the whole project. Having said this, what is to be done in the emergency situation? The research associates have pressed for no action (probably to protect themselves), but this is untenable for both ethical and scientific reasons. Leaving an animal with an untreated, "badly infected" hind limb for two weeks is simply unacceptable morally, as the pain and suffering are likely to be quite severe. From a scientific point of view, leaving the animal septic is equally unacceptable. The infection process and the attendant inflammatory and other physiological changes have biological consequences, rendering this animal incommensurable with others on the project. In addition, the pain and distress attendant to the infection are significant stressors, also affecting innumerable variables very likely to be germane to the research project. Thus leaving the animal untreated is not a live option, either ethically or scientifically.

What of treating the animal? Here it is important to consult a competent laboratory animal veterinarian to answer the question of whether treatment is likely to skew the results of the experiment in unpredictable ways. If it is, then there is no reason to treat the animal, since even in the best of circumstances, given that the leg is badly infected, the animal is likely to suffer for the period of time it takes for treatment to work. If, on the other hand, the treatment is irrelevant to what is being investigated, then treating the leg is a possibility. In order to choose, if such is the case, between treatment and euthanasia, one must now weigh the animal's suffering during the treatment. If we have reason to believe that treatment will be quickly efficacious and dramatic in removing suffering, that is a viable option. If, on the other hand, the treatment is going to be slow in alleviating the animal's suffering, I would lean toward euthanasia. In assessing how long the animal should be allowed to suffer, I would suggest using anthropomorphic criteria. This will help keep the committee from being cavalier about allowing the animal to a suffer "for a few days." Whenever one is in such a position, one should recall the wisdom of the old Jewish joke that defines major surgery as surgery I get, minor surgery as surgery you get.

Case

70

Anorexic Client Not Feeding Her Dog

Question

A seven-year-old golden retriever is presented to your clinic with a complaint of chronic weight loss. The dog weighs only fifty-eight pounds and appears to have lost at least twenty pounds since you administered its rabies booster seven months ago. You observe that the owner, a young woman, also appears to have lost a lot of weight. When you comment on this, she changes the subject. You hospitalize the dog and run a series of tests, all of which are within normal limits. The dog eats ravenously while hospitalized and gains three pounds. You discharge the animal with strict instruction regarding feeding, and schedule a follow-up exam in two weeks. When the dog returns, it weighs only fifty-five pounds. The owner assures you she has adhered to the diet.

What should your response be?

Response

Again, this case should be required reading for all preveterinary students who wish to enter veterinary medicine because they "don't want to deal with people." Here all the signs point to the owner's psychological problems being responsible for the animal's weight loss, rather than any metabolic problem or disease process in the dog. If this is indeed the case, this situation demonstrates that, once again, a veterinarian's human skills can be as important as his or her medical skills in resolving problems for the animal.

Such situations are far from unique or even scarce. In fact, one successful small-animal veterinarian I know feels so strongly about the relevance of client psychopathology to veterinary practice that he has sought extensive training in psychology and urged such training upon members of his local association. Further, many rural veterinarians have told me that, as the only professional in their area, they are often sought out by clients for advice more appropriately in the province of psychologists or marriage counselors. At Colorado State University our veterinary students are taught to look for signs of depression or suicidal tendencies in grieving clients.

In the face of such situations it is not unreasonable for a veterinarian to establish a good professional relationship with a clinical psychologist and/or psychiatrist in his or her area, so that one may refer troubled clients or at least seek professional advice on how to handle them. As this case illustrates, such a liaison can benefit not only the clients, but also the animals in the clients' charge. Although this case is a companion-animal situation, the same sort of thing can occur with horses and farm animals, for example, if a depressed owner ceases to provide care.

But suppose one has no such rapport with a mental health professional. How should the veterinarian proceed? Were I the clinician, I would call the woman into my office and frankly state my concern that she is having eating problems and projecting them onto the animal. I would offer to use my connections to assist her in finding counseling. Since many anorectics have a distorted body image, she might well deny that there is a problem. (The way the case is structured in fact indicates that she will probably dismiss my statements.) If this occurs, I would ask her to leave the dog with me for a few weeks and document the weight gain on the diet I prescribed. I would then confront her again. If she continues to protest that she did follow the diet, or if she did not allow me to take the dog, I would contact the anticruelty authorities. My obligation to the animal militates against letting her starve it, even if she is mentally ill. In most if not all jurisdictions, failing to provide adequate nutrition counts as cruelty. Just as it is immoral to allow a mentally ill person to beat an animal, it is immoral to permit starvation. Indeed, being confronted by the authorities may be the only way to force her to seek help for herself.

I am grateful to Dr. Ernie Chavez for dialogue.

Case

71

Improving Rural Euthanasia

Question

After twenty years in mixed-animal practice, you have observed widely varying practices concerning on-farm euthanasia of unwanted dogs and cats. From the shepherd who routinely shoots every stray dog that crosses the farm, to the dairy farmer who takes a few litters of kittens out to the pond every summer, you have been witness to many differing disposal techniques. Many of these procedures appear less than humane. You have tried offering a free euthanasia service to your regular clients; however, coordinating the capture of these often semiferal animals with your visits seldom occurs. Leaving an injectable solution for euthanasia on the farm seems too risky.

What should you do?

Response

This case is less a question about the logistics of euthanasia, which it appears to be at the outset, than it is about client attitudes, at least in the instances cited. To the shepherd, the dogs that cross his property line are threats to be disposed of in any way possible and expeditious, even as western sheep ranchers view coyotes. Thus euthanasia, in the sense of a good death, is no part of his mental set. The issue is the elimination of a hated enemy and competitor. For this reason sheep ranchers do not cavil at poisoning coyotes, running them down with dogs (that tear them apart), killing pups, shooting from the air, and so on. Given that mind-set, a suggestion from the veterinarian to the shepherd to try trapping stray dogs so that they can be given a lethal injection or adopted out would be greeted with derision and incredulity.

In fact, I knew such a farmer. He kept a number of dogs that he treated very well, even with affection. But he ruthlessly shot any dogs that crossed his property line, even those belonging to his neighbors, and notched his rifle stock after doing so.

So the issue here is changing the shepherd's mind-set, or at least beginning to do so. One suggestion he might be willing to entertain is the use of nonlethal bullets or shells—for example, those containing rock salt, which sting but do not (usually) injure or kill. On the other hand, he is more likely to argue that such a tack will simply postpone the inevitable or pass the threat to his sheep onto a neighbor's. In most areas, what he is doing is legal, and few sheep ranchers who have seen what dogs can do to lambs, especially packs of dogs, will be willing to settle for something less than killing.

If the fate of these dogs is inevitably death, there are worse, slower, and more stressful ways to die than by a well-placed gunshot. On the other hand, if the shepherd regularly wounds the animals, or uses insufficient firepower to kill cleanly, there is a true issue of euthanasia here. Although society may mandate the shepherd's right to kill such animals, it would resist their suffering. If the shepherd's skill is limited, the veterinarian might suggest the use of a tranquilizer to knock the animal out. Then the shepherd can at least place a humane killing shot, a method in fact approved by the AVMA. But, fundamentally, the issue for the veterinarian is overcoming ingrained, long-standing cultural attitudes, and getting the shepherd to see the dog not as evil, but as a living creature that at least ought not to suffer.

The dairy farmer who drowns kittens regularly represents a totally different situation for a variety of reasons. First of all, the kittens are totally under his control, unlike the feral dog. Second, society would unequivocally reject the drowning of these harmless, helpless animals. Third, he could easily cage the animals until such time as the veterinarian visits the farm, or even bring them to the clinic. You, in turn, could probably adopt them out, or foster them—if not, you could at least give them a painless death. Once again, education is called for on the part of the veterinarian to overcome ignorance, or ingrained attitudes, or both. A powerful argument on your side involves pointing out that drowning the kittens would most certainly be actionable under anticruelty laws. Using this veiled threat as a lever, you could even *demand* that he turn the kittens over to you.

The key part is that each of these rural situations may be different. Some may indeed be simply a matter of logistics, but others represent a real clash of values and ingrained customs and habits. Even if leaving a euthanasia solution with a client were not problematic, it would have no relevance to the shepherd. Perhaps the most important things the veterinarian can do in all of these cases is explain the difference between euthanasia and killing, underscore the social commitment to the former, and endeavor to get the clients to "recollect" their own aversion to unnecessary suffering.

I am grateful to Michael Rollin for dialogue on this case.

Case

72

Second Commentary on Stray Tattooed Beagle

Question

(New information on this case prompted a second publishing, which follows.)

Your veterinary clinic advocates and performs the tattooing of clients' animals. You recommend this procedure as a permanent form of identification. New clients arrive with a stray beagle, which is already tattooed. The tattoo was not administered at your clinic. Apparently, the dog had wandered around the clients' neighborhood for a week before they decided to adopt it. You advise the clients that the tattoo indicates previous ownership. They respond by saying that they called the local Society for the Prevention of Cruelty to Animals (SPCA), and there had been no report of lost beagles. The clients do not want to take the dog to the SPCA, where it will be eligible for adoption if unclaimed after five days. Your local veterinary association states that your responsibility ends with notifying a new owner of the tattoo and its significance; you are not to actively pursue locating the original owner. You have been tattooing pets in good faith, assuring clients that it is a real safeguard against loss or theft. You now feel you have been misleading your clients.

What is your next course of action?

Response

In my previous commentary on this case (Case 66), I focused on the social need for a uniform system of identification for lost animals. I frankly did not see an issue of confidentiality. I am therefore grateful to those who have raised the latter question.

Even twenty-five years ago, when veterinary ethics (like all professional ethics) was largely a matter of intraprofessional etiquette, the issue of confidentiality was an exception to the general disregard of serious ethical issues. This has been true probably because, in addition to confidentiality's being a fundamental human moral concern regulating our interactions in ordinary life, it is absolutely presuppositional to any professional role in society. Because professionals—doctors, lawyers, veterinarians—often are privy to the most intimate secrets that clients possess, it is essential that they keep clients' counsel. To take a trivial example, a urologist would not last long if he gossiped about who came in with gonorrhea. Similarly, veterinarians often come to know things about clients that can, if divulged, harm them—for example, that a given farm is in financial difficulty.

All too often, however, veterinarians assume that confidentiality is an absolute obligation to clients that cannot be overridden under any circumstances. A moment's reflection reveals the patent falsity of such a supposition. Physicians are legally (because morally) obligated to report suspected child abuse, though a child is certainly brought to the physician with a presumption of confidentiality. Veterinarians are also legally (because morally) obliged to report certain diseases, regardless of the fact that such reporting plainly violates confidentiality.

Clearly, then, there are moral imperatives that can outweigh the presumption of confidentiality. And it appears to me that the circumstances of the case in question clearly fit that description. The beagle is not a puppy; the presence of the tattoo suggests a caring owner. It is thus safe to assume a significant bond between the dog and the original owner. The new owners, on the other hand, have just acquired the dog. Were I the veterinarian, I would feel it my duty to explain to the new owners the pangs of loss and grief the original owners were probably experiencing. After all, they themselves already care for the animal after a very short while. It is for this reason, I would add, that I encourage tattooing. Thus I would enlist these clients' help in making a full-scale effort to locate the original owner. If they were willing to do so, there is no issue. If they were not, I would point out the onus on me to do so, or else one subverts the whole purpose of identification! Ideally, they would agree. If they did not, I would make an effort to locate the owner based on the tattoo. The worst that could happen is that I might lose them as clients. Allowing them to keep the dog without a sincere effort to locate the original owner both diminishes the seriousness of the bond between animals and owners and undermines much-needed efforts to establish a viable system of permanent identification linking companion animals and their households. Any veterinary association that opposed such an effort on the part of a practitioner would surely lose massive credibility in the court of public opinion, were the case to become known.

Case

73

Bull Mastiff with Osteosarcoma

Question

You diagnose an osteosarcoma in the left front leg of a two-year-old bull mastiff. There is no evidence of metastasis, based on chest radiographs. Your experience with front limb amputations on large breed dogs has been that significant arthritis commonly occurs in the remaining front limb within two years of amputation.

Is amputation of the affected limb an acceptable treatment in this dog?

Response

This case raises a very interesting issue, which bespeaks deep cleavages among veterinarians in North America and, even more dramatically, across national boundaries. That issue is, in essence, whether there is a place for oncology in veterinary medicine. When I visited a European veterinary school, I was informed that both the school and the profession in this particular country did not believe in veterinary oncology—standard treatment of tumors is euthanasia as soon as quality of life is compromised. In sharp contradistinction to this stance, my own veterinary school runs a very complete oncology service that has pioneered in control of osteosarcoma, including limb-sparing procedures. Often amputation is utilized in our service as a therapeutic modality.

Underlying this case is a widespread, dogmatically held belief that large breeds, at least, cannot function on three legs, especially when a foreleg is amputated. In the experience of our oncology service, this supposition is clearly false. Indeed, as early as 1979 Withrow and Hirsch surveyed owners who had elected amputation but had expressed a variety of concerns about the procedure, including the animal's appearance, expense, problems with mobility, the animal's suffering, adaptability of the animal, and so on. In the responses, 100 percent of the clients indicated that their concern had been unfounded. Subsequent studies with a much larger number of cases confirmed this early report (Carberry and Harvey, 1987).

According to Dr. Stephen Withrow, arguably one of the best and most experienced veterinary oncologists in the world, the concern expressed in this case is totally unwarranted. In his extensive clinical experience only 1 percent of dogs with osteosarcoma "can't make it on three legs." Further, the dog that is going to develop crippling arthritis on three legs would almost invariably do so on four legs as well. In fact, although Dr. Withrow never assures clients that the cancer will not reappear after amputation, the one assurance he does provide is that the animal will almost certainly succeed on three legs. The one exception to this assertion is, of course, a situation wherein the dog is already experiencing crippling arthritis prior to amputation, but this is extremely unlikely in a two-year-old animal of the sort described in this case. Withrow stresses that one should look to clinical evidence of arthritis rather than to radiographic evidence when making an amputation decision, as large dogs (and large people) will show radiographic evidence of arthritis well before there are any clinical signs.

On the strength of this evidence, it is clear that amputation is a viable therapeutic modality. My personal experience confirms this—I had a ten-year-old Great Dane that functioned beautifully after a forelimb amputation for a number of years before succumbing to the osteosarcoma. The issue, in my view, is not rejecting amputation a priori. It is, rather, the need to monitor the animal's quality of life carefully after amputation. If the dog in the case described begins to display clinical arthritis that causes uncontrollable pain and suffering two years later, one should think in terms of euthanasia. But even if this occurs, the dog will have enjoyed two years of good-quality living. We also now have good drugs for arthritis pain.

Incredible as it may sound, I have observed (and played Frisbee with) a medium-size dog that functioned admirably with both forelimb and hind limb missing on the left side. Many veterinarians keep videotapes of amputee animals in order to show clients that the animals can live full and happy lives. In my view amputation should not signal an end to an animal's life any more than it should signal an end to a human's life.

I am grateful to Drs. Greg Ogilvie and Steve Withrow for dialogue and references.

Case

74

Financially Stressed Client and Annual Physical

Question

A single mother from out of town, on a limited fixed income, comes to you with her middle-aged dog. She routinely receives reminder notices telling her that her dog needs an annual check-up and vaccinations, heartworm test, fecal examination, dental work, and, recently, a vaccination against Lyme disease.

She's read the CVMA advertisements in *Chatelaine*, and elsewhere, telling her that the dog needs these things, but as much as she and her kids love Rover, they don't consider him "part of the family." They actually consider him, well, a dog. Many of her friends in similar financial straits never take their animals for their "annual physical check-ups," and apart from kitty or puppyhood shots and the occasional rabies vaccination, their animals remain equally healthy and robust.

This woman does not herself qualify for an annual physical check-up, being told by her physician and this province that it represents a waste of time and valuable medical resources. Nor does this veterinarian.

She wonders aloud whether or not the one hundred dollars or so might not be better spent on dental work for herself or, say, getting shoes for her kids.

What should you tell her?

Response

I confess to having some difficulty in identifying a significant ethical issue in the situation described. Presumably, the question is whether the veterinarian ought to do a "hard sell" on the woman and aggressively attempt to get her to part with her one hundred dollars for the regimens mentioned.

To me, the answer is clear. Although I am well aware that we live in an age wherein a business model is ubiquitous in our lives, from prenuptial agreements to the industrialization of agriculture and the aggressive selling of caskets, I resist its wholesale application to professions. (I once had a real estate agent ask me my occupation. When I said "college professor," she enthusiastically replied, "Aha! So you're in sales also!") I concur with Plato's argument in *The Republic* that we should conceptually separate our role as professional from our role as wage earner, at least as an ideal. Thus I detest administrators who tell me to treat students as consumers or customers, for that invariably means pandering to them.

From a professional perspective, we must thus ask if the regimen described is necessary, and it seems clear that it is not. Perhaps it is desirable, but this client is clearly doing without some necessities and is missing much that is desirable. If she cannot afford Cadillac medicine, she should not be made to feel guilty for it.

Were I the veterinarian, I would spend a few minutes educating her on what to watch for concerning the health of her animal. For example, I would discuss the danger of heartworm in her area. I would then express my willingness to work with her to resolve pressing health problems with her dog, either by allowing her to pay me over time, if necessary, or by my accepting barter or doing the work for cost. Aside from being the right thing to do, such an attitude on my part is sure to generate much goodwill for me in the community, though there is, to be sure, always the danger of attracting chiselers.

The bottom line is that her attitude is sensible and "feet on the ground"; she has a good sense of husbanding her resources, yet is not putting the animal in danger. Assuring that she does not should be the veterinarian's primary professional goal. I would not sleep well if I pressed her to spend the hundred dollars.

Case

75

Botched Caesarean Section

Question

A long-standing client, a breeder of champion springer spaniels, arrives out-of-hours with a bitch in labor. The dog has been whelping for six hours and one stillborn puppy has been delivered. Your new associate examines the dog and decides to do a caesarean section. Four additional dead puppies are delivered, and the dog is discharged the next day with instruction to administer oral antibiotics for five days. After three days the dog is returned because of inappetence and a vaginal discharge. Your associate changes antibiotics and discharges the dog. Two days later the dog is returned, severely dehydrated and unable to stand. The abdomen is tense, and abdominal radiographs reveal a fetus in the body of the uterus. You attempt to stabilize the dog for surgery, but it expires within hours of admission. You believe your clinic is responsible for the death of this dog, and you contact your lawyer. She advises you not to admit liability, not to apologize for the dog's death, and to refer any inquiries to her. You believe a mistake was made and want to be honest with this client.

What should you do?

Response

As I remarked in another case, our lives are increasingly driven by fear of lawsuits. Though it is tempting, and partly accurate, to blame lawyers for this state of affairs, greater blame must accrue to society in general for what one may call "wimpification." In my youth, if I fell in a Safeway parking lot, I (or my family) would tend to blame my own clumsiness, not Safeway. And suing a restaurant chain—let alone successfully—because I spilled their hot coffee in my lap would have been the stuff of low comedy. Today, however, people do sue, and juries award absurd amounts to such people instead of laughing them out of court.

Not only is this wimpy, it is dishonorable and socially evil. We are working to create a generation of people who take no responsibility for anything—they are being taught to blame "society" or teachers for their academic failure, parents for their social failure, genetics for their vices and addictions. This, in turn, inevitably ruptures the social fabric and accelerates social devolution in the direction of a "war of each against all," as Thomas Hobbes put it.

How can we stop this litigiousness? Only, I would argue, by taking responsibility for our actions and hoping that such behavior spreads. Indeed, taking responsibility is alive and well in small rural communities. I recently visited a small ranch community in South Dakota, where I was fed lunch by a neighbor of my host. After we left, my host remarked that he had been custom feeding for that neighbor for thirty years "on a handshake." If we wish to create this sort of social *Gemeinschaft,* we must begin with our own actions and circumstances.

What does all this have to do with the current case? Very simply, the situation as described is a paradigmatic instance of malpractice. The surgeon clearly did not fully exteriorize the uterus and thus missed one of the puppies—a patent error. Further, my veterinary colleagues inform me that the surgeon very likely made a poor choice in antibiotics, else the bitch would not have died.

On the other hand, the error made by the surgeon is precisely the sort of mistake one is likely to make early in one's career—and, it is to be hoped, never again. And that is what I would say to the client. I would admit culpability, make restitution, and attempt to deal with her the way I would want to be dealt with. Of course, she might still sue me, but at least I would feel that I had taken an honorable tack, rather than hiding behind an attorney.

For that matter, this approach seems to me prudential as well as ethical. Not to apologize and not to admit liability, as the lawyer suggests, is to spit in the client's face and ask for a lawsuit. The situation is very clear, and it wouldn't be hard for the client to find veterinarians to testify that a mistake was made. Further, word will inevitably spread in the community, especially if the client is angry, adversarial, and disposed toward revenge. Even pragmatically, then, it seems to me much better to admit blame, rather than to aggrieve and antagonize the client further.

I am grateful to Drs. Lynne Kesel and Wendell Nelson for dialogue on this case.

Case

76

Farmer Asking Advice of "Experts"

Question

One of the best dairy farms in your area uses your services irregularly. The university-educated owner consults several "expert" veterinarians from out of province. When talking with the owner one evening after a dystocia, you learn that this producer routinely treats fevers in lactating cows with banamine, while saving the milk; mixes Rumensin in the milking cow ration without a prescription; and purchases modified-live vaccines in large vials, using them for four to five weeks after mixing to reduce the cost per vaccination. When you ask where all these off-label recommendations originated, he tells you they come from his out-of-province veterinarians. He laughs about the joke by one veterinarian concerning the large number of chickens in Wisconsin now being fed monensin sodium (Rumensin, Elanco). He mentions that another consultant veterinarian told him that no one checks for flunixin meglumine (Banamine, Schering Plough) in milk, so the ninety-six-hour withdrawal period is meaningless. This producer wants to produce a wholesome product and is acting on the advice of "experts."

What should you tell him?

Response

For many years, following the superb insights provided by Paul Feyerabend in his seminal work *Science in a Free Society* (1978), as well as my own life experiences, I have been mistrustful of experts and specialists. It is the "experts" who tell people that they will never walk again, often creating self-fulfilling prophecies. It was "experts" who told us that there was no danger in nuclear power, no possible escape of killer bees, no danger of contracting AIDS through the skin. (I heard one such expert from CDC [Centers for Disease Control] say reassuringly to a group of citizens who were fearful of AIDS research being undertaken in their community that he would "bathe" in the AIDS virus with no fear.) And it was "experts" who missed the end of the Soviet Union until they saw reports on CNN.

In addition to almost inevitably failing to see the big picture (due to the tunnel vision inherent in knowing more and more about less and less), experts invariably have values that differ from those the rest of us hold and, in particular, may fail to see the value of democratic decision making, and the good of society as a whole.

Such is patently the case in this situation. Here we have veterinarians who not only do not see the growing social issues associated with food safety, but also do not have a vision broad enough to recognize the potential harm they may bring to their own profession.

If one asks any agriculturist what is the greatest challenge facing animal agriculture as we enter the twenty-first century, the answer will be quick and unequivocal: It is food safety. This trend has been driven by a series of disasters involving bacterial contamination of animal products, and drug and antibiotic residues in meat and milk, to say nothing of the terrifying advent of prions. Regulators and veterinarians struggle to protect public health and safety, improve accountability, and reassure the public that they need not fear the food supply.

Enter our "experts" from out of town. With cavalier disregard for both safety issues of substance and issues of public perception, they disdain published rules for dosing, use, and withdrawal, and mock the ethical requirement of a well-established professional relationship between veterinarian and client as a necessary condition for the latter's prescribing drugs in an extralabel way. At the very least, then, they risk worsening the compromised reputation of animal agriculture. At worst, they are endangering human health. In addition, they are imperiling the future of veterinary medicine. U.S. veterinary medicine came very close to losing the privilege of extralabel drug use through congressional action precisely because of the proliferation of situations in agriculture of the sort described in this case.

This, then, is what I would tell the dairy farmer. To replace Banamine, if he insists on shipping the milk, I would suggest ketoprofen (trade name Anafen), an anti-inflammatory, antipyretic, and analgesic drug that will work as well as Banamine but requires zero withdrawal time in milk.

Case

77

Confidentiality in the Case of a Client Selling Sick Animals

Question

A dairy client of yours sells his farm as an ongoing operation. Over the last several years there have been serious disease problems in the herd, including *Staphylococcus aureus* mastitis, classical mucosal disease, and abortions due to both bovine viral diarrhea virus and *Neospora* spp.

The problems are continuing with the new owner, who wonders if he is doing something wrong or if he bought these problems with the farm. The original owner of the farm has moved out of the province. Your obligations to your new client appear to conflict with your confidentiality obligations to the previous owner.

What should you do?

Response

This case is very reminiscent of Case 5, in which I discussed a situation wherein a veterinarian was working with a farmer to eradicate bovine viral diarrhea from his herd. He recommended to the farmer that the chronic shedders be shipped to slaughter; instead, the veterinarian finds out later that the farmer has sold these cows to another of the veterinarian's clients without revealing that the animals were shedders.

In that case I argued that, though there is a general presumption of respect for confidentiality, that presumption could be, and indeed was, overridden by two special circumstances. First, failure of the veterinarian to break confidentiality would result in significant harm to the innocent party, namely the buyer, and his herd. Second, the original client had acted in a grossly immoral way, wantonly ignoring the harm that would result by his failure to heed the veterinarian's advice.

Although the current case appears similar at first glance, there are some important dissimilarities that prevent us from simply applying the logic of the earlier case here.

Most important, perhaps, is the fact that the veterinarian's breaking of confidentiality in this case will not prevent harm to the purchaser or the animals—the harm has already been done. At the very best the veterinarian will provide ammunition to the purchaser if he wishes to sue the seller. But breaking confidentiality will do nothing whatever to rectify the situation *medically*.

To deal with the situation as it stands, the veterinarian could simply begin by stressing that rectification of the problem requires drastic solutions, perhaps repopulation of the herd, and later ensure that the client understands the severity of the situation, deflecting attention away from the origin of the problem. If the client says, "Okay, let's do whatever it takes to fix the problem," the veterinarian can concentrate on managing the diseases in the future, and de-emphasize past history. Thus, the issue of breaching confidentiality has been circumvented.

It is very likely, however, given human nature, that the client will persist in exploring the history of the trouble, essentially wanting to know if he has purchased a "lemon" or if he has made some fundamental errors in management, in effect forcing the veterinarian to focus on the history. At this point, the principle of caveat emptor becomes morally relevant—in a deep sense the buyer behaved very shortsightedly in not having the herd health-checked, though this of course does not exonerate the seller of having been duplicitous. Obviously the veterinarian should not simply come out and say, in essence, "The seller got you, stupid!" On the other hand, it would be perfectly appropriate to remark, if pressed, that because the seller was a client of yours, you are not in a position to discuss the medical history. This is right and true. But by the same token, if the farmer has any sense at all, he will get the message.

I am grateful to Michael Rollin and Dr. Frank Garry for very helpful dialogue.

Case

78

Conflict in Obligations to a Peer and a Client

Question

A client brings his cat to you for a second opinion. He is employed by another veterinarian in the town where you work. His employer examined the cat, performed blood work, took radiographs, and told him there were no serious problems. Your examination reveals a number of clinical signs that require more sophisticated diagnostic procedures and referral to a specialist. You tell the client that you will call the original veterinarian and discuss the case. The client is adamant that confidentiality be maintained. He is sure that he will be fired if his employer realizes he has sought a second opinion from a neighboring veterinarian. You know this colleague well enough to believe that she might behave in this manner. Your provincial code of ethics dictates that you contact the original veterinarian in cases wherein second opinions are sought. The specialist may also want to speak to the original veterinarian, although the client believes he can direct all communication from the specialist to you.

Do you follow the code of ethics or your client's wishes?

Response

Historically, codes of ethics for professions have in fact been codes of etiquette or intraprofessional niceties, designed to keep members of a profession from cutting each other's throats or harming the image of the profession in the eyes of the public it serves. Often codes of ethics have had precious little to do with social ethical concerns. The AVMA Code of Ethics twenty years ago, for example, had numerous entries regarding the restriction of advertising (including a discussion of how large one's sign could "ethically" be), and none regarding the euthanasia of healthy animals! Not only did that code of ethics fail to address most of the genuine ethical issues raised by the practice of veterinary medicine, it was in fact at odds with the ethics of the larger society, as evidenced by the fact that U.S. courts struck down the code's restrictions on advertising.

The key point is not to bash codes of ethics—they do serve an essential purpose. But they should not be viewed as the final word on genuine ethical issues, and even if they are presumptively taken as binding on all professionals, that presumption can (and must) be overridden in the presence of moral pressures exerting greater force in a given situation.

Such is the case in the situation described. The purpose of the rule in the provincial code is to prevent fratricidal warfare (or at least bickering) between peers, which can make individual veterinarians (and the profession as a whole) appear divided and mean-spirited in the eyes of the public. Generally, it is probably a good idea for a clinician from whom a second opinion is sought to discuss the case with the original veterinarian, if for no other reason than to check and corroborate the client's account of the case and the first veterinarian's diagnosis and recommendations, as well as to discover relevant information about the client's likelihood of following a regimen, exaggerating symptoms, and so on.

In this case, however, the situation is extraordinary. Aside from conflicting with the presumptive ethical obligation to respect the client's confidentiality, adherence to the code of ethics puts the client at risk, that is, endangers his employment. On the other hand, failure to notify the first veterinarian does not put her at any risk, as the pet owner–employee will certainly keep his counsel regarding whatever errors of omission or commission she may have made in order to protect his job! He is obviously interested only in getting his cat diagnosed and treated, not in bringing forward recriminations or lawsuits against his employer.

Were I the veterinarian, I would thus respect the client's confidentiality. I would explain the situation to the specialist to whom I was referring the case and ask him or her to respect the client's desire for confidentiality and address any questions to me. Thus I believe that obligation to the client and to the animal trump my presumptive obligation to my fellow clinician, as the latter will suffer no harm in virtue of my failure to contact her, while the client and perhaps the animal will suffer if I do insist on letting her know the situation.

Case

79

Reporting a Dog Being Used to Carry Drugs

Question

A client brings a dog to your clinic for follow-up care after it has been treated at an emergency clinic. The puppy is still semicomatose. The owner tells you that the pup ate 3 grams of hashish the previous day. The puppy recovers in your clinic and passes a broken balloon. You suspect the dog was used to transport illegal drugs.

Does client confidentiality prevent you from reporting the owner to the police? Is this incident considered animal abuse (which you can report), considering that the owner did not intend abuse and sought immediate veterinary attention?

Response

The issue of confidentiality and when it should be breached has been discussed on many occasions in this book. This is quite proper, since the question arises, with some frequency, in any professional's life, and there is no set way of deciding when one ought or ought not violate one's presumptive moral commitment to keeping one's counsel. By looking at a range of cases, however, we can refine our moral sensitivities regarding the sorts of situations wherein the presumption of confidentiality may, or even should, be overridden.

Given that confidentiality is so essential to any professional relationship with a client, be the professional a veterinarian, physician, dentist, attorney, psychologist, or so on, it cannot be violated merely because the practitioner unwittingly witnesses something illegal or immoral. Thus, if while visiting a client during his wife's absence you find him entertaining a chorus girl, you certainly shouldn't report this to his wife. On the other hand, if you find a kidnapped child locked in his barn, confidentiality should clearly not take precedence.

One ought not conclude from the foregoing discussion that merely witnessing an illegal act justifies violating confidentiality. What is also required, at least as a necessary condition for such violation, is the certainty that only by disclosure can you prevent far greater harm to innocents. Were you to find dozens of boxes of illegally imported Dutch tulip bulbs in a client's garage, I wouldn't argue that such a situation justifies overriding the presumption of secrecy. Similarly, even if the client were smuggling diamonds in his dog's rhinestone collar, I would not break confidence—professionals simply encounter too much questionable behavior to report any but the most egregious. Such smuggling endangers no one.

The importation of illegal drugs is, of course, a good deal more socially dangerous than smuggling cigars or diamonds, but let us suppose in this case that the drug is hashish, as the client said (concern for the dog presumably led him to tell you the truth, so that you could treat the toxicity expeditiously). Here we are not dealing with a hard drug or one typically leading to clear danger to innocents who consume it. Thus, if I were to find out that the dog was being used to carry hashish in his collar, presumably only enough for the owner's personal use, I would feel no onus to report it.

The moral gestalt changes, however, when the dog is being forced to swallow the balloon in order to transport the drug. In essence, the animal's life and health are put at significant risk, as indeed the situation clearly evidences. So the situation is morally the same as one wherein an owner fights a dog, or deprives an animal of food and water. One's duty to the innocent animals takes precedence. Force-feeding a potentially lethal balloon filled with hashish is as much cruelty as force-feeding any toxic substance would be—if it is not abuse, it is at least cavalier negligence. Whether or not you report the incident, despite your moral entitlement to do so, depends on your reading of your relationship with the client. If the threat of reporting can be used to prevent the client from behaving badly toward the animal in the future, and you can verify this at regular intervals, that is a morally viable option. If, however, you believe that you cannot accomplish this "in house," I see no problem with reporting the owner to the authorities who deal with cruelty. The potential for further abuse of the dog clearly outweighs the presumption of confidentiality.

Furthermore, I can imagine, and sympathize with, veterinarians who would automatically report any illegal drug under any circumstances for fear of affecting their own drug license by failing to report. If one's license is indeed placed in peril by failure to report, the presumption of confidentiality is outweighed.

Case

80

An Elderly Client Seeking "Unnecessary" Medical Advice

Question

An older client of yours has begun arranging weekly appointments for his four-year-old cocker spaniel. Each week he describes a new problem. You have never been convinced on any of the examinations that there was a serious illness. On several occasions you have suggested that he take the dog home and see if the problem recurs. He is always openly dissatisfied with this approach. He prefers that you do some tests or prescribe a treatment. This behavior began shortly after his wife died. The hospital staff think these regular visits are amusing. You feel guilty charging for your services.

What should you do?

Response

When I began to teach veterinary ethics in 1978, I was fortunate enough to be paired with Dr. Harry Gorman as co-teacher. Dr. Gorman was probably the most accomplished veterinarian I have ever known—past president of the AVMA, inventor of the artificial hip joint, head of the aerospace program's use of animals. Harry's most pronounced characteristic, however, was his boundless empathy with suffering beings, whether animals or humans. During the years we taught together, I was privileged to learn a great deal about veterinary medicine from him that one could not get from textbooks.

One of the first things he taught me was that a veterinarian is far more than an animal doctor. This is especially the case, he stressed, in rural areas, where the veterinarian may be the only professional for one hundred miles and may be called upon for legal advice, marital counseling, psychological help, human medical advice, all under the ostensible guise of treating the animal. "It's part of the job," he told me, "That's why a veterinarian needs to be more of a people person than a physician does." (Harry certainly was, which accounts for the indelible mark he left on students, clients, and peers.)

At any rate, the veterinarians I have most respected have instantiated Dr. Gorman's dictum. For example, when I discussed the current case with Dr. Walt Weirich, the eminent Purdue surgeon and a friend for twenty years, he instantly sparkled with recognition. "I had a situation like that in the early seventies," he said. "The old man brought his dog in every week like clockwork for a recheck of an ear infection—for ten years. There was never any reason to believe that animal was reinfected. He just wanted someone to talk to besides other lonely, retired people. I enjoyed him and looked forward to his visits."

"How did you handle the fees?" I queried.

"Oh, I just charged him the minimum—three dollars in those days—each time for a recheck," he replied.

This, I think, is the answer to our case. Here the veterinarian has an opportunity to brighten someone's life immeasurably by spending a few minutes chatting with him. No one is harmed, and the client can clearly afford the weekly minimum examination fee, which is doubtless a good deal less than he would pay a psychologist or "bereavement counselor," and also doubtless much more enjoyable, and far less erosive of his self-concept. You can always provide innocuous placebos, such as vitamins or nutritional supplements, and thereby "do no harm." You, in turn, lose nothing and can probably use at least some of the time to educate the client—and perhaps, indirectly, his elderly peers—on various aspects of pet care, behavior, and nutrition. No one loses. There is nothing to feel guilty about.

If I see a problem at all here it is with the "hospital staff," who see the visits as "amusing." If they are so lacking in empathy and understanding, I would question their people skills and ability to relate to clients. If they are treating the client with contempt, I would read them the riot act. At the very least, I would meet with them and explain, in clear terms, that there is nothing funny about the client's needs and that, if they are lucky enough to reach old age, they could well be in a similar position.

I am grateful to Dr. Walt Weirich for dialogue. I dedicate discussion of this case to the memory of my mentor, Dr. Harry Gorman.

Case

81

A Cat Who Fractures Both Legs after a Surgical Procedure

Question

A cat was brought to your clinic to be declawed. Anesthesia (xylazine and ketamine) and surgery were routine. Following the surgery, the cat was returned to her cage, as is the normal procedure. She had a very stormy recovery from the anesthetic, and a towel was placed over the front of the cage to quieten her. Unnoticed by the staff, she wedged her front legs between the bars of the cage and broke both legs at midradius. You offered to do all the surgery and follow-up on the fractures at no charge. The owner declined your offer and requested euthanasia and cremation.

Do you charge for:

1. *The surgery?*
2. *The euthanasia?*
3. *The cremation?*
4. *All of the procedures?*
5. *None of the procedures?*
6. *All of the procedures at a discounted price?*

Response

It appears that the cat experienced an extremely dramatic and violent reaction to ketamine, as some animals do. In such a case it would probably have been wiser for the staff to keep the animal under fairly close surveillance, rather than to cover the cage. Perhaps cognizant of the clinic's moral responsibility for what occurred, even in such a freakish incident, or else aware that an angry client can do immeasurable damage to a veterinarian's reputation via the grapevine, the clinician has rightly offered to repair the damage at no cost to the client. Assuming a clean break and the extraordinary bone-healing capacity of cats, the cat is likely to return to normalcy in six weeks with no major difficulty.

At this point, however, a morally problematic dimension is introduced—the client refuses to allow the fracture repair. The client's reasons for this refusal must be known before analysis of the case can be completed. There are at least three possible reasons for the client's demand for euthanasia. First, the client may believe that the animal will be crippled or will be in great pain. Such a client mind-set about dysfunction often arises vis-à-vis limb amputation in the case of osteosarcoma, and many veterinarians counter this response with videotapes of dogs that do splendidly on three or even two legs. Concern about the animal's pain and suffering is probably not as easily countered, especially if the client anthropomorphically identifies with the cat, but here too a good clinician should be able to convince the owner that excellent pain control modalities exist. Nonetheless, the client may continue to fear for the animal's quality of life and demand euthanasia. Were I convinced this was the case and, despite my best efforts at persuasion, could not convince the client to allow me to keep the animal through repair and subsequently to return it or adopt it out, I would reluctantly agree to euthanasia and would not charge for anything, provided I was convinced that the client was acting purely out of concern for the animal.

A second and related reason for the request for euthanasia might be that the client is aged or infirm and feels unable to provide the requisite postsurgical attention. If such is the case, I, as the veterinarian, would suggest that a family member—or perhaps one of the veterinarian's staff—could see the animal through convalescence and return to normalcy.

If the client still wishes euthanasia and cremation, despite my offer, I would explain that I would charge for the euthanasia and cremation, but that I would not charge for the surgery and convalescent care or for the original procedure, if she or he agrees to take the animal after it is healed. My rationale would be that I do not wish to participate in putting down a potentially healthy animal. Perhaps the economic incentive, coupled with absolving the client of responsibility for convalescence, will encourage the client to rethink euthanasia.

A third reason might be that the client does not wish to deal with a "defective" or "imperfect" animal—in other words, elects euthanasia for reasons of convenience. If I could not convince such a client to let me recover and adopt out the animal, I would certainly charge for what is, in effect, a paradigm case of convenience euthanasia, though I would not charge for the initial procedure.

In sum, the veterinarian should assume responsibility for the fracture. If the client, for anything other than purely moral reasons, rejects trying to save the cat, I would certainly charge for the euthanasia and cremation.

Case

82

Can Annual Vaccinations Be Justified?

Question

Sporadic reports have drawn associations between the use of certain vaccines in dogs and cats and disorders such as vaccine-associated sarcomas or certain autoimmune diseases. In the case of rabies vaccine, manufacturers assure veterinarians that the three-year product is efficacious.

Can veterinarians justify annual vaccinations for diseases that can be controlled by the use of multiyear vaccines?

Response

The issue of animal vaccinations has a venerable history in veterinary medicine. For a long time, such vaccinations were sources of income and practice builders. Further, they were rationalized as a way of bringing people and their animals into one's clinic for general checkups. Recent scientific advances have called this practice into serious question.

In the first place, we know that vaccination is not a costless panacea. In a remarkable series of articles entitled "Intuitive Immunology," appearing in the New Zealand veterinary Journal *Vetscript* in 2004 and 2005 written for veterinarians, immunologist Kent Dietemeyer has explained that vaccines need to be used judiciously, if only because activation of the immune system involves not inconsiderable degrees of what he calls "immunological stress," stressors on the organism resulting from activation of the immune system. These include repartitioning of nutrients, increased glucocorticoid levels favoring fat deposition rather than muscle growth, increasing energy metabolism, and other physiological costs. Deitemeyer convincingly argues that vaccination should be used judiciously (like antimicrobials), not as a way of compensating for bad animal management by humans, good management being the first line of defense against disease. Overuse of vaccines can lead to emergence of new production disease, in what Deitemeyer calls the "Red Queen effect."

There is, in fact, increasing evidence that overvaccination can actually be conducive to disease development, not only as a consequence of immunological stress, but also more directly. Early evidence implicated frequent vaccination in the development of injection-site sarcomas in cats, and autoimmune hemolytic anemia in dogs, both of which can be fatal. It has thus become a science-based consensus that, for most companion animal diseases, annual boosting is not necessary. Immunity for rabies, for example, appears to last at least three years, and perhaps a good deal longer. Thus, a boost every three years suffices to maintain immunity to the disease, while significantly reducing other disease risk.

What does all this mean to the average clinical practitioner? To the food animal practitioner, it continues the trend introduced by the imperative to cut back on antimicrobials; namely, manage animals in a more healthy way, aimed at hygiene and stress reduction, not medical intervention. To the pet practitioner, it means developing new ways of bringing in clients. One such strategy that has proven effective involves dentistry, promulgated by having a free dental examination day once or twice a year on a Saturday. Alternatively, one can hold a behavior clinic periodically to draw in new clients, recalling that most animals that die of "convenience euthanasia" do so for reasons of behavior problems. As pets grow more and more important in peoples' lives, it should become easier to attract people to seek veterinary care and advice.

Case

83

An Organic Farmer Who Won't Use Antibiotics for Foot Rot

Question

You are the veterinarian for a very successful organic dairy farm with a rapidly expanding market. The owner is extremely diligent regarding your recommendations concerning preventative medicine practices to maintain health and productivity in the herd. In many ways, he has helped restore your own confidence in such practices.

During a regular herd health visit, you observe a severely lame cow. You examine her and determine that she is suffering from foot rot. You recommend treatment with penicillin, but the owner replied that he needs her in the milking line and is treating her topically. He says that with root trimming and topical organic disinfectants, she should recover in two to three weeks. You are fairly certain she would recover in two to three days with penicillin therapy.

How should you respond?

Response

One of the most odious, sanctimonious, and outright stupid locutions in the modern vernacular is "zero tolerance." I call it stupid, because it is the primary enemy of common sense and the flexing of ideas requisite to fit new and emerging situations. As a paradigm case, consider the little girl, an honor student in elementary school, whose mother packed a fruit knife in her lunchbox to allow the child to peel her orange. With the mindless rectitude so often found in school officials, the administrators invoked the school's "zero tolerance" policy regarding weapons and expelled the little girl. In the same way, security people at airports will confiscate nail clippers but allow passengers to carry on large, glass bottles that are breakable at will and, as any bar fighter knows, are far superior to nail clippers as weapons.

The rules for organic agriculture smack of similar mindless mantra chanting, as this case makes plain. The concept of organic agriculture is a highly laudable one—a major step, potentially, towards restoring our ancient husbandry and stewardship contract with agricultural animals and with the earth. Enter the ideologues, who blur the distinction between using tons of antibiotics prophylactically to promote growth and cover-up for bad husbandry and using a two-day course of antibiotics to treat foot rot efficiently and expeditiously.

Foot rot is significantly painful to the cow. One of my colleagues, a large animal practitioner, tells me it is like walking on a needle. Furthermore, if not treated expeditiously, the animal can lose a foot. In addition, the condition is highly contagious. The same expert told me that the presence of foot rot is usually an indication of bad management and bad husbandry.

Thus, we have a situation involving major suffering, possibly related to poor management, threatening the rest of the herd, yet treatable in two to three days. But the producer clearly embraces a zero tolerance mind-set and insists on using an inferior treatment.

In the producer's defense, it is possible—and indeed probable—that rules of organic certification drive the zero tolerance. But, if that is the case, the producer needs to have made provisions for this sort of emergency. For example, some organic beef producers, when faced with this sort of situation, move the animal to their nonorganic production line and use an antibiotic. Some dairy producers do also. Possibly, this producer runs only organic animals, in which case, the reasonable move is to sell the cow to a nonorganic producer (presumably at some loss), so that the animal is not left to suffer for three weeks.

Ironically, consumers often equate organic with welfare friendly, to the benefit of organic producers. Failure to address the current sort of situation will soon banish that idea.

Case

84

Using Wood Chippers to Kill Chickens

Question

Correspondence in a veterinary journal has concerned the use of a wood chipper to dispose of laying hens following the end of their production cycle or as an emergency measure in the case of an exotic disease outbreak. It is likely that such a device kills birds instantly.

Is there anything wrong with such a practice?

Response

Some years ago, I experienced a situation exemplifying the flip side of the issue facing us. While visiting another country, I had a meeting with the executive board of the group representing equine veterinarians in that country. We discussed many ethical issues facing equine medicine in our respective countries, and eventually we engaged the issue of euthanasia for injury at the racetrack. I was horrified to learn that their veterinarians dispatched such animals with succynilcholine, a paralytic depolarizing the neuromuscular junction, resulting in an agonizing terrifying death by suffocation via paralysis of the diaphragm. Though I am not clear whether or not these practitioners understood what was going on physiologically, they defended their practice on aesthetic grounds, since the public did not wish to witness a gunshot—in fact, a far more humane procedure.

Now we are discussing a procedure that is allegedly humane, involving instant death, but one which is as aesthetically disturbing as could be. If it is true that the animals do not suffer, the chicken euthanasia is far superior to the equine one just described, but it is still problematic.

Though not definitive, public sensibilities are highly relevant to methods of euthanasia. Not only must euthanasia create quick and painless death, it must not shock, horrify, or brutalize practitioners or observers. The problem with using the chipper is that it violates the latter set of concerns. As one of my students put it, "It may not hurt the animals, but it certainly hurts people." How so? Because it is horrible to observe and surely desensitizing to those who do it. We must ask ourselves, would we do it to companion animals? Would we allow our children to watch it? Would society accept it as a method of capital punishment, if one could demonstrate scientifically the instantaneous loss of consciousness?

It is bad enough that industrialized agriculture has commodified animals and replaced husbandry with industry. Should we now further evidence a view of animals that see them as logs to be chipped? And in an ironic reversal of the horse situation, where it never even occurs to the public that the animals are not going to sleep peacefully, the public will never believe that being ground up alive doesn't hurt, thereby further eroding the image of agriculture in the public mind and further potentiating the social demand for legislated regulation of agriculture.

Case

85

Should Shelters Place Animals in Less than Perfect Homes?

Question

Some animal welfare organizations recommend euthanasia of unwanted or feral animals. The alternative of leaving the animals to roam free or of placing them in less than ideal homes (for example, kittens placed in livestock barns) is deemed unacceptable. These organizations believe that euthanasia is preferable to life in a less than what they consider perfect environment.

If "ideal" homes are not available for all unwanted or feral domestic animals, are environments with higher risks of morbidity and mortality acceptable alternatives to euthanasia?

Response

Over the years, I have had many disagreements with humane societies. Though undoubtedly well meaning, they often rigidly follow *idées fixes*, even when one can marshal powerful arguments against those positions. I have detailed some of my objections previously. These included questioning the spay-neuter "gonad hunting" mantra in the face of the fact that most animals euthanized are not unwanted puppies and kittens but are adolescent males, and that some humane societies have to import litters to meet demand. I have also expressed concern that the brightest, most responsible people, who probably get the best animals, zealously adhere to spaying and neutering, thereby compromising the gene pool. Further, I have been impressed with veterinarian and former humane society president Dr. David Neil's point that the humane society is guilty of pursuing "preventive death"—killing the animals so that nothing bad will happen to them. In addition, some humane societies make adopting animals so difficult and uncomfortable for people that many potential adopters are turned off or turned away.

Many years ago, Professor Alan Beck, Purdue University, and Dr. Michael W. Fox, former vice president of the Humane Society of the United States and of the International Humane Society, studied the ecology of urban stray dogs for over a year, observing their behaviors and survival strategies. At the end of the study, one dog that was taken off the street and checked by a veterinarian who found the animal to weigh thirty-four pounds, to be in good health, and to have worms. After deworming, the animal was placed in a good home. After a year, the animal was checked again and was found to weigh thirty-one pounds, to be in good health, and to have worms! In other words, "preventive death" for such an animal, had it been unadoptable, would have been unwarranted for humane reasons. And this is even truer of feral cats. While one can argue that control of such feral animals is a public health necessity, there are counterarguments supporting the claim that feral animals prevent disease spread by rodents. In any case, humane societies exist for purposes of animal welfare, not public health.

Obviously, not all potential homes are better than euthanasia—I would not advocate placing an animal with an abusive person or with a collector or hoarder who is known not to take care of the animals. But I have certainly known barn cats and warehouse or factory dogs and cats that lived quite well and enjoyed significant human companionship, being "everyone's" pet. Were we to apply the stringent criteria that some humane societies use for the adoption of animals in order to foster children, many children would be homeless.

In short, I would argue that a chance of a life, where an animal enjoys proper food, water, shelter, and companionship, albeit not under perfect ideal conditions, is considerably better than preventive death. Let us remind ourselves of the many cases of hoboes who, while themselves scruffy and disreputable, are accompanied by bright, alert, well-fed, and, to all appearances, happy dogs. In many cases of such relationships, both parties are better off, with the person deriving friendship, companionship, and some sense of responsibility from having something to love and be loved by, and the animal enjoying a bohemian life that few could argue is worse than death.

Case

86

Why Should We Worry about Animal Suffering Right before Death?

Question

Animal scientists and veterinary researchers strive to minimize the length of time and amount of discomfort that occurs in food or laboratory animals at the time of euthanasia or in food animals at slaughter. The times compared between techniques are nearly always measured in seconds.

Considering other welfare issues associated with laboratory and food animals that last for minutes, hours, or days, is this attention to a few seconds appropriate? Do not most animals, including humans, suffer for a few seconds before they die?

Response

This question raises a fascinating point: Why does society provide scrupulous rules to prevent relatively momentary suffering in animals being killed for food and research, while overlooking the much greater suffering that the same animals may experience in *life* if they are food or research animals? One can only speculate in response to an issue that concerns our collective moral psychology, but some points seem illuminating.

In the first place, we have no clear-cut answer to the all-important question of whether death harms an animal. Insofar as we can rationally reconstruct the views of most people, or at least structure a view they would assent to, it is commonly believed that animals live in the moment, in the now, with no long-term futural projects of the sort that give meaning to human life—wanting to finish one's novel, see one's grandchildren graduate, visit Ireland again, or leave one's family secure and provided for. Such "projects," according to the philosopher Martin Heidegger, are uniquely constitutive of human life. Animals lacking language cannot project beyond the very proximal future. Hence, killing them painlessly does not harm them.

Having said this, no one can be certain that this is truly the case. If it is not the case, then taking an animal's life is not trivial in terms of the harm caused. If it is the case, we naturally feel that an animal's last moments should be, if not positive, at least not horrible. In other words, given our uncertainty about death, we approach it with profound concern. I recall team-teaching a course in the proper use of laboratory animals. One week, we taught euthanasia, using animals (rats) that needed to die for a research protocol. I recall the profound experience of uncertainty and regret I experienced when my colleague injected them with pentobarbital, and I watched the little life-flame flicker and die. I recall feeling "Who am I to do this, given the struggle these little creatures had engaged in to survive?" My only consolation, for want of a better word, was that they went to sleep peacefully, unaware that what they struggled to preserve had ended.

Aristotle once said, "Count no man happy until he is dead." Perhaps we impute something like this to animals. It is important to us that the summation, or consummation, of their lives not involve fear, horror, pain, or suffering as the final encapsulation of their lives, particularly given that we cannot provide compensation or remedy after death. The finality of killing makes us tread lightly.

Concern for these last moments is, in my view, an affirmation of decency in the face of inflicting irreversible termination of the creatures whose lives seem to be metaphysically their own, not ours to dispose of. This is a primordial emotion, more primordial than the reflective hope that society will continue to develop its reflective concern about how we in fact make these animals expend their lives.

Case

87

"Good" versus "Natural" Death

Question

Humane destruction of runt pigs in the farrowing crate or nursery pen is commonly performed by means of "blunt trauma." This technique is safe for the operator, is economical, and requires no special instruments. When performed properly, it results in an instantaneous loss of consciousness and rapid death. Nevertheless, it can be an extremely unpleasant task for the dedicated stockperson.

Is it wrong to allow a runt pig to die a natural death?

Response

There is an ever-increasingly pervasive view in society that what is natural is good. This seems to be a belief that undergirds society's intoxication with natural remedies, so that we spend billions each year on untested herbs, nostrums, and supplements of dubious or no proven value to health.

When asked to define "the natural," most advocates of it are stymied. Indeed, I devoted my first book to demonstrating that it is difficult, if not impossible, to draw a clear-cut distinction between what is natural and what is "conventional" or "artificial." To pose one obvious conundrum: If humans are part of nature, human behavior must be natural, even behavior like bridge building or city planning, which are schematized as artificial.

Nonetheless, we use *natural* as a term of approval. Natural foods are good, even though unprocessed linseed oil is poisonous. Such a use of the term is absurd, even ignoring our inability to define *natural*. Smallpox, cancer, and acquired immunodeficiency syndrome (AIDS) are surely "natural" (whatever that means), yet not good; telephone, cars, and many medicines are products of human artifice, yet are viewed by many as good.

A natural death is probably often not a good death, vide drowning, starvation, dehydration, or being eaten by sharks or destroyed by cancer. This is why euthanasia for suffering animals is seen as a powerful tool veterinary medicine has and human medicine lacks. This is also why veterinary medicine has devoted much attention to studying true euthanasia. Through this sort of study, we have learned that killing by using succinylcholine does not provide a good death, nor does being beaten to death or electrocuted. We currently believe that for a method of death to be "good," it must lead to rapid unconsciousness, be painless, and not offend the sensibilities of those who cause the death or observe it.

Judged by these criteria, this case presents us with a false dichotomy. Neither the blunt trauma nor letting the animal die of starvation or dehydration count as providing the animal with a good death, an objection our social ethic takes very seriously. If humans are to take animal life for their benefit, performing such an act should not force the operators to be traumatized or the animals to suffer.

We are responsible for the animals whose lives we choose to take. If they are to die at our hands, they should die without pain, fear, or anxiety, or as close to that ideal as we can achieve, regardless of the cost. In any case, it only takes a few pennies worth of pentobarbital to assure that the runt piglet truly goes to sleep and does not die a natural but lingering death, just as we in the United States use pentobarbital for effecting good death in humane societies or pounds. Allowing humane societies in the United States the use of pentobarbital twenty-five years ago was a major triumph for animal welfare, and there is no reason the same thing could not be allowed by farmers.

A quarter of a century ago, killing in shelters and pounds in the United States was done by high-altitude chambers, which if imperfectly used and maintained, as was usually the case, did not produce a good death. Veterinarians led the change to allow technicians and trained personnel at pounds to use pentobarbital under the veterinarian's license. To my knowledge, there has been little or no abuse of these drugs. There is no reason why a barbiturate-derived euthanasia solution cannot be dispensed for such uses as described in this case.

Case

88

Is It Wrong to Modify Animals to Fit Production Systems?

Question

Livestock farming imposes certain restrictions on the natural behaviors of animals. Some welfare advocates have proposed that animals with reduced natural behaviors should be selected for breeding so that welfare is improved. For example, by selecting more submissive sows, the aggressive encounters involved in establishing a social hierarchy could be reduced. Such a selection process could improve the welfare of group-housed sows.

Is there an ethical problem with breeding "natural" behaviors out of domestic animals?

Response

I have addressed this issue in numerous books and articles in reference to genetic engineering of animals: If animals are miserable in confinement, is it morally acceptable to engineer them so that they are, in fact, happy in the system wherein we compel them to live? I believe that the same answer is relevant whether one uses artificial selection or genetic engineering, assuming that the latter modality does not cause unanticipated negative welfare consequences.

As a specific example, consider the chickens kept in battery cages for efficient, high-yield egg production. It is now recognized that such a production system frustrates numerous significant aspects of chicken behavior under natural conditions, including, for example, nesting behavior (violates the *telos* or nature of the animal), and that frustration of this basic need or drive results in a mode of suffering for the animals. Let us suppose that we have identified the gene or genes that code for the drive to nest. In addition, suppose we can ablate that gene or substitute a gene (probably *per impossibile*) that creates a new kind of chicken, one that achieves satisfaction by laying an egg in a case, or suppose we create a pig that prefers not to move. Would that be wrong in terms of the animal ethic that is emerging in society?

If we identify an animal's *telos* as being genetically based and environmentally expressed, we have now changed the chicken's *telos*, so that the animal that is forced by us to live in a battery cage is satisfying more of its nature than is the animal that still has the gene coding for nesting. Have we done something morally wrong?

I would argue that we have not. Recall that a key feature, perhaps *the* key feature, of what I have called the new social ethic for animals is concern for preventing animal suffering and augmenting animal happiness, which I have argued involves satisfaction of *telos*. I have implicitly argued that the primary pressing concern is the former—the mitigating of suffering at human hands—given the proliferation of suffering that has occurred in the twentieth century. I have also explicitly argued that suffering can be occasioned in many ways, from infliction of physical pain to prevention of satisfying basic drives. So, when we engineer the new kind of chicken that prefers laying in a cage and we eliminate the nesting urge, we have removed a source of suffering. Given the animal's changed *telos,* the new chicken is now suffering less than its predecessor and is thus closer to being happy, that is, satisfying the dictates of its nature.

Why then does it appear to some people to be prima facie somewhat morally problematic to suggest tampering with the animal's *telos* to remove suffering? In large part, I believe, because people are not convinced that we cannot change the conditions rather than the animal. If people in general do become aware of how animals are raised, as occurred in Sweden and animal activists are working to accomplish elsewhere, they will doubtless demand, just as the Swedes did, a change in the raising conditions, not a change in the animals. (It is far more sensible to raise the bridge than lower the river, just as it is more reasonable to alter clothes than to surgically remodel a body.) And it is quite plausible to change conditions, since we raised chickens for millennia outside the confinement deprivational conditions.

In the end, to breed or engineer pigs or chickens to fit confinement life is continuous with what we have always done with domestic animals—select them to live with us. If there is anything horrifying in the case under discussion, it is an aesthetic revulsion born of disgust at our own behavior: "Have we really gone so far over the edge in how we treat animals that we must radically modify the animal for the sake of cheap meat?"

Case

89

How Do Veterinarians Respond to Clients with Too Many Animals?

Question

As a veteran mixed animal practitioner in a medium-sized rural town, you have seen a number of cases where owners take on more responsibility in caring for animals than they can manage. From the woman with over one hundred cats in an apartment to the older, mixed-livestock farmer who is unwilling to retire, animals may receive less than adequate care, despite the best intentions of the owner. These dedicated clients of yours often make significant personal sacrifices to care for their pets and livestock.

Your most recent case is a widower with health problems who cares for twenty-three horses and eighteen miniature donkeys. The specific need of some of the geriatric animals together with the constant need for hoof trimming and parasite control have recently led to some animal welfare concerns. You have spoken to the owner several times about decreasing the numbers, but he is reluctant because these animals are his family and he just couldn't bear to let any of them go.

How should you respond to your client's reluctance to reduce the number of animals in his care?

Response

Animal control officers, humane society workers, pound employees, cruelty investigators, and veterinarians have long recognized the phenomenon raised in this case. Formerly called "collectors," people who adopt or rescue large numbers of animals are now designated "hoarders." Such individuals—usually middle-aged and female (Wirth and Beck, 1981)—are widely believed to be "crazy" by the mainstream animal welfare professionals listed above.

The distinction is usually made between hoarders and rescuers. Rescuers are committed to not euthanizing animals and their approach has precipitated a major war between members of the humane movement who operate "no kill" shelters and those whose shelter operation involves euthanasia of unadoptable (or unadopted) animals. While this distinction is sometimes blurry, we can mark a real conceptual difference by describing hoarders as those who take in more animals than they can properly care for even at the level of minimal decency. The homes of hoarders are often littered with excrement, animal feed, cans, and sick or dying animals, with the person unable to afford enough help to keep the area livably clean, or to pay for veterinary attention.

To me, spending one's life trying to save as many animals as possible from an untimely death is not crazy; it is no crazier than members of Amnesty International trying to do whatever possible to stop political prisoners being incarcerated and tortured or pacifist groups attempting to stop defense spending. In a way, one can call all high idealism crazy, since the goal of such idealists is never fully achievable in the real world. But that does not make the attempt ignoble or unworthy of praise.

On the other hand, if the animals are not being properly nourished, watered, fed, or housed, such behavior falls foursquare under the traditional definition of legal cruelty, specifically *neglect*.

The well-being of the animals should always guide veterinarians who encounter situations like the one described. If a person is compromising his or her lifestyle to take care of a large number of animals, that is not the veterinarian's business. But if the animals are malnourished or their hooves are untrimmed, or if their diseases or injuries are untreated, that does fall within a veterinarian's moral purview. If such neglect is occurring, it makes sense for the veterinarian to raise the issue forthrightly with the client, delivered with a healthy dose of Aesculapian authority. The veterinarian should point out what is needed and help the client to plan for proper management, even as herd-health practitioners do. If the client won't listen or limit the number of animals he or she is attempting to save, without the financial wherewithal to do so properly, the veterinarian should strongly advise "trimming the herd." If the client systematically fails to listen or improve the situation and the animals are suffering, the case becomes another cruelty situation where it is the veterinarian's responsibility to bring in the authorities to rectify the situation, despite the client's putative good intentions or, at least, get the client's attention by raising that possibility.

Case

90

Should a Veterinarian Wear Company Logos?

Question

Should independent veterinarians wear clothing that advertises for feed companies, pharmaceutical companies, or their products, while performing professional duties?

Response

There is, of course, a semiotic as well as function to dress; nuns do not wear miniskirts. When I began my traveling lecture twenty-five years ago, I found that if I wore a sport shirt to universities, I was called Bernie; if I wore a sports jacket, I was called Mr. Rollin; if I wore a suit, I was Dr. Rollin. If I wore a suit on the streets of New York City, I might as well have a sign flashing "victim, victim, victim." If I wear a Harley-Davidson t-shirt in New York City, no one bothers me, not even panhandlers. One semester when I taught veterinary students, I wore a tie and jacket to class each week, but I also wore a biker ring with a skull on it. Some 75 percent of my student evaluations commented on that ring, mostly informing me that it was "unprofessional." (How, I wondered, did my students know what professional philosophers wear?)

For more than two decades, people have inexplicably paid fifty dollars for t-shirts emblazoned with uninspiring logos like The Gap, Benetton, and DKNY. What message is being sent? What received? Why should I pay to advertise; I should be paid. Why do men wear Viagra ball caps? Is it to communicate that they have overcome a handicap?

What do all these ruminations have to do with the issue at hand? In my view, there is no ethical difference between wearing a dress shirt or t-shirt emblazoned with Nike versus Pfizer or Merck. People are so inured to the fashion of wearing logos that I can see little harm in it. Few, if any, veterinarians will be moved to promote a product because the company representative gave them a hat. Few, if any, clients will suspect the veterinarian of promoting Pfizer's interests over theirs merely because the veterinarian is wearing a hat with the company's logo.

Certainly, there is a continuum along which, at a certain point, it becomes improper to take a gift from a company—free weekend getaways, free trips, cases of whiskey—but I hardly see any slippery slope from twenty-five-cent pens to airline tickets and, thus, don't see the t-shirt or hat wearer as embarking on the road to perdition.

A veterinarian colleague has argued to me that the issue here is one of professionalism. If you are selling ivermectin to clients, it is odd to wear an ivermectin t-shirt, implying that you are biased in favor of the company in question. If you have a reason to believe that this is the message being received by the clients, by all means, discontinue dressing in such attire. But most clients, I believe, are not paranoid and would recognize that you are wearing one of the few, rather limited, veterinary perks that you got at a convention.

In any case, what is "professional" in attire varies with cultural changes. Fifty years ago, a male veterinarian or physician wearing a ponytail or tattoo would stop conversation, and a nun without a habit was a mini-scandal. Both clients and practitioners should learn to look beyond external trappings. If you are nervous about wearing such clothing, don't. Or ask clients what they think.

Case

91

Technicians Performing Management Procedures on Farm

Question

Should veterinarians employ individuals to perform livestock "processing" procedures, such as dehorning, castrating, vaccinating, implanting, and checking pregnancy using ultrasound, on farms in the absence of on-site veterinary supervision?

Response

When I first read this question, I was struck by the fact that I had already addressed virtually the same issue (Case 31). Puzzled, I phoned Dr. Tim Blackwell to determine if I was missing something, or if the duplication had been overlooked. Dr. Blackwell informed me that, in fact, new circumstances had emerged that I could not have been aware of a decade ago.

I argued that, when people hire a veterinarian, they are, in part, paying for the veterinarian's expertise in case unusual circumstances arise in the course of a putatively routine procedure. Twenty-five years ago, Dr. Bill Tietz, then dean of the Colorado State University, College of Veterinary Medicine, explained to me that one can quickly teach a high school student how to spay and castrate by rote, but that does not mean that he or she should be allowed to do so on their own, for they have no grasp whatever of physiological principles, principles of anesthesia, asepsis, and so on. If anything unexpected should occur, they are laypeople. When one hires a genuine professional, one rightly expects that he or she has such expertise! Thus I argued in 1993 that no technician should be allowed to perform a procedure that could conceivably go wrong in the absence of direct veterinary supervision.

I still stand by this principle, but certain social factors have changed the playing field. Whereas, in the past, recent graduates could be presumed to be willing to take up the arduous work of doing a routine procedure under bad conditions, such as inclement weather, today's graduates are not as eager to do so. This is true across all professions. I know of an oncologist who refused to see an elderly patient suffering from complications of chemotherapy, referring her instead to his nurse, until a veterinarian friend of mine, diagnosing serious anemia in the old lady, threatened the oncologist with legal action! The work ethic has been eroded and, far worse, professional schools do not select for people having a work ethic, choosing to utilize safe (lawsuit-avoiding) criteria, such as grade point average, which are "objectively" defensible.

The result is that many young professionals—veterinarians included—do not feel obliged to perform "scut work," duties that recent graduates would have taken for granted thirty years ago. I hear complaints from practitioners all over North America that, if they mention nights or weekend work in the course of interviewing a recent graduate, he or she will often walk out of the interview. So now the farm animal practitioner is faced with a dilemma; he or she may be over fifty, suffer from a bad back, and not be capable or desirous of any longer doing what they have done for thirty years. On the other hand, recent graduates, to whom such work was historically axiomatic, no longer wish to do it. In an effort to escape such a dilemma, increasing numbers of veterinarians are training "pit crews" of technicians to do such jobs.

In my view, this is a poor solution unless the veterinarian is on-site. The bottom line is that the client is paying for professional expertise and is not getting it. Many ranchers already believe that they can do what a veterinarian does much more cheaply, and the question under discussion buttresses that mischievous view. So what should be done?

In the short term, in my view, the veterinarian should always be present and directly supervising such technicians. In the long run, veterinary schools must move away from using grades as the sole or dominant criterion for admission and face the hard legal problems of using more subjective criteria. For example, people from a farm background, with a proven willingness to do such work, should be actively recruited. Some will not be A students, but many are likely to be A practitioners.

Case

92

Extralabel Drug Use

Question

A large amount of testing is required by veterinary pharmaceutical companies to license medications to treat specific diseases in specific species. The testing is required to demonstrate efficacy, safety, dosage, and withdrawal times, among other things. Licensed veterinarians, however, may prescribe medications in an extralabel manner (including changes to the indications, species, and dosages), based on their own understanding of pharmacology and disease pathogenesis.

Can veterinarians defend their right to prescribe in this manner?

Response

Drug companies are driven by the need to produce profits for their stockholders. The cost of discovery and validation of new drugs for safety and efficacy is enormous, both in terms of money and time. For this reason, these companies are unwilling to make such an investment if a market big enough to justify the expenditures does not exist. While certain select veterinary drugs, such as ivermectin and carprofen, do create huge profits, many do not. The market for mouse analgesics, for example, is limited to research animals used in painful (usually surgical) protocols. Researchers with thousands of mice will not pay for expensive regimens. The market for tiger analgesics is considerably smaller. Food animal producers cannot pay ten dollars per daily dose for cutting-edge antibiotics.

As of 1997, the number of companies doing animal health research on drugs in Canada had shrunk from twenty-one to seven. According to the Animal Health Institute in the United States, only 1 in 7500 compounds succeeds in gaining approval over a period of ten to twelve years, at a cost of $250 million. Clearly drugs serving limited markets will not be forthcoming.

Veterinarians who wish to use only drugs approved for their particular species of interest thus face a huge obstacle: Such drugs are rarely available. It is for this reason that legislatures have granted veterinarians the privilege of using drugs in an off-label way—for example, in a manner that has not yet been approved for the species in question.

Usually this means using human drugs in an animal species, but it may mean using a drug licensed for use in cattle, in a pig, or a water buffalo or licensed for use in dogs or cats.

Such use is not just shooting in the dark. Safety and efficacy of human drugs are tested first in a number of animal species before clinical trials; if we can extrapolate from animals to humans, logic dictates that we can go in the other direction. In fact, when, in the mid-1980s, U.S. federal law mandated pain control for laboratory animals, such extrapolations were the basis for most analgesic use.

Furthermore, as we understand drug action in a clearer way, we can make reasonable extrapolations from established information. For example, we know that pain in pigs is not controlled well by opiates, so the chances are that a new opiate will yield dubious results.

The point is that the alternative to extralabel drug use is doing nothing at all. The position of the Canadian Veterinary Medical Association (CVMA) (2004) on the extralabel use of drugs is to encourage Canadian veterinarians to prescribe veterinary approved drugs when available. The position states, "The extra label use of drugs must be based on a valid veterinarian/client/patient relationship. Inherent with this is the responsibility to assure safe application to the animal and education of the client in a manner that will contribute to the safety and wholesomeness of foods of animal origin. Veterinarians can adhere to these principles through dedication to continuing education on pharmaceutical issues, and by obtaining the most up-to-date information from the pharmaceutical companies, veterinary colleges, and regulatory agencies."

In the United States, the Animal Drug Use Clarification Act was passed in 1994. This law specifies that to use a drug in an off-label way, a veterinarian must have a valid veterinary/client relationship and not use the drug in animal feed. Certain drugs (e.g., clenbuterol and chloramphenicol) may not be used at all in food animals. Further, the Secretary of Health and Human Services may specify safe levels of residue for drugs used in food animals and require a method of detecting residues; proper labeling and record keeping are required by legislation passed in 1997.

Some years ago, a number of veterinarians were cavalier about the use of antibiotics for growth promotion in feeds. This led Congress perilously close to banning extralabel drug use, which would have virtually destroyed veterinary medicine. Thus veterinarians should be careful not to violate the public trust in this area, lest a major tool be removed from them.

Case

93

Animal Welfare versus Animal Rights

Question

The recent passing of animal rights legislation in some jurisdictions has lead to debates on whether or not it is possible for any animal to possess "rights." The argument most often given is that only humans have rights. People are responsible for the welfare of animals in their care, but this is not the same as giving rights to animals.

Is there a difference between being responsible for the well-being of an animal and giving that animal the right to be well cared for?

Response

Organized veterinary medicine and most animal users, particularly in agriculture, have consistently failed to understand emerging social ethics for animals. They have mistakenly equated advocating the abolition of animal use in society with a belief in animal rights. In fact, on the one hand, a person can believe in the legitimacy of the use of animals by humans in society and still believe that animals have rights, and on the other hand, a person can deny the legitimacy of such use without believing in rights. This misunderstanding puts veterinary medicine in conflict with society, since the overwhelming majority of citizens (over 80 percent) believe that animals have rights (Kane and Parsons, 1989). It then jars society when veterinarians deny that animals have rights and affirm that they only have "welfare."

Widespread belief in animal rights emerged as a creature of radical changes in animal use in the mid–twentieth century. For most of human history, the overwhelming use of animals in society was for agriculture—food, fiber, locomotion, and power. And the key to successful agriculture was respecting animals' natures, putting them into environments for which they were biologically suited, and augmenting their natural ability to survive and thrive with protection from predation and provision of food during famine, water during drought, medical attention, and so on. This approach was called *husbandry* (from the Old Norse phrase for "bonded to the household") and is optimized in the Twenty-third Psalm's depiction of the shepherd: "The Lord is my shepherd, I shall not want. He maketh me to lie down in green pastures, he leadeth me beside the still waters, he restoreth my soul." We want no more from God than the shepherd provides to his sheep!

As long as this contract of "we take care of the animals, they will take care of us" obtained, society needed no additional ethic or laws save prohibition of cruelty to animals, for self-interest was the greatest stimulus for proper animal treatment, and the anticruelty ethic covered the sadist and psychopaths unmoved by self-interest. No traditional husbandry agriculturalist would have put one hundred thousand chickens in one building, for all would have died in weeks.

Technology broke this ancient contract when it allowed us to put animals into environments and uses that didn't impair their productivity but harmed their well-being. We could now put square pegs into round holes and suppress with technological fixes the loss of revenue. Because of antibiotics, vaccines, air-handling systems, et cetera, we could raise one hundred thousand chickens in one building or pigs in crates. Similarly, the rise of significant funding for biomedical research at mid-century broke the contract; we inflicted disease, pain, fractures, wounds, et cetera, on animals with great benefit to ourselves and to other animals, but with no compensatory benefit to the subjects.

When society became aware that the proper treatment of animals was no longer natural and integral to their successful use, as was the case in husbandry, people began to demand that such proper use be guaranteed in the law. In our social ethic for humans, such protection for human nature against individuals being submerged for the sake of the general welfare is prescribed in the Bill of Rights and in other legal rights deduced therefrom. In the same way, society began to demand legal protections or rights for animals to protect them against exploitation for the sake of profit and productivity or medical advancement. Animal protection laws beyond cruelty have proliferated, and this is the mainstream sense of "animal rights." Animal rights is simply the demand for legal protection for fundamental aspects of animal need and nature in the face of high technology-based loss of husbandry in agriculture and infliction of suffering in research, neither of which counts as deliberate cruelty. Animal rights is the form that animal welfare concerns have taken since the mid–twentieth century.

For the sake of its own social credibility, veterinary medicine should cease to deny that animals should have rights, when most of society sees such protection as essential.

Case

94

Raw Diet

Question

The feeding of raw meat and bone diets is being promoted by many people, including some veterinarians, with an almost evangelical zeal.

As a small animal practitioner, you have seen many dogs on these diets that appear to be in excellent general health. Also, you have had clients report that some chronic problems, such as allergic skin disease, have resolved since their pet has been on the diet.

Based on conventional standards of nutrition, you know that these diets are not balanced, especially for growing dogs. Also, the potential for zoonotic disease from the raw foods and for complications from ingesting bone is very real.

Although not convinced that these diets are appropriate pet foods, you have begun to wonder if some processed commercial diets are lacking nutritional factors that may be present in raw diets. You also question whether the large proportion of processed grain found in commercial diets is biologically appropriate for dogs and cats, which are basically carnivores.

Raw diets appear to be increasing in popularity; *therefore, how should a veterinarian respond to questions regarding the appropriateness of these diets?*

Response

We live in an age of faddishness in lifestyles; how else can one explain the $29 billion spent per year on unproven nostrums and remedies? In the United States, thanks to Utah Senator Hatch's bill exempting nutritional supplements from Food and Drug Administration surveillance, we are free to consume untested, non-quality-controlled weeds and herbs from the Orient, many of which have been shown to be toxic. We align our furniture with the energy lines of the universe, tie ourselves in yoga knots, wear magnetic bracelets, and consume homeopathic remedies that cannot possibly work, if what we know of chemistry is correct. We consume all meat diets, no meat diets, grapefruit diets, and caveman diets, and we switch from killer butter to margarine and back to butter. Do we owe our pets any less? Apparently not.

For some years, hucksters have been pushing the "raw diet" of raw meat and bones for dogs. Never mind an absence of scientific evidence; if hearsay is good enough for us, it is good enough for our pets. After all, it is natural, and what is natural is good (never mind that aflatoxins, botulinum toxin, and snake venom are also natural, as is anthrax). Aren't dogs descended from wolves, and don't wolves eat raw food? Actually, there is evidence that wolves in the wild don't eat so well, are not always well nourished, and carry formidable parasite loads. In addition, they consume far more than raw meat, including vegetation and predigested food in their prey's intestines. Just because evolutionarily dogs are derived from wolves does not mean they are wolves. In fact, there is anthropological evidence that domestic dogs have been eating cooked food for over three hundred thousand years and thus cannot be compared with their wild ancestors. Cooked meat is in fact more easily digested by dogs.

There is a good deal of evidence in fact that dogs do not do well on a raw diet. Raw meat can infect animals with parasites, toxoplasma, *Salmonella* spp., *Escherichia coli*, and *Campylobacter* spp. These can present zoonotic disease risks. The diet can eventuate in irritable bowel syndrome, significant nutritional deficiencies, and vitamin A toxicity. Choking and bloody diarrhea can be a problem when such raw food as chicken and turkey bones are fed and splinter. Raw foods also grind down teeth prematurely. For most of dog's evolutionary history, dogs ate what we ate, that is, cooked table scraps; commercial dog food is only about a hundred years old. And dogs and cats are living longer now than they did twenty years ago. All of which suggests that present-day feeding regimes are all right. We have many choices now, including diets aimed at special problems (e.g., urinary) and at young and old animals. Medical professionals, human and veterinary, are probably undertrained in nutrition. Nutritional education can be improved for both laypeople and medical professionals. In the meantime, common sense goes a long way.

Case

95

Using an Elastrator on Older Bulls

Question

A new marketing campaign for a castration device emphasizes its use for the banding of bulls at a later age. One advantage cited for this device is its ability to castrate bulls within 120 days of market, thereby allowing the producer to benefit from the natural growth-promoting effects of testosterone for a longer period of time. Several clinics and sales barns in your area are advocating this new technique. You have reservations regarding the use of the procedure at this age, as there is a possibility of greater distress for bulls castrated at heavier weights. However, your reservations have also been interpreted as your concern that this new technique will cut into your sales of implants.

How should you respond?

Response

Many people involved in the cattle business (including some older veterinarians who went to school when pain was not much discussed) believe that bloodless castration is also painless. On the contrary, of all methods of castration with which I am familiar (knife, burdizzo, chemical, immunological, and banding), banding is probably the most painful. Anyone who doubts this should wind a rubber band or elastrator tightly on his or her finger and let it remain there for *hours*, not days, and the nature of the pain will be eloquently demonstrated.

Moreover, there is no reason to believe that castration is any less painful in a newly born calf than in an older animal, despite the fact that British law allows castration without anesthesia only before an animal reaches eight weeks of age, though it is easier to control bleeding in a young animal and thus early castration generates fewer complications.

Nor is castration very sensible from a production point of view. As one Wyoming rancher told me: "First we cut off the animal's testicles and get dinged by the public for being inhumane. Then we place the testicles in their ears [implants] and get dinged by the public for adulterating the food supply. And to add insult to injury, the implants don't work as well as the testicles." A friend of mine could market intact animals one to two months earlier than castrates, thereby saving a good deal of feed, being able to advertise the product as humane and hormone-free, and getting top dollar. Research done at Colorado State University and elsewhere has shown that people cannot distinguish young bulls from steers in taste and tenderness tests!

Both the grading system and producer ignorance perpetuate castration. (Some producers do not even believe one can feed bulls!) Veterinarians are perfectly positioned to dispel such ignorance and to help producers penetrate niche markets.

In any event, a veterinarian should always try to mitigate animal pain, for example, by using anesthesia and analgesia for castration, as is legally mandated in northern Europe. He or she certainly should not perpetuate the most painful method, banding, whether it is more painful in older animals or not. Nor should he or she fear gossip impugning his or her motives, since as the influence of People for the Ethical Treatment of Animals on fast food restaurants and grocery chains has shown, society will not tolerate such painful practices much longer, and the industry needs to be seeking alternatives.

I dedicate this column to the memory of Dr. Frank Loew, who would certainly have endorsed the message it contains.

Case

96

Finding Animals for Continuing Education

Question

Veterinarians must stay abreast of new surgical, medical, and diagnostic techniques to provide the best possible care for their patients. One method of ensuring competency in new or unfamiliar procedures is to practice new procedures on animal cadavers. In certain jurisdictions, humane societies refuse to allow cadavers to be used for such purposes, because it is not within their mandate to do so. You have considered the possibility of adding an addendum to the clinic's euthanasia consent form to allow clients to consent to such use. However, there is some hesitation to do this for fear of how clients may perceive or respond to such a request.

Is there a method by which private practitioners can obtain suitable cadavers in an ethical, timely, and financially practical manner?

Response

The use of animals for practice procedures and training of veterinarians has had a historical evolution worth reflecting upon. Veterinarians trained in the 1940s have told me of going to pounds on Fridays as senior students and acquiring live dogs on which to practice surgical procedures over the weekend. In the 1970s, surgery was taught by using unwanted animals repeatedly in successive survival procedures. In "multiple survival surgery" training, an animal could be used eight or more times before finally being allowed to expire in a terminal operation with no provision for aftercare, and at some schools, they were used for a semester. Procedures often included fracturing a femur or even a mandible.

At Colorado State University, training by use of multiple survival surgery was abolished in the late 1970s for ethical reasons; it was replaced first with single survival surgery, where students were graded on aftercare as well, and later with terminal procedures, with students learning aftercare on client animals in clinical situations. Other schools followed suit. By the 1980s, even though pain had largely been eliminated from the teaching of surgery, many people objected to taking a life, even painlessly, for the purpose of becoming a veterinarian, arguing that physicians did not do terminal surgery on humans. Such students were generally provided with alternatives, such as models, cadavers, and spay-neuter work on human society animals, and today some schools have altogether eliminated terminal surgeries for training. It is common to affirm that there are many paths to learning the same material and that students using alternate training methods are no worse surgeons than those doing terminal procedures.

In the case of continuing education for veterinarians, society has moved in the direction of opposing the use of pound and shelter animals for such procedures, and even of opposing the use of cadavers and unadoptable animals killed in pounds and shelters. In some places, purpose-bred animals costing as much as five hundred to six hundred dollars must be purchased for terminal procedures. As long as animals are being killed in pounds and shelters, however, this seems to be a waste of life and of money. While reasonable people can debate the use of such animals for terminal surgery, banning the use of cadavers is totally irrational in my view, and provides a good example of how far the social pendulum can thoughtlessly swing in thirty or fewer years!

It is time for organized veterinary medicine to explain that veterinarians in practice need to update their skills, and that a reasonable way to do so is on cadavers of animals that have been killed not for the sake of education, but because of social irresponsibility or because the animals are unadoptable. As long as millions of animals meeting that description are killed, it seems paradigmatically wasteful to forbid their use as cadavers to help veterinarians learn to improve their treatment skills or to require the use of live or dead purpose-bred animals. It is especially important to stress the elimination of pain and of taking life in the training of veterinary surgeons. Providing society with both a historical perspective on this issue and an explanation of the training needs required to help veterinarians help people's animals could serve to blunt the current tendency of society to worry about the bodies of dogs and cats while ignoring the fact that we often take their lives for no good reason. Acquiescence to mindless faddishness should be resisted. Using live animals as they were used thirty years ago was wrong, whether society cared or not. Not using cadavers today is also wrong. Veterinarians should lead in rational, ethical humane approaches to animal use, not just follow.

In the case of euthanized client animals, veterinarians should prepare brochures explaining the problem and allow interested clients to approach them. I would not myself explicitly raise the issue to a client with a terminally ill animal, as some people do care about the bodies of their animals and could see your request as being insensitive. There is precedent here in cadavers used in human medical schools.

Case

97

Should Veterinarians Support Activist Groups?

Question

Many producers and veterinarians consider animal rights groups out of touch with modern animal agriculture. They see these groups as being threats to their livelihood, lawbreakers, distorters of facts, and bad for modern livestock farming. They overlook the groups' success at, for example, improving the handling of animals at slaughterhouses and increasing the living space for caged layer hens. Producers and veterinarians, as advocates for livestock, should expectedly be applauding their success.

Should veterinarians give support to an animal rights group or is there a better way to improve the welfare of farm livestock?

Response

There is no simple, all-encompassing answer to this question; the response will clearly be situation-specific. Let us recall that it was radical groups in the United States that informed the public of the need for reform of animal research. The distribution by People for the Ethical Treatment of Animals (PETA) of the infamous University of Pennsylvania videotapes documenting atrocities by researchers unquestioningly galvanized public support for federal legislation, which all sides now admit makes for better research and better animal care. For many years, the National Institutes of Health used these tapes to educate their own researchers.

The confinement agriculture industry has been just as guilty as many activists of distortion: Compare advertisements run for many years by a major broiler company showing chickens pecking in a barnyard and averring that the company raises "happy chickens," when, in fact, the birds were raised in high confinement. Not very long ago, organized veterinary medicine in the United States argued that there are no major issues with U.S. agricultural systems, only a few bad managers. I would be hard-pressed to find any farmers among the thousands of agriculturalists I have addressed who would make such a statement.

In short, radical groups have no monopoly on exaggeration, distortion, and self-serving rhetoric. Much as we may temperamentally eschew activists, they help to move social recognition of new issues. In the 1970s, when I argued that science and medicine ought to acknowledge, recognize, and manage animal pain, a high official in the scientific community phoned my university and said that I was a "viper in the bosom of biomedicine" and should be removed from teaching veterinary students. Six years later, to his credit, this official publicly acknowledged his error and, in fact, became one of my references and a cherished friend. Without people on the fringes challenging the status quo, we would not resist complacency.

I have long argued that veterinarians are the natural movers of animal welfare in society, as evidenced by the fact that society in the United States and Britain charge veterinarians with guaranteeing laboratory animal welfare. That society is concerned about farm animal welfare is unquestionable: A May 2003 Gallup poll showed that 75 percent of U.S. citizens want the well-being of farm animals guaranteed by legislation (Gallup, 2003). The vast majority of the public, however, does not accept the vegan-like answer given by activists. They want animal products, but they also want assurance that animals live decent lives. Organized veterinary medicine has not been helpful in resolving this tissue of issues. Veterinarians should examine all opinions on farm animal welfare and then lead in suggesting and implementing rational solutions; I have heard for twenty years that the industry itself wants leadership from veterinary medicine. If relevant information—for example, on forced molting—comes from radical groups, we should be grateful to them for supplying the information. The operative question is not "Who supplies the relevant knowledge"? but rather "Is it true, and if so, how can we fix it?"

Case

98

Auditability of Animal Welfare

Question

In the past, humane societies and veterinarians have struggled to reach consensus on what constitutes animal neglect or animal abuse. Today, several different groups are creating "welfare audits" for livestock operations. Some of these groups want veterinarians to perform the welfare evaluations. It has been argued that these audits reflect the viewpoints of the authors. For example, one auditing system may start with the assumption that battery cages or veal crates do not promote good welfare, while another audit system may accept these housing options. Critics view these audits as marketing schemes rather than a means to promote acceptable animal welfare.

Can the welfare of domestic livestock in modern production systems be scored accurately?

Response

An accurate response to this query requires the realization that the concept of "animal welfare" is value-laden; that is, it contains a range of value judgments and is not simply empirical. It is thus not surprising that widespread disagreements exist as to what considerations count as welfare and to what extent they need to be provided. While we will probably all agree that good health is part of welfare, health itself is in part valuational—compare the World Health Organization's definition of human health as "a state of complete physical, mental, and social well-being" and not merely absence of disease. Compare, too, the old CAST Report (1981) concept of animal welfare as being defined by the animal meeting its production purpose!

Obviously, for many producers adequate welfare would still be defined by the animals being able to produce, while for many animal advocates, an animal not actualizing its basic biological and psychological nature (e.g., a sow in a sow stall) would not count as enjoying adequate welfare however productive it might be.

The fact that the concept contains value judgments does not mean that it cannot be objectively audited. Suppose we define human welfare in part in terms of a set of basic needs that must be met to a certain level. If we accept this notion and agree on the implicit value judgments contained within it, we can objectively decide which societies provide for these needs and which don't. In other words, we can objectively audit various societies.

With animal welfare, we therefore need some notion of what society in general would value as at least minimally required for animals to be kept acceptably. The problem is determining such a consensus view in the absence of legislation. If we look to what has occurred in Europe with farm animal welfare, for example, and assume that similar views will eventually emerge in North America, something like the Brambell Commission notion of animal freedoms seems to guide European thought, coupled with the animal enjoying the ability to display its natural behavioral repertoire. Clearly this is auditable.

Regrettably, the industry seems unwilling to embrace what I have called the new social ethic for animals, and is thus playing Russian roulette with legislation. It would be wiser for producers to preserve their freedom and begin to operate in accord with that ethic in the absence of legislation than to risk well-intended but overly restrictive laws.

In the interim, one can certainly audit accord with industry-accepted standards for housing, veterinary care, transport, and slaughter. Temple Grandin has developed such a system that McDonald's uses with their suppliers. There exist clear cases where these standards are not being met, for example, in the Glatt Kosher Iowa slaughterhouse exposed by PETA.

In sum, welfare is auditable provided one reaches a consensus between industry and society on what animal welfare means. Currently, such a consensus is not yet codified, but minimal standards adopted by government and industry are auditable, which is better than nothing.

Case

99

Producer Unwilling to Euthanize Sick Pigs

Question

You are called to examine a problem with infectious arthritis on a six-hundred-sow, farrow-to-finish swine farm. The manager explains that he has had lameness problems in the past. The problem is worse now and no longer responds to therapy. You arrange for several lame pigs to be sent to the diagnostic laboratory for testing. There are ten to fifteen additional pigs of various ages in the barn with enlarged, painful joints. In your experience, these chronically infected pigs do not respond to therapy. You tell the owner that these pigs are unlikely to be profitable and should be euthanized. He tells you that he is in the business of raising pigs, not killing pigs. In your experience, this reluctance to euthanize animals is common, even among the best stockpeople. They are reluctant to kill an animal that they have tried, but failed, to nurse back to health. They sometimes say they might kill a pig if you could suggest a method that is humane and not overly risky to those performing the euthanasias.

What should be your response?

Response

This is a very interesting case, in that the producer takes a very strong ethical stand, but one that is, in my view, significantly misguided. When the producer says that he is "in the business of raising pigs, not killing them," it sounds, at first blush, like the sort of strong position favoring the sanctity of animal life that some vegetarians and anti-vivisectionists might take. Indeed, I am familiar with a number of sanctuaries that take in farm animals and let them live out their normal lives instead of being slaughtered for food.

But a moment's reflection reveals that the producer cannot possibly be taken as espousing such a right-to-life position, since his livelihood depends on killing pigs at approximately 250 pounds, or six months of age. Perhaps, then, he means that, as a producer whose raison d'être and livelihood is raising slaughter pigs, he cannot accept their premature killing. But, if this is what he means, he is being irrational, as you have already shown him that such pigs are unlikely to be profitable, so from the perspective of rational self-interest, it makes no sense to keep them alive.

What he probably means is that, as a husbandry person, he does not like to give up on an animal. (In fact, I know many cattlemen, deeply imbued with the husbandry ethic, who, out of sense of obligation to the animal, will spend more than the animal is worth to cure it.) But in this case, such an ethic does not apply, since you have already told him that such chronically infected pigs do not respond to therapy, so there is little point in spending the money, even if he is inclined to do so.

Having made these points, and if the producer is indeed responding to a husbandry ethical imperative, I, as the veterinarian, would point out that part of husbandry and good stockmanship is not letting animals suffer unnecessarily. Thus, euthanasia is the only rational solution in this situation.

It remains only for the veterinarian to suggest a cost-effective, humane modality for euthanasia (I will assume that food safety issues are irrelevant here, as the pigs are unlikely to be consumed). And it appears to me that there are plenty of choices. The most plausible is pentobarbital, which all veterinarians should probably carry in their trucks. Alternatively, many farm veterinarians carry a captive bold pistol, which would also be an inexpensive method. In addition, the veterinarian should discuss the captive bolt for on-farm euthanasia with the client, to avoid causing him prohibitive expense for euthanasia if he must call a veterinarian each time.

This case is also valuable in demonstrating the degree to which any veterinarian must be an accomplished ethical thinker and communicator. Failure in this area dooms the animal to prolonged suffering.

Case

100

Veterinarians and Laws Banning Pitbulls

Question

You work in a companion animal practice in a large suburban center. Three years ago, the city enacted a bylaw that banned the ownership of pitbull terriers, Staffordshire terriers, crosses of either breed, or any dog resembling either of the two breeds. Anyone owning such a dog at the time the bylaw was enacted was allowed to keep the dog, but no new dogs fitting the descriptions above would be permitted within the city limits. Two years ago, unaware of the bylaw a family with three young children and a six-year-old, registered pitbull terrier moved across the country to this city. The dog has been a patient of yours for the last two years and has never shown any signs of aggressive behavior. The owners present you with a notice from the city that the dog must be taken outside the city or be destroyed; it is not allowed within the city limits. The owners ask you to write a letter to the appeals committee that is authorized to grant exceptions to the bylaw. Your recommendation will likely weigh heavily with the decision makers. You do not want to be responsible for another serious dog bite injury in this area nor do you want to see this family lose a pet that, as far as you can ascertain, has never shown any aggressive tendencies, unlike many of the dogs under your care.

How should you respond?

Response

It appears that society perennially runs something like a "monster-dog-of-the-year" contest, wherein certain breeds are designated as vicious human-killers, providing us with a thrill of fear whenever we see a member of that breed. When I was young, it was German shepherds that struck terror into our hearts; later, it was Doberman pinschers, then rottweilers, then pitbulls and pitbull crosses. Society has grown progressively crazier in a variety of areas, including the prosecution of frivolous lawsuits, such as against McDonalds (blaming the company for the hot coffee a customer spilled and burned himself with); the rise of everyone claiming victim status; or the demonization of other creatures. Society's response to these perceived threats have also become crazier, with the advent of laws banning the ownership of these breeds, as in this case. Former veterinary dean, Frank Loew, a man of profound common sense, has referred to the paranoia evidenced by such responses as "canine racism."

The issue, in my view, is not the breed of dog so much as the people who wish to acquire a dog with a killer reputation. In fact, although pitbulls have indeed traditionally been used as fighting dogs, they were bred to be aggressive toward other dogs, not to their handlers or other humans, because people needed to be able to intrude into a dogfight without evoking an attack response. Similarly, people who want to own vicious dogs will own them, regardless of what breed they are. Almost any animal can be made mindlessly aggressive by agitating it, tying it to a short lead, disallowing positive human contact, using a poor genetic selection, and employing training methods that evoke paranoia or hostility. "Adorable" poodles, terriers, and St. Bernards can be a good deal more aggressive than pitbulls. I have, in fact, owned many dogs that were viewed by society as killers, including pitbulls and rottweilers, and have found them to be more trustworthy around children than my highly malevolent Chihuahua.

In the end, dogs, like people, should be looked at as individuals, not stereotyped in what can be a self-fulfilling prophecy. In fact, in this case, the veterinarian knows this dog as an individual and has no reason to believe that it fits the aggressive cliché. He or she actually has reason to believe it does not. It is morally incumbent upon him or her to write the letter stating what he or she knows, to save both the animal and the owners anguish. Taking the argument one step further, veterinarians should aggressively battle laws that stereotype animals at the expense of their individuality.

Case

101

Giving Analgesics to Mask Pain in Horses

Question

A long-time client of yours has a fourteen-year-old pleasure horse that she rides occasionally in twenty-five-mile endurance rides. The horse has been sore after the last few of these rides and your lameness examination reveals early navicular disease. Your client asks you for analgesics to help the horse to remain competitive. Many of her friends who are endurance riders routinely give anti-inflammatory and analgesic drugs before and after each competition. You know that the more the horse is used in this manner, the faster the navicular bone will degenerate. You also know that the horse will likely go to slaughter when it can no longer be used for endurance riding.

Is it ethically acceptable to provide analgesia under these circumstances? (You wonder this on the morning after the old-timers' hockey tournament, as you pop two aspirin to relieve the ache in your shoulder.)

Response

Immanuel Kant pointed out that one of the fundamental dictates of moral law is to treat objects of moral concern as ends in themselves, not merely as means. Obviously, we do treat others as means, as we call a plumber to unclog a drain. Clearly, we are primarily interested in the plumber as a means to getting the water to flow freely. But that does not mean that we can treat him as a mere tool and toss him casually into the garage, as one would a plunger, when he is done.

This is an extremely valuable notion and has, for example, been used as a way to articulate sexual ethics. It is often said, today, that what determines the morality of sexual behavior is whether or not one treats one's partner as an end in himself or herself, with an awareness of his or her needs, not merely a means to one's own gratification.

The animal ethic that has developed over the past three decades is couchable in these terms. Whether an animal is a companion animal viewed as a member of the family or an animal destined to serve as food, it is argued that it is wrong to lose sight of the animal's needs and treat it simply as a means to our selfish ends. This is why many countries are rejecting industrialized confinement agriculture since the systems fail to meet the animals' needs for space, sociality, play, and so on. And it is no response to this moral thrust to say that ignoring the animals' needs and natures keeps food prices low.

Well before the advent of this new ethic for animals, many horse owners felt such an obligation to the animals that served them faithfully. A fortiori, in a world where California passed a law forbidding horse slaughter as a felony in order to serve notice that horses are companion animals, not livestock, one would hope that horse owners would be inclined to see their animals as more than tools.

In this case, the horse has served the owner well for fourteen years and is now no longer fit for endurance riding. One would hope that the owner is sufficiently bonded morally to the animal not to trash it, but to let it live out its life without hard use. The use of analgesics to mask the pain will lead to the horse's inevitable breakdown and consequent destruction.

The overwhelming majority of veterinarians see themselves as, ideally, more like pediatricians with the primary obligation to the animal patient, not as garage mechanics fundamentally obligated to the owner. And clearly, it is not in the animal's best interest to mask the pain. Were I the veterinarian, I would utilize my considerable Aesculapian authority to help the owner recollect, in Plato's felicitous phrase, her obligation to the animal as an end in itself. Once again, we find the veterinarian serving as an animal advocate, whose skills at awakening moral awareness in the client are as important as his or her strictly medical skills.

To medicate the animal to mask pain, while assuring further deterioration of its health and function, is a violation of one of the fundamental principles of all medical ethics: Primum non nocere—first of all, do no harm. It is inimical to respect for the animal as an end in itself and totally violates what is called "bond-centered practice." And it is as crass and insensitive to the animal's needs as any profit-driven animal use most horse owners would deplore.

In short, I would counsel the owner to allow the animal to live out its life as soundly as possible. If she refused to do so, I would sever my relationship with her; her custom is not worth the moral stress that comes from actions so inimical to my fundamental values.

Case

102

Are Animals Raised in Confinement Happy in Confinement?

Question

One argument for keeping wild or domestic animals in close confinement is that those animals have never known a less restrictive environment. Exotic animals born in zoos; mice, beagles, and monkey raised in laboratory colonies; and livestock reared under intensive farming operations are assumed to be content, provided they have never lived under less restrictive conditions. It is also argued that zoos, laboratory colonies, and farmers select for adaptation to confinement rearing.

Are these views justified?

Response

In my view, this argument is made from desperation and is being advanced in a vain attempt to defend the indefensible, severe confinement of animals under unnatural conditions. Unfortunately, both the argument and its opposite counterpart enjoy a long history inversely proportional to their probability.

In essence, this argument affirms that animals are strictly products of their experiences, as is rooted in Locke's tabula rasa notion, which is that people and animals are born as blank slates, genetically predetermined, and that all mentation and behavior are products of learning. This notion was hardened into an unquestioned ideology by American Behaviorists and Russian Marxists. In defense of this view, Russians declared Darwinian biology persona non grata; behaviorists simply ignored it!

In direct contrast to the ideology just described is genetic determinism, as defended by the Nazis and such ethologists as Konrad Lorenz (a Nazi sympathizer). In his view, learning has no ability to counter the genetic blueprint—inferiors will remain inferior and beget inferiors.

Common sense recognizes, of course, that both of the above views are totally implausible. We are to some extent a product of our genes but also of the environment that we grow up in or are raised in. So, too, with animals. Animals have natures that are genetically determined—birds gotta fly, fish gotta swim—but the exact form this takes is subject to environmental modification. A dog's inborn hunting urge can be channeled into chasing a Frisbee.

The problem with severe confinement in agriculture, laboratories, and so on is that it totally disallows even the most basic aspects of an animal's nature to be fulfilled. Not only can a sow in confinement not build a nest, she cannot even *move*—this for an animal that would cover a mile a day foraging under extensive, natural conditions and that has bones and muscles that create a built-in urge for movement.

Common sense is supported by empirical data. My colleague, Temple Grandin, has taken pigs that have lived their whole lives in confinement and are tenth- or twentieth-generation confinement animals, and turned them loose (Grandin, personal communication, 2000). Big surprise: They immediately head for a mud wallow to cool off. Similarly, Levine (1989) has shown that monkeys possess innate fear of snakes and heights. Such urges are inborn, not learned—"hard-wired" in today's jargon. Social animals cannot be happy in twenty-four-hour daylight; animals built to move can never be happy in severe confinement. Effort is far better spent in working to accommodate animal nature than in denying its existence.

Case

103

Elderly Couple Adopting Many Animals

Question

You are called to a home in the country to examine a dog with blood in its urine. The owners, an elderly couple, have decided to change veterinary clinics. They take you out to the barn where they have approximately twenty dogs and fifteen cats in various pens, cages, and box stalls. All the animals appear healthy and have good hair coats. When you enter the barn, most of the dogs begin to bark, rattle their cages, or jump against the stall doors. You examine the dog with the urinary problem, collect samples for laboratory testing, and provide symptomatic treatment. You learn through your conversation with the owners that they have been "rescuing" dogs and cats for years. Many of the animals they take in are unlikely to be adopted. All are well to overfed, neutered, and receive veterinary attention when needed. Two collie crosses receive twice-daily topical treatments for lick granulomas and one cat is tranquilized in efforts to reduce its tendency towards self-mutilation. The noise in the barn is deafening and you are anxious to leave. While driving back to the clinic, you wonder if this couple is doing a good thing or a bad thing.

Response

In Case 89, I noted a distinction between the sorts of people who are committed to saving animals from death, "hoarders" (or "collectors") and rescuers. Hoarders mindlessly collect as many animals as they can, even when they lack the space or resources to care for them. A hoarder may have one hundred cats, many of which are sick, in an excrement-littered apartment and be unable to afford veterinary care. The situation described here, however, is closer to the other end of the spectrum. We are told that the animals are well fed and appear healthy and that scrupulous attention is given to treating disease and calling for veterinary attention when needed.

Plainly, we are not dealing with the question of whether a terrible life is better than no life, nor are we working with an economically impossible situation or with a mentally ill person. The people in this case seem to be morally motivated, all the more so because they provide homes for allegedly unadoptable animals, spending whatever is necessary.

What is most problematic about this situation is that it could be made better with relatively little expenditure. For example, one could easily build access to the outdoors for these animals; ideally, a setup in which they could go in and out at will. The owners probably do not realize that noise is a physical stressor and has even been shown to increase the incidence of mammary tumors, though it is also a problem wherever one keeps a group of dogs, even in expensive boarding kennels.

Your job, as veterinarian in this situation, is to share your expertise with the owners to the benefit of the animal. You might suggest ways to improve the housing and husbandry, so as to provide exercise and outdoor access and alleviate boredom to cut down on self-mutilation and some kinds of lick granuloma. You might also discuss methods of muffling the sound. You could propose a way to ration the animals' diets, and you should advise on sanitation and disease control. You also can help to determine if the animals are, indeed, unadoptable.

Equally important, you can assist the owners in assuring the authorities (and their neighbors) that the situation here is not pathological but, rather, is the case of an elderly couple trying to fill a void in their lives by doing something to help others.

Finally, I am not sure what "unadoptable" means or that anyone should presume to have that knowledge, a priori. I am familiar with people who adopt physically and mentally disabled children, blind and geriatric dogs, and aggressive dogs. Unadoptable is not a judgment to be made in the absence of attempts to adopt, which may have been limited in this case.

Case

104

The Ethics of Killing Healthy Animals

Question

Veterinarians have refused to euthanize a companion animal when the reason for euthanasia is that the owner no longer needs or desires the animal's companionship. Most working animals, on the other hand, are killed when they can no longer work or when they are no longer profitable.

On what should the decision to keep or kill the animal be based? Is it a matter of species, economics, or the type of service that the animal provides?

Response

The answer to this question is not to be found in our social consensus ethic, which is essentially silent on any matter of right-to-life for other than humans. Thus, such decisions are left to a veterinarian's personal ethic, his or her own view of right and wrong, good and bad, justice and injustice, as these apply to animals. It may well be that, in the future, the veterinary profession will collectively adopt some ethical principles regarding these matters as part of professional ethics, but, as yet, it has not done so, and, in fact, veterinarians (as well as humane societies) are split evenly on convenience euthanasia of healthy companion animals.

The one exception to the above generalization lies in the area of laboratory animals. Most societies that have laws or rules governing the treatment of laboratory animals mandate early endpoints (euthanasia) for animals used in experiments entailing pain and distress, and, in some countries, euthanasia is mandatory for animals experiencing intractable pain. Such laws set the legal standard of veterinary practice and, at least, tell us that a suffering animal, regardless of the purpose for which it is used, is entitled to a "good death" to end that suffering.

But what of a healthy animal—dog, cat, horse, bird, zoo animal—that is not suffering? What principles, in such a case, might guide a conscientious veterinarian? I do not believe that any of the considerations listed in the question provide an adequate moral guide for the veterinarian, for neither species, use, nor economics provides morally relevant reasons to veterinarians who believe, in response to what, elsewhere, I have called the Fundamental Question of Veterinary Medicine, that their primary obligation is to the animal rather than the owner, and that part of their primary job is to save life. To go against one's own moral commitments on such an issue is to invite what we have called moral stress, arising out of discordance between what one believes one ought to do and what one is in fact doing. Moral stress, as I have noted before, is highly erosive of physical and mental well-being, as well as job satisfaction. To such a veterinarian, only the amelioration of suffering provides a good reason for killing.

Thus, to such a practitioner there is *never* a good reason for killing a healthy animal. Such a veterinarian should, therefore, work to find alternatives to killing. For example, in the equine area, veterinarians have worked with others to find homes for animals that are incapable of performing their humanly designated function, such as racing, but are still capable of reasonable quality of life. Some horses no longer able to race can be used in riding programs or returned to live out their lives on "retirement" farms.

For veterinarians who do not, in their personal ethic, see animal life as morally requiring preservation, the issue is clear; animals may be killed at an owner's behest. The only issue for them is assuring that death is indeed painless. Such veterinarians are morally culpable, if they save the owners money at the expense of animal suffering, as when for reasons of cost, infusion of disinfectant is used for killing horses. By and large, the AVMA guidelines for euthanasia provide valuable guidance in avoiding "bad deaths."

Appendix

We gratefully acknowledge the *Canadian Veterinary Journal* for allowing us to reprint these cases and thereby reach a significant veterinary audience outside of Canada.

Case	Commentary Title	Vol.	No.	Issue	Year	Page
01	Cow with cancer eye	32	1	January	1991	5
02	Substandard husbandry for sheep	32	2	February	1991	68
03	Fracture fixation	32	3	March	1991	139
04	Farmer using illegal growth promotant	32	4	April	1991	202
05	Client sells known BVD shedders	32	5	May	1991	268
06	Client requests dog euthanasia because she is moving	32	6	June	1991	328
07	Farmer requests a fetotomy	32	7	July	1991	390
08	Suspected dogfighting	32	8	August	1991	456
09	Docking and cropping of Dobermans	32	9	September	1991	522
10	Leaving a sow untreated	32	10	October	1991	584
11	Euthanasia of cat who sprays	32	11	November	1991	648
12	Euthanasia of treatable horse for insurance	32	12	December	1991	714
13	Euthanasia of grieving dog	33	1	January	1992	7
14	Supernumerary teat removal	33	2	February	1992	84
15	Breeder seeking euthanasia for puppy with overbite	33	4	April	1992	220
16	Veterinary anatomist spaying farm cats	33	5	May	1992	296
17	Breeder asking for anesthetics so she can crop ears	33	6	June	1992	358
18	Penicillin residue in milk	33	7	July	1992	422
19	Marketing heartworm regimen	33	8	August	1992	486
20	Dairy farmers using unauthorized feed additive prescribed by a veterinarian	33	10	October	1992	629
21	Veterinarian's responsibility when a dog is suspected to be overly aggressive	33	11	November	1992	696
22	Painful research designed without analgesia	33	12	December	1992	776
23	Clients who insist on continuing treatment for failing cancer dog	34	1	January	1993	10
24	Tail docking in dairy cattle	34	2	February	1993	72
25	Killing of neonatal buck kids	34	3	March	1993	136
26	Veterinarian discovers violations in religious slaughter	34	4	April	1993	201
27	Using information about alternative surgical training in hiring	34	5	May	1993	264
28	Pig farmer asking for euthanasia solution	34	6	June	1993	326
29	Feeding kittens to snakes	34	7	July	1993	388

30	Veterinarian seeking maternity leave	34	8	August	1993	459
31	Surgical procedures performed by a technician	34	9	September	1993	519
32	Veterinary liaison with pet store chain providing poor animal care	34	10	October	1993	586
33	Freeze-firing racehorses	34	11	November	1993	646
34	Performing cat castration on the farm	34	12	December	1993	712
35	Irresponsible veterinarian-breeder	35	1	January	1994	6
36	Annual rabies vaccination	35	2	February	1994	72
37	Government policy regarding export of breeding swine	35	3	March	1994	136
38	Improperly labeled prescriptions swallowed by child	35	4	April	1994	202
39	Referral practice "stealing" clients	35	5	May	1994	262
40	Confidentiality and a breeder perpetuating a line of dogs with seizures	35	6	June	1994	332
41	Should veterinarians be required to report animal abuse?	35	7	July	1994	408
42	Two cases of found dogs	35	9	September	1994	536
43	Should a biting dog be adopted out?	35	10	October	1994	598
44	Euthanizing sick animals without their owner's permission	35	11	November	1994	679
45	Partner's misdiagnosis	35	12	December	1994	745
46	Heavy metal toxicosis and slaughter for food	36	1	January	1995	9
47	Conflict of interest	36	2	February	1995	74
48	Rabies vaccine for livestock	36	3	March	1995	178
49	Female veterinarian receiving unwelcome attention	36	6	June	1995	353
50	Female veterinarian offended by colleagues' humor	36	7	July	1995	410
51	Client refuses euthanasia for sick cat	36	8	August	1995	471
52	Should veterinarians prescribe drugs to increase productivity?	36	9	September	1995	535
53	Previous practitioner leaves sponge in dog's peritoneum	36	10	October	1995	599
54	Illicit importation of boar semen	36	11	November	1995	674
55	Misreading of radiograph	36	12	December	1995	739
56	Cattery serving as source of FIP	37	1	January	1996	7
57	Injured, unowned animal	37	2	February	1996	74
58	Writing prescriptions for branded drugs in return for financial incentive	37	3	March	1996	149
59	Negligence of an emergency clinician in treating trauma	37	4	April	1996	201
60	Poor air quality in swine barn	37	5	May	1996	262

61	Supplementing income with prescription drugs	37	6	June	1996	330
62	Client's request to euthanize his dog after his death	37	7	July	1996	393
63	Confidentiality and an employee's history of drug abuse	37	8	August	1996	456
64	Convenience euthanasia of a dog without proper permission	37	9	September	1996	519
65	Veterinarian who ignores roundworms in puppies	37	10	October	1996	585
66	Stray tattooed beagle	37	11	November	1996	648
67	Prescribing and selling pharma-ceuticals	37	12	December	1996	713
68	Suspected poisoning	38	1	January	1997	6
69	Euthanasia of research animal without researcher's permission	38	3	March	1997	136
70	Anorexic client not feeding her dog	38	5	May	1997	263
71	Improving rural euthanasia	38	6	June	1997	334
72	Second commentary on stray tattooed beagle	38	8	August	1997	472
73	Bull mastiff with osteosarcoma	38	9	September	1997	536
74	Financially stressed client and annual physical	38	10	October	1997	603
75	Botched caesarean section	38	11	November	1997	682
76	Farmer asking advice of "experts"	38	12	December	1997	745
77	Confidentiality in the case of a client selling sick animals	39	2	February	1998	72
78	Conflict in obligations to a peer and a client	39	3	March	1998	136
79	Reporting a dog being used to carry drugs	39	4	April	1998	200
80	An elderly client seeking "unnecessary" medical advice	39	5	May	1998	264
81	A cat who fractures both legs after a surgical procedure	39	6	June	1998	337
82	Can annual vaccinations be justified?	46	1	January	2005	19
83	An organic farmer who won't use antibiotics for foot rot	46	3	March	2005	203
84	Using wood chippers to kill chickens	45	1	January	2004	9
85	Should shelters place animals in less than perfect homes?	45	4	April	2004	291
86	Why should we worry about animal suffering right before death?	45	6	June	2004	457
87	"Good" versus "natural" death	45	10	October	2004	806
88	Is it wrong to modify animals to fit production systems?	45	11	November	2004	899
89	How do veterinarians respond to clients with too many animals?	42	11	November	2001	853

90	Should a veterinarian wear company logos?	43	7	July	2002	494
91	Technicians performing management procedures on farm	43	8	August	2002	583
92	Extralabel drug use	43	10	October	2002	749
93	Animal welfare versus animal rights	43	12	December	2002	913
94	Raw diet	44	6	June	2003	449
95	Using an elastrator on older bulls	44	8	August	2003	624
96	Finding animals for continuing education	44	11	November	2003	867
97	Should veterinarians support activist groups?	44	12	December	2003	955
98	Auditability of animal welfare	44	5	May	2005	396
99	Producer unwilling to euthanize sick pigs	42	1	January	2001	8
100	Veterinarians and laws banning pitbulls	42	4	April	2001	258
101	Giving analgesics to mask pain in horses	42	6	June	2001	420
102	Are animals raised in confinement happy in confinement?	42	9	September	2001	676
103	Elderly couple adopting many animals	43	5	May	2002	327
104	The ethics of killing healthy animals	42	12	December	2001	908

REFERENCES

American Academy of Pediatrics, Committee on Children with Disabilities. 2001. Counseling families who choose complementary and alternative medicine for their child with chronic illness or disability. *Pediatrics* 107(3):598–601.

American Veterinary Medical Association (AVMA). 1982. Executive Board Minutes, July 14–15, 1982, p. 11.

———. 1993. 1993 Report of the AVMA Panel on Euthanasia. *Journal of the American Veterinary Medical Association* 202:229–249.

Anand, K.J.S., and P.R. Hickey. 1992. Halothane-morphine compared with high-dose sufentanil for anesthesia and postoperative analgesia in neonatal cardiac surgery. *New England Journal of Medicine* 326:1–9.

Animal Legal and Historical Center. Michigan State University, College of Law, East Lansing, MI. www.animallaw.info/articles/ovuspetdamages.htm

Arkow, Phil. 1994. Child abuse, animal abuse, and the veterinarian. *Journal of the American Veterinary Medical Association* 204(7):1004–1006.

Austin, J.L. 1965. *How to Do Things With Words.* New York: Oxford University Press.

Beauchamp, Tom, and Leroy Walters. 1978. *Contemporary Issues in Bioethics.* Belmont, CA: Wadsworth.

Benson, G.H., et al. 1989. Laboratory animal analgesia. In *The Experimental Animal in Biomedical Research*, ed. B.E. Rollin and M.L. Kesel. Boca Raton, FL: CRC Press.

Benson, J., and B. Rollin. 2004. *The Well-Being of Farm Animals: Challenges and Solutions.* Ames, IA: Blackwell Publishing.

Bentham, Jeremy. 1961. An introduction to the principles of morals and legislation. In *The Utilitarians.* Garden City, NY: Doubleday.

California Veterinary Medical Association. 2004. http://www.cvma.net/doc.asp?ID=2405

Canadian Veterinary Medicine Association (CVMA). http://www.canadianveterinarians.net

Carberry, C.A., and H.J. Harvey. 1987. Owner satisfaction with limb amputation in dogs and cats. *Journal of the American Animal Hospital Association* 23:227–232.

CAST (Council of Agricultural Science and Technology). 1981. Scientific Aspects of the Welfare of Food Animals. Report No. 91.

Daly, C.C., E. Kallweit, and F. Ellendorf. 1988. Cortical function in cattle during slaughter: Conventional captive bolt stunning followed by exsanguination compared with shechita slaughter. *Veterinary Record* 122:325–329.

Davis, L. 1983. Species differences in drug disposition as factors in alleviation of pain. In *Animal Pain: Perception and Alleviation*, ed. R.L. Kitchell and H.H. Erickson. Bethesda, MD: American Physiological Society.

Donham, K.A., B. Haglind, R. Rylander, and Y. Peterson. 1989. Environmental and health studies of workers in Swedish swine buildings. In *Principles of Health and Safety in Agriculture*, ed. J.A. Dosman and S.W. Cockcroft. Boca Raton, FL: CRC Press.

Donham, K.J., and K.E. Gustafson. 1982. Human occupational hazards from swine confinement. *Annals of the American Conference of Governmental Industrial Hygienists* 2:137–142.

Ferrell, B.R., and M. Rhiner. 1991. High-tech comfort: Ethical issues in cancer pain management for the 1990s. *Journal of Clinical Ethics* 2:108–115.

Feyerabend, Paul. 1978. *Science in a Free Society.* London: NLB.

Fox, Michael A. 1986. *The Case for Animal Experimentation.* Berkley: University of California Press.

Gallup. 2003. http://www.gallup.com; http://www.animalrights.net/archives/year/2003/000193.html

Grandin, T., and J.M. Regenstein. 1994. Religious slaughter and animal welfare: A discussion for meat scientists. In *Meat Focus International,* March: 115–123. CAB International. Wallingford, Oxon., U.K.

Harrison, Ruth. 1964. *Animal Machines.* London: Vincent Stuart.

Hendrick, M.J., M.H. Goldschmidt, F.S. Shafer, Y. Wang, and A.P. Somiyo. 1992. Postvaccinal sarcomas in the cat: Epidemiology and electron probe microanalytical identification of aluminum. *Cancer Research* 52:5391–5394.

Hrobjartsson, A., and T.C. Gotzsche. 2001. Is the placebo powerless? An analysis of clinical trials comparing placebo with no treatment. *New England Journal of Medicine.* 344(21):1594–1602.

Kane and Parsons. 1989. *Parents* poll on animal rights, attractiveness, television, and abortion. *Parents.* (Kane and Parsons is a New York firm.)

Kant, Immanuel. 1959. *Foundations of the Metaphysics of Morals,* trans. Lewis White Beck. New York: Liberal Arts Press.

Katz, Jon. 2003. *The New Work of Dogs: Tending to Life, Love, and Family.* New York: Villard.

Kellert, Stephen, and A. Felthous. 1985. Childhood cruelty towards animals among criminals and noncriminals. *Human Relations* 38:1113–1129.

Kilgour, R. 1978. The application of animal behavior and the humane care of farm animals. *Journal of Animal Science* 46:1478–1486.

Kitchell, Ralph L., and Howard H. Erickson, ed. 1983. *Animal Pain: Perception and Alleviation.* Bethesda, MD: American Physiological Society.

Kitchell, R., and M. Guinan. 1989. The nature of pain in animals. In *The Experimental Biomedical Research,* Vol. 1., Chapter 12, ed. B.E. Rollin and M.L. Kesel. Boca Raton, FL: CRC Press.

Levine, S. 1989. Stress and cognition in laboratory animals. In *The Experimental Animal in Biomedical Research,* ed. B.E. Rollin and M.L. Kesel. Boca Raton, FL: CRC Press.

Lumb, William, and E. Wynn Jones. 1973. *Veterinary Anesthesia.* Philadelphia: Lea and Febiger.

McMillan, F. 1999. The placebo effect in veterinary medicine. *Journal of the American Veterinary Medical Association* 215(7):992–998.

McMillen, F. 1998. Comfort as the primary goal in veterinary medicine. *Journal of the American Veterinary Medical Association* 212:1370–1374.

Markowitz, H., and S. Line. 1989. The need for responsive environments. In *The Experimental Animal in Biomedical Research,* ed. B. Rollin and M. Kesel, 153–173. Boca Raton, FL: CRC Press.

Merchant, J.A., and K.J. Donham. 1989. Health risks from animal confinement units. In *Principles of Health and Safety in Agriculture,* ed. J.A. Dosman and S.W. Cockcroft. Boca Raton, FL: CRC Press.

Merillat, L.A. 1906. *Principles of Veterinary Surgery.* Chicago: Alexander Eger.

Michigan State News. 1989. Director addresses health research. February 27, p 8.

Mill, John Stuart. 1961. Utilitarianism. In *The Utilitarians.* Garden City, NY: Doubleday.

Morton, D.B., and P.H.M. Griffiths. 1985. Guidelines on the recognition of pain, distress, and comfort in experimental animals and an hypothesis for assessment. *Veterinary Record* 20:431–436.

National Research Council. 1992. *Recognition and Alleviation of Pain and Distress in Laboratory Animals.* Washington, DC: National Academy Press.

Page, G.G., S. Ben-Eliyahu, and J. Lebeskind. 1993. Morphine attenuates surgery-induced enhancement of metastatic colonization in rats. *Pain* 54:21–28.

Panel Report on Euthanasia. 1986. *Journal of the American Veterinary Medical Association* 133:252–268.

Panel Report on the Colloquium on Recognition and Alleviation of Animal Pain and Distress. 1987. *Journal of the American Veterinary Medical Association* 191(10):1186–1191.

Papageorges, Marc. 1995. The unification theory of all radiographic fumbles. Paper presented at the 47th Annual Convention of the Canadian Veterinary Medical Association, "Scientific Presentations," July 12–15, Victoria, B.C.

Plato. 1965. *The Meno: Text and Criticism,* ed. A. Sesonske and N. Fleming. Belmont, CA: Wadsworth.

Plato. *The Republic,* Book I, Chapter 3.

Ramey, D., and B.E. Rollin. 2001. Ethical aspects of proof and alternative therapies. *Journal of the American Veterinary Medical Association.* 218(3):343–345.

———. 2004. *Complementary and Alternative Veterinary Medicine Considered.* Ames, IA: Blackwell Publishing.

Religious slaughter: Stunning called for. 1985. *Veterinary Record* 117:97–98.

Reynells, Richard D. 1996. Animal welfare and rights: Public perception of the poultry industry. Speech delivered before the 1996 Poultry Institute, University of Florida, Gainesville, FL, October 9, 1996.

Rights, wrongs, and ignorance. 2002. Editorial. *Nature* 416:351.

Robinson, E.A. 1921. *Collected Poems.* New York: MacMillan.

Rollin, Bernard E. 1978. Updating veterinary ethics. *Journal of the American Veterinary Medical Association* 173:1015–1018.

———. 1981. *Animal Rights and Human Morality,* first edition. Buffalo, NY: Prometheus Books.

———. 1983. The concept of illness in veterinary medicine. *Journal of the American Medical Association* 182:122–125

———. 1986. Euthanasia and moral stress. In *Loss, Grief and Care*, ed. R. DeBellis. Binghamton, NY: Haworth Press.

———. 1989. *The Unheeded Cry: Animal Consciousness, Animal Pain and Science.* Cambridge University Press.

———. 1991. Social ethics, veterinary medicine and the pet overpopulation problem. *Journal of the American Veterinary Medical Association* 198:1153–1156.

———. 1992. *Animal Rights and Human Morality*, second edition. (First edition, 1981.) Buffalo, NY: Prometheus Books.

———. 1993. The new ethic for animals and the equine industry. In *Proceedings of the Thirty-Seventh Annual Convention of the American Association of Equine Practitioners.* Lexington, KY: American Association of Equine Practitioners.

———. 1995. *Farm Animal Welfare.* Ames: Iowa State University Press.

———. 1997. Pain and ideology in human and veterinary medicine. *Seminars in Veterinary Medicine and Surgery* (Small Animal): *Pain* 12(2):56–61.

———. 1998. *The Unheeded Cry: Animal Consciousness, Animal Pain and Science.* Ames, Iowa: Iowa State University Press.

———. 1999. Some conceptual and ethical concerns about current views of pain. *Pain Forum* 8(2):84–86.

———. 2000. The Ethics of Pain Control in Companion Animals. In *Animal Pain*, ed. J. Ludo. Utrecht, Netherlands: Van Der Wees.

———. 2001. Dogmatisms and Catechisms. *Anthrozoös* 14(1):4–11.

———. 2006. *Animal Rights and Human Morality*, third edition. Buffalo, NY: Prometheus Books.

Rollin, B.E., and M.L. Kesel. 1989. *The Experimental Animal in Biomedical Research.* Boca Raton, FL: CRC Press.

Rosenthal, Robert. 1966. *Experimenter Effects in Behavioral Research.* New York: Appleton.

Schoen, A., and S. Wynn. 1998. *Complementary and Alternative Medicine: Principles and Practice.* St. Louis: Mosby.

Siegler, M., and H. Osmond. 1974. *Models of Madness, Models of Medicine.* New York: Harper Colophon.

Singer, Peter. 1975. *Animal Liberation.* New York: New York Review of Books.

Taylor, P. 1985. Analgesia in the dog and cat. *Practice* 7:5–13.

Taylor, Robert E. 1992. *Scientific Farm Animal Production.* New York: Macmillan.

Thomas Aquinas. 1956. *On the Truth of the Catholic Faith. Summa Contra Gentiles.* Garden City, NY: Doubleday.

Thurman, John C., William J. Tranquilli, and Gordan J. Benson. 1996. *Lumb and Jones' Veterinary Anesthesia.* Baltimore, MD: Williams and Wilkins.

Visscher, Maurice B. 1982. Review of *Animal Rights and Human Morality. New England Journal of Medicine* 306: 1303–1304.

Walco, G.A., R.C. Cassidy, and N.L. Schechter. 1994. Pain, hurt and harm: The ethics of pain control in infants and children. *New England Journal of Medicine* 331:541–544.

Warren, C.P.W. 1989. Overview of Respiratory Health Risks in Agriculture. In *Principles of Health and Safety in Agriculture*, ed. J.A. Dosman and S.W. Cockcroft. Boca Raton, FL: CRC Press.

Wemelsfelder. 1989. Boredom in Laboratory Animals. In *The Experimental Biomedical Research*, Vol. 1, ed. B.E. Rollin and M.L. Kesel. Boca Raton, FL: CRC Press.

Wilson, J.F., B.E. Rollin, and J.L. Garbe. 1988. *Law and Ethics of the Veterinary Profession.* Yardley, PA: Priority Press.

Wirth, D., and A. Beck. 1981. Multiple ownership of animals in NYC. *Transaction and Studies of the College of Physicians of Philadelphia* 3(4):280–300.

Withrow, S.J., and V.M. Hirsch. 1979. Owner response to amputation of a pet's leg. *Veterinary Medicine: Small Animal Clinician* March:332–334.

Wood-Gush, D.G.M. 1983. *Elements of Ethology.* London: Chapman and Hall.

Wood-Gush, D.G.M., and Alex Stolba. 1981. Behavior of pigs and design of a new housing system. *Applied Animal Ethology* 8:583–585.

INDEX